Clinical Reproductive Medicine and Health

Clinical Reproductive Medicine and Health

Editor: Cameron Baker

AMERICAN
MEDICAL PUBLISHERS
www.americanmedicalpublishers.com

AMERICAN
MEDICAL PUBLISHERS
www.americanmedicalpublishers.com

Cataloging-in-Publication Data

Clinical reproductive medicine and health / edited by Cameron Baker.
p. cm.
Includes bibliographical references and index.
ISBN 979-8-88740-009-9
1. Reproductive health. 2. Human reproduction--Endocrine aspects.
3. Human reproduction. 4. Fertility, Human. 5. Embryology, Human.
I. Baker, Cameron.
RG133 .C55 2023
613.9--dc23

American Medical Publishers,
41 Flatbush Avenue,
1st Floor, New York,
NY 11217, USA

ISBN 979-8-88740-009-9 (Hardback)

Contents

Predictors of Premature Rupture of Membranes among Pregnant Women in Rural Uganda: A Cross-Sectional Study at a Tertiary Teaching Hospital

Simon Byonanuwe,[1] Emmanuel Nzabandora,[1] Baltazar Nyongozi,[1] Theophilus Pius,[2] David Santson Ayebare,[3] Collins Atuheire,[4] Wilson Mugizi,[5] Martin Nduwimana,[6] Maxwell Okello,[1] Yarine Fajardo,[1] and Robinson Ssebuufu[7]

[1]*Department of Obstetrics and Gynaecology, Kampala International University Teaching Hospital, Uganda*
[2]*Department of Medical Laboratory Science, Kampala International University Teaching Hospital, Uganda*
[3]*Interdisciplinary Research & Development Center Limited, Mbarara, Uganda*
[4]*Department of Public Health, Kampala International University-Western Campus, Uganda*
[5]*Postgraduate Studies & Research Directorate, Kampala International University-Western Campus, Uganda*
[6]*Department of Paediatrics, Kampala International University Teaching Hospital, Uganda*
[7]*Department of Surgery, Kampala International University Teaching Hospital, Uganda*

Correspondence should be addressed to Simon Byonanuwe; byonsimon@gmail.com

Academic Editor: Kai-Fai Lee

Background. Premature rupture of membranes (PROM) is a common condition in developed and developing countries and poses a serious threat to the maternal and fetal well-being if not properly managed. This study delineated the prevalence and predictors of PROM in the western part of Uganda so as to guide specific preventive measures. *Methods.* A cross-sectional study design was conducted in the months of September 2019 to November 2019. A total of 334 pregnant women above 28 weeks of gestation admitted at the maternity ward of KIU-TH were consecutively enrolled. Interviewer-administered questionnaires were used to obtain the data. Descriptive statistics followed by binary logistic regression were conducted. All data analyses were conducted using STATA 14.2. *Results.* Of the 334 pregnant women enrolled, the prevalence of PROM was found to be 13.8%. The significant independent predictors associated with lower odds of PROM were no history of urinary tract infection (UTI) in the month preceding enrollment into the study (aOR = 0.5, 95% CI: 0.22-0.69, $p = 0.038$) and gestational age of 37 weeks or more (aOR = 0.3, 95% CI: 0.14-0.71, $p = 0.01$) while history of 3 or more abortions (aOR = 13.1, 95% CI: 1.12-153.62, $p = 0.05$) was associated with higher likelihood of PROM. *Conclusions.* Majorly urinary tract infections, low gestational age, and abortions influence premature rupture of membranes among women. There is a great need for continuous screening and prompt treatment of pregnant women for UTI especially those with history of 3 or more abortions at less than 34 weeks of gestation.

1. Introduction

PROM is defined as the spontaneous rupture of the fetal membranes prior to onset of labour [1]. It may occur when the fetus is 37 weeks or more of gestation (term premature rupture of membranes (TPROM)) or before 37 weeks of gestation (preterm premature rupture of membranes (PPROM)) [2]. PROM generally affects between 5 and 15% of all pregnancies worldwide with a relatively higher incidence in Africa [3–5]. About 3% of the pregnancies are complicated with preterm premature rupture of membranes [6, 7]. For several years, PROM has been the subject of several clinical and epidemiologic studies and is considered one of the great obstetrical syndromes responsible for spontaneous preterm birth and its related complications such as respiratory distress syndrome, intraventricular haemorrhage, and

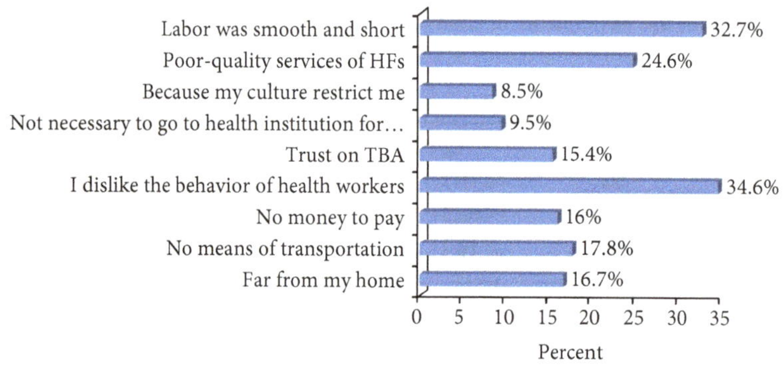

FIGURE 6: Reasons for preferring home delivery ($n = 200$) in Jimma Arjo District, Oromia, Ethiopia, 2018. *More than one possible answer was used.

pay for transportation and health service-related costs 68 (16%), and the least mentioned reason was having trust on TBA 58 (15.4%) (Figure 6).

Regarding assistance of the last childbirth at the health institution, 182 (59.7%) were assisted by midwives, followed by health officers 72 (23.6%) and nurses 36 (11.8%). From those mothers who gave their last birth at home, 95 (47.3%), 73 (36.3%), and 26 (12.9%) of them were assisted by their neighbors, mothers-in-law, and their mothers, respectively (Table 3).

TABLE 3: Last delivery assistance among the woman respondents, in Jimma Arjo District, Oromia, Ethiopia, 2018.

Variables	Frequency (n = 506)	Percent
Assistant at home delivery		
Mother	26	12.9
Mother-in-law	73	36.3
Women from my neighbor	95	47.3
TBA	7	3.5
Assistant at HI delivery		
Midwife	182	59.7
Nurse	36	11.8
Health officer	72	23.6
Doctor	15	4.9
Next delivery place		
Health institution	326	64.4
Home	180	35.6
Husband's choice of place of delivery		
Health institution	298	58.9
Home	208	41.1

3.4. Factors Affecting Choice of Childbirth Place. In bivariate logistic regression analysis, variables with p value < 0.25 which were added in the final multivariate logistic regression model were age of respondents, residence, educational status, husband education, monthly household income, information of delivery in a health institution, ANC visits, obstetric difficulties, distance to the nearby health institution, means of transportation, and time spent to reach health institution.

Accordingly, a multivariate logistic regression analysis was done and the result showed that mothers who completed secondary education were 4.4 times more likely to choose health institution as childbirth place compared to those who cannot read and write (AOR = 4.4 (1.47, 13.42) at 95% CI). Similarly, women whose husband completed secondary education were 4 times more likely to choose health institution as delivery place compared to a husband who cannot read and write (AOR = 4 (1.43-11.60) at 95% CI). Compared to mothers who had first ANC visit, those mothers who had 2-3 times ANC follow-up were also 4 times more likely to choose health institution as a delivery place (AOR = 4 (1.95, 8.52) at 95% CI). It was also found that a woman who have ever encountered obstetric difficulties and who had access to vehicles to reach health institutions was more likely to choose institutional delivery with adjusted odds ratio of (6, (2.08, 17.60) at 95% CI) and (2.8 (1.23, 6.46) at 95% CI), respectively (Table 4).

4. Discussion

This study revealed that 200 (39.5%) of the total respondents chose home delivery, whereas the rest (60.5%) chose institutional delivery. This finding is almost similar with the study done in Jimma Zone, Southwest Ethiopia, in which 35.38% of the mothers chose home delivery [20]. However, it is inconsistent with EDHS 2016 where home delivery accounts 81.2% [4].This could have resulted from the fact that EDHS is a large-scale national data, while this study was conducted only in a single district.

The reasons mentioned for preferring home delivery were smooth and short labor (32.7%), uncomfortable behavior of health workers (34.6%), no means of transportation (17.8%), and no money to pay for transportation and health service (16%). Though the magnitude differs, similar reasons were also mentioned in the study conducted in Dega Damot woreda in which no money to pay for transportation and health service (113 (50.7%)), no means of transportation (134 (60.1%)), and smooth and short labor (106 (47.5%)) [19] were mentioned as reasons. This may indicate that the reasons for preferring home delivery are common everywhere except some differences that exist due to socioeconomic, time, and related differences.

TABLE 4: Multivariate analysis of selected variables ($n = 506$) with women's choice of delivery place in Jimma Arjo District, East Wollega Zone, Oromia Regional State, Ethiopia, May 2018.

Variables	Choice of birthplace Home, *n* (%)	HI, *n* (%)	COR, 95% CI	AOR, 95% CI
Residence				
Rural	189 (48.5)	201 (51.5)	1	1
Urban	11 (9.5)	105(90.5)	9 (4.68, 17.23)	2 (0.46, 7.99)
Educational status of the mother				
Cannot read and write	75 (49.7)	76 (50.3)	1	1
Read and write	87 (50.9)	84 (49.1)	0.9 (0.58, 1.40)	0.8 (0.36, 1.86)
Primary education (1–8)	7 (20.6)	27 (79.4)	3 (1.31, 6.72)	1.8 (0.57, 5.93)
Secondary education	22 (24.7)	67 (75.3)	3 (1.71, 5.43)	4.4 (1.47, 13.42)
Diploma and above	9 (14.8)	52 (85.2)	9 (3.67-22.27)	3.8 (0.92, 16.05)
Husband education				
Cannot read and write	60 (58.8)	42 (41.2)	1	1
Read and write	76 (53.1)	67 (46.9)	1.6 (0.91-2.76)	2 (0.77, 5.50)
Primary education (1–8)	27 (42.2)	37 (57.8)	2.5 (1.29-4.91)	1.8 (0.57, 5.60)
Secondary education	25 (24)	79 (76)	3.47 (1.96, 6.15)	4 (1.43, 11.60)
Diploma and above	12 (12.9)	81 (87.1)	12 (5.73, 26.59)	4 (1.17, 13.38)
Information about the benefit of delivery in health institution				
Yes	185 (38.8)	292 (61.2)	1.7 (0.80-3.59)	3.8 (0.98-14.35)
No	15 (51.7)	14 (48.3)	1	
ANC visits (362)				
1	73 (52.9)	65 (47.1)	1	1
2-3	31 (16.8)	153 (83.2)	5.5 (3.33-9.24)	4 (1.95, 8.52)
≥4	16 (40)	24 (60)	1.7 (0.82-3.45)	1.2 (0.45, 3.27)
Obstetric difficulties (like prolonged labor, hemorrhage)				
Yes	6 (7.1)	79 (92.9)	11 (4.80-26.38)	6 (2.08, 17.60)
No	194 (46.1)	227 (53.9)	1	1
Estimated distance to the nearby HI				
<2 km	15 (13.9)	93 (86.1)	4 (2.22-8.09)	0.9 (0.23, 3.94)
2-5 km	90 (51.1)	86 (48.9)	0.8 (0.60-1.29)	1 (0.81, 3.03)
>5 km	95 (42.8)	127 (57.2)	1	1
Means of transport				
On foot	113 (32.9)	230 (67.1)	1	1
Traditional transportation	39 (43.3)	51 (56.7)	1.5 (0.90, 2.34)	1.3 (0.62, 3.09)
Vehicle	48 (65.8)	25 (34.2)	3 (1.92, 5.26)	2.8 (1.23, 6.46)
Time spent to reach HI				
<1 hr	8 (11.8)	60 (88.2)	5.8 (2.73, 12.54)	2 (0.44, 12.49)
1-2 hrs	192(43.8)	246 (56.2)	1	1

Regarding factors affecting choice of delivery place, in this study, it was found that mothers with the level of secondary education and whose husbands' educational status was diploma and above were more than 4 times more likely to choose institutional delivery compared to those who cannot read and write. This is similar with the study done in Dega Damot district of Amhara and Ahferom district of Tigray, Ethiopia [19, 21]. This could have resulted from the reason that an educated husband is expected to have better knowledge and awareness about the advantages of institutional deliveries and seeking modern health care than those who are not.

It was also found that mothers who had 2-3 ANC visits during the last pregnancy were 4 times more likely to choose health institution compared to women who had a single ANC visit. This finding is consistent with a study finding of Sekela district in which mothers who have ANC visits were 4 times more likely to deliver in health facilities than those who did not have ANC visits [22, 23]. This indicates that the more the number of ANC visits, the more opportunity

4

Influence of Lifestyle and Environmental Factors on Semen Quality in Ghanaian Men

Richard Michael Blay,[1] Abigail Duah Pinamang,[2] Augustine E. Sagoe,[3] Ewurama Dedea Ampadu Owusu,[2] Nii Koney-Kwaku Koney,[1] and Benjamin Arko-Boham[1]

[1]*Department of Anatomy, University of Ghana Medical School, College of Health Sciences, University of Ghana, Korle Bu, Accra, Ghana*
[2]*Department of Medical Laboratory Sciences, School of Biomedical and Allied Health Sciences, College of Health Sciences, University of Ghana, Korle Bu, Accra, Ghana*
[3]*Central Medical Laboratory, Immunology Unit, Korle-Bu Teaching Hospital, Korle Bu, Accra, Ghana*

Correspondence should be addressed to Benjamin Arko-Boham; barko_boham@chs.edu.gh

Academic Editor: Robert Gaspar

Introduction. Male infertility is known to contribute about half of all infertility cases. In Ghana, the prevalence of male infertility is higher (15.8%) than in females (11.8%). Sperm quality is associated with the likelihood of pregnancy and known to be the cause of male fertility problems 90% of the time. Exposure to certain environmental factors reduces semen quality in men. The study examined the effects of environmental and lifestyle factors on semen quality in Ghanaian men. *Materials and Methods*. This was a cross-sectional study involving 80 apparent healthy adult males in their reproductive age. Participants were males referred to the laboratory (Immunology Unit of the Korle-Bu Teaching Hospital) for semen analysis test and/or culture and sensitivity. Participants were made to fill out a questionnaire which entailed selected environmental factors (accidents or trauma, exposure to chemicals, radiation, and heat) and lifestyle habits (including alcohol consumption, smoking, and whether participants sat more or less than 4 hours per day). Semen samples were then collected by masturbation into sterile containers and analysed in accordance with WHO guidance for semen analysis within 60 minutes after ejaculation and collection. *Results*. About 69% of participants had semen pH within the normal range compared to 15% whose pH were lower than 7.2. There was a significantly high number of immotile sperm cells (p value = 0.017) in participants who sat for more than 4 hours as compared to those that sat for less than 4 hours in a day. Active sperm motility and viability showed significant increase (p value = 0.002 and 0.009, respectively) in participants who kept their cell phones in their side pockets. Smoking produced a twofold decrease in sperm count as smokers had a significantly lower sperm count ($12.28 \pm 10.95 \times 10^6$/ml) compared to the smoke-free ($23.85 \pm 22.14 \times 10^6$/ml). For exposure to STDs, no significant differences were recorded among study groups concerning semen quality. *Conclusion*. Sperm quality in Ghanaian men is associated with lifestyle habits. Smoking and sitting for long hours influenced sperm motility and count, respectively. Knowledge of the factors that influence sperm quality in this geographical region can contribute to informed decisions on effective management of infertility in Ghanaian men.

1. Introduction

Male infertility is known to contribute to about half of all infertility cases and is usually the most difficult form to treat [1]. The prevalence of infertility may be higher in males than in females, indicating the importance of studying the male contribution to infertility [2]. Sperm count and concentration are strongly associated with the likelihood of pregnancy and known to be the cause of male fertility problems 90% of the time [3]. The rapid decline in global fertility rates in recent decades has occurred alongside decreasing sperm count and quality suggesting that decline in fertility may be due to decreasing sperm quality [4–6]. Meta-analysis studies show that there has been a 57% reduction in sperm concentration around the globe over the past 35 years, 32.5% decline over the past 50 years in Europe, and a 72.6% decline found in Africa over the past 50 years [7]. Although several factors may affect male fertility and sperm quality, industrialization and economic growth have been shown to be a significant contributor due to increased exposure to pollutants, changes in diet, and lifestyle [8, 9]. Recent studies show that exposure to certain environmental factors such as noise pollution and lifestyle habits such as sitting for more than 6 hours per day, tobacco use, alcohol, testicular heat stress, radiation, and obesity all reduce semen quality in men [10, 11]. A systematic review [9] of literature in association with lifestyle factors and male infertility over the last 10 years using PubMed showed that smoking, alcohol, obesity, diet, psychological stress, advanced paternal age, genital heat stress, and sleep disturbances may all adversely impact sperm quality. Another report [12] also showed evidence that diet, extreme physical activity, and body mass index (BMI) may also have adverse effects on male fertility. Furthermore, there is evidence that low sperm quality, occupational exposure, and unhealthy lifestyle habits in men may be associated with recurrent pregnancy loss (RPL) in their partners [13] suggesting far-reaching effect of environmental exposure and lifestyle on the reproductive health of men. Work and life stress factors that are perceived to be high in modern populations are also associated with sperm concentration, motility, and morphology [14]. Yang et al. [15] reported that smoking and consumption of caffeinated drinks and fried foods were significantly associated with poor semen quality. Other studies have also suggested that prolonged use of mobile phones and the wearing of tight underwear also impact negatively on semen parameters and DNA integrity [16].

The mechanism by which lifestyle and environmental factors reduce the quality of sperms is not fully understood; however, there are studies that suggest disruption of endocrine function, aberrant DNA methylation in sperm cells, abnormal seminal plasma zinc levels, and morphological damage to sperms [17–21]. A recent publication has shown several genes linked to fertility, and mutations to these single genes lead to low sperm quality [22]. To understand decreasing fertility rates and factors that lead to genetic and physiological aberrations resulting in low sperm quality, this study examined the influence of environmental and lifestyle factors on parameters of semen quality in Ghanaian men.

2. Materials and Methods

The study was approved by the Ethics and Protocol Review Committee of the School of Biomedical and Allied Health Sciences, College of Health Sciences, University of Ghana (Ethics Identification Number: SBAHS-MD./10468875/AA/5A/2016-2017). Informed consent was obtained from participants prior to study enrolment.

2.1. Study Participants. This was a cross-sectional study conducted at the Immunology Unit of the Korle-Bu Teaching Hospital (KBTH), Accra. The study participants were adult males in their reproductive years referred to the Immunology Unit of the Central Laboratory of the KBTH for semen analysis. To be eligible, a participant should have been referred to the Unit by a qualified medical officer. These are males seeking medical attention for difficulties with conception with their spouses. In addition, eligible participants should not have ejaculated at least 3 days prior to the day of investigation. All those who did not meet these criteria were excluded from the study.

2.2. Data Collection on Lifestyle Factors. A structured questionnaire which had previously been pretested was administered to consented and enrolled participants. Participants responded to close-ended questions bordering on their lifestyle such as smoking habit, alcohol intake (daily, weekly, or occasionally), the type of underwear, approximate number of sitting hours per day including occupation and the use of cell phones and the site of common storage on the body, and environmental factors, including exposure to X-ray and participants' history on sexually transmitted diseases (STDs). Participants were classified as smokers (exposed) if they indicated they did smoke either daily or occasionally and nonsmokers (unexposed) if they never smoked.

The face validity approach was used to validate the questionnaire. In doing that, the structured questionnaire was first reviewed by an expert in male reproductive health, after which the questionnaire was piloted in a selected population.

2.3. Sample Collection. Participants were asked to fill out a questionnaire which entailed selected environmental factors and lifestyle habits. Selected environmental factors included accidents or trauma, exposure to chemicals, radiation, and heat. Lifestyle habits investigated included number of hours spent sitting, alcohol consumption, and smoking. Semen samples were then provided by participants using masturbation method into sterile containers for analysis.

2.4. Semen Analysis. Semen samples were analysed in accordance with World Health Organisation (WHO) guidelines and reference values [23] for semen analysis within 60 minutes after ejaculation. Macroscopic examination was performed to determine parameters such as pH, volume, colour of semen, liquefaction, and consistency. Microscopic examination was also performed to determine sperm count, sperm morphology, and sperm motility.

2.5. Macroscopic Examination. Semen appearance, using colour, was noted, and the volume was measured using a graduated Pasteur pipette. The semen was then allowed to drop from the Pasteur pipette by gravity, and the length of the thread was observed for liquefaction. Semen pH was determined using a pH strip. According to the WHO Manual [23], normal ranges for volume and pH are 1.5 ml-5 ml and 7.2-8.0, respectively.

2.6. Microscopic Examination. To assess sperm motility, a drop of semen was delivered onto a treated clean glass slide

TABLE 3: Effect of lifestyle on semen parameters in Ghanaian men.

Lifestyle	Volume	pH	Active motility (%)	Sluggish motility (%)	Immotile (%)	Viability (%)	Count ($\times 10^6$/ml)
				Semen parameters			
				Alcohol			
Yes	2.23 ± 1.16	7.94 ± 0.41	23.75 ± 20.20	26.60 ± 18.36	42.14 ± 27.66	44.64 ± 25.74	25.00 ± 22.14
No	2.52 ± 1.20	7.77 ± 0.50	22.75 ± 25.22	22.73 ± 15.62	50.67 ± 31.35	38.55 ± 28.23	21.68 ± 21.44
p value	0.295	0.108	0.847	0.323	0.214	0.334	0.516
				Smoking			
Yes	2.48 ± 1.10	7.78 ± 0.39	12.85 ± 17.04	22.85 ± 22.14	48.57 ± 34.84	27.85 ± 27.05	12.28 ± 10.95
No	2.41 ± 1.20	7.84 ± 0.48	24.08 ± 23.84	24.20 ± 16.19	47.60 ± 30.01	41.91 ± 27.27	23.85 ± 22.14
p value	0.877	0.741	0.147	0.839	0.936	0.198	0.036*
				Hours of sitting			
≤4 hours	2.39 ± 1.26	7.81 ± 0.50	26.02 ± 24.95	24.18 ± 17.14	41.42 ± 30.12	42.24 ± 27.52	23.03 ± 20.75
>4 hours	2.46 ± 1.07	7.87 ± 0.44	18.48 ± 20.42	23.93 ± 16.03	57.58 ± 28.07	38.22 ± 27.43	22.54 ± 23.47
p value	0.791	0.590	0.145	0.948	0.017*	0.526	0.923

*Statistically significant p value < 0.05.

TABLE 4: Effect of exposure to environmental factors on semen parameters in Ghanaian men.

Environmental factors	Volume	pH	Active motility (%)	Sluggish motility (%)	Immotile (%)	Viability (%)	Count ($\times 10^6$/ml)
				Semen parameters			
				STD exposure			
Yes	2.32 ± 1.02	7.87 ± 0.45	18.90 ± 21.01	28.10 ± 21.86	42.50 ± 30.97	40.25 ± 26.03	20.22 ± 19.73
No	2.45 ± 1.24	7.82 ± 0.48	24.50 ± 24.22	22.75 ± 14.45	49.41 ± 30.02	40.83 ± 27.90	23.60 ± 22.30
p value	0.632	0.662	0.328	0.215	0.379	0.933	0.565
				X-ray exposure			
Yes	1.98 ± 0.87	7.88 ± 0.48	34.44 ± 28.77	33.33 ± 23.97	20.00 ± 18.02	58.33 ± 26.80	34.55 ± 24.63
No	2.47 ± 1.21	7.82 ± 0.48	21.66 ± 22.54	22.91 ± 15.29	51.19 ± 29.70	38.45 ± 26.81	21.35 ± 20.92
p value	0.158	0.724	0.124	0.076	0.000*	0.039*	0.084
				Site of mobile phone storage			
Side pocket	2.41 ± 1.24	7.82 ± 0.48	25.26 ± 24.45	24.95 ± 16.48	46.69 ± 29.73	43.83 ± 27.19	24.16 ± 22.32
Other places	2.45 ± 0.87	7.8 ± 0.43	10.83 ± 10.83	19.16 ± 17.29	53.33 ± 33.66	22.91 ± 21.79	15.33 ± 15.62
p value	0.884	0.741	0.002*	0.269	0.486	0.009	0.109

*Statistically significant p value < 0.05.

inactive men [29]. Increased fat mass in men reduces plasma testosterone levels and also increases gonadal temperatures due to increased fat tissue around the testes [30]. Furthermore, it is reported that resistance exercises may reduce inflammation and oxidative stress in physically active men, thereby improving semen quality [31]. Studies on exercises and sperm quality have shown inconsistent results, and as such, more reliable and reproducible experiments will have to be designed [32, 33].

We examined the influence of cigarette smoking on semen quality owing to the fact that smoking has been associated with several pathological changes, and retrospective studies have shown smoking to lower semen volume, sperm count, and motility [34–36]. Our results showed that men who reported to smoke had a twofold decrease in sperm count. Smoking may reduce sperm quality due to the effect of nicotine and reduced concentration of zinc in semen [37]. In 2016, a study by Asare-Anane et al. [38] showed that smoking reduced semen volume, pH, viability, morphology, and sperm count, with the effects on count, viability, and morphology more pronounced in men who smoked more sticks per day. They suggested that smoking may decrease sperm quality by reducing testosterone levels in smokers. Put together, the data suggests that cigarette smoking reduces sperm quality through multiple pathways including reduced testosterone levels and zinc concentration in semen.

Our study found no significant differences in sperm parameters of participants who consumed alcohol and those that did not. This is in contrast to previous studies that reported that habitual consumption of alcohol reduced sperm quality [39, 40]. On the other hand, a systematic review of studies on alcohol intake and semen quality showed that moderate drinking did not affect semen parameters, but daily consumption affected semen quality [40]. Our results did not show significant differences in semen parameters mainly due to the fact that our data compares occasional consumption versus no consumption [40]. Whereas the study categorized responses into exposure to alcohol and nonexposure, more reliable results may be obtained by differentiating between moderate and daily or high levels of alcohol intake. Nevertheless, the present data shows that occasional alcohol consumption may not negatively impact semen quality.

We also investigated the effect of mobile phone usage and exposure to mobile phone radiations on semen and sperm quality by taking into consideration the site of common storage of the mobile phones on the body. The side pockets were thought to be closest to the groin and therefore may expose the testes and other related structures to the greatest radiation insult, but on the contrary, our study showed phone storage in the side pocket may increase sperm motility and viability. Previous studies have reported reduced motility and morphology of sperms due to radiation, thermal effect, and increased oxidative stress caused by the use of mobile phones [41]. The contradictory results may be due to huge disparity in the percentage of participants that stored mobile phones in side pockets (85%) compared to those that reported to store mobile phones in the breast pocket and other places like in handbags. Moreover, our study did not take into account the type of mobile device as well as the length of time the participants had been using the device. Future studies must take into account these factors. Another limitation of the study may be that semen samples were collected from men referred to the laboratory indicating possible underlying fertility issues as well as the fact that semen collection was done once as opposed to possibly collecting multiple samples for analysis.

5. Conclusions

Sperm quality in Ghanaian men is associated with lifestyle habits. Smoking and sitting for long hours in a day influenced sperm motility and count, respectively. Knowledge of the factors that influence sperm quality in this geographical region can contribute to informed decisions on effective management of infertility in Ghanaian men.

Acknowledgments

We acknowledge the Korle-Bu Teaching Hospital and College of Health Sciences for the support for this study as well as laboratory technicians from the Immunology Unit of Korle-Bu Teaching Hospital.

References

[1] D. S. Irvine, "Epidemiology and aetiology of male infertility," *Human Reproduction*, vol. 13, Suppl 1, pp. 33–44, 1998.

[2] P. O. M. Maison, C. K. Gyasi-Sarpong, and A. K. Koranteng, "The pattern of male infertility in Kumasi, Ghana," *African Journal for Infertility and Assisted Conception*, vol. 2, no. 1, p. 3, 2017.

[3] R. B. Leaver, "Male infertility: an overview of causes and treatment options," *British Journal of Nursing*, vol. 25, no. 18, pp. S35–S40, 2016.

[4] H. Levine, N. Jørgensen, A. Martino-Andrade et al., "Temporal trends in sperm count: a systematic review and meta-regression analysis," *Human Reproduction Update*, vol. 23, no. 6, pp. 646–659, 2017.

[5] P. Sengupta, S. Dutta, and E. Krajewska-Kulak, "The disappearing sperms: analysis of reports published between 1980 and 2015," *American Journal of Men's Health*, vol. 11, no. 4, pp. 1279–1304, 2017.

[6] P. Sengupta, E. Borges Jr., S. Dutta, and E. Krajewska-Kulak, "Decline in sperm count in European men during the past 50 years," *Human & Experimental Toxicology*, vol. 37, no. 3, pp. 247–255, 2017.

[7] P. Sengupta, U. Nwagha, S. Dutta, E. Krajewska-Kulak, and E. Izuka, "Evidence for decreasing sperm count in African population from 1965 to 2015," *African Health Sciences*, vol. 17, no. 2, pp. 418–427, 2017.

[8] N. E. Skakkebaek, N. Jørgensen, A.-M. Andersson et al., "Populations, decreasing fertility, and reproductive health," *The Lancet*, vol. 393, no. 10180, pp. 1500-1501, 2019.

[9] D. Durairajanayagam, "Lifestyle causes of male infertility," *Arab Journal of Urology*, vol. 16, no. 1, pp. 10–20, 2019.

[10] J. Jurewicz, M. Radwan, W. Sobala, P. Radwan, M. Bochenek, and W. Hanke, "Effects of occupational exposure - is there a link between exposure based on an occupational questionnaire and semen quality?," *Systems Biology in Reproductive Medicine*, vol. 60, no. 4, pp. 227–233, 2014.

[11] K. Leisegang and S. Dutta, "Do lifestyle practices impede male fertility?," *Andrologia*, vol. 24, Article ID e13595, 2020.

[12] R. P. Hayden, R. Flannigan, and P. N. Schlegel, "The Role of Lifestyle in Male Infertility: Diet, Physical Activity, and Body Habitus," *Current Urology Reports*, vol. 19, no. 7, 2018.

[13] W. Ruixue, Z. Hongli, Z. Zhihong, D. Rulin, G. Dongfeng, and L. Ruizhi, "The impact of semen quality, occupational exposure to environmental factors and lifestyle on recurrent pregnancy loss," *Journal of Assisted Reproduction and Genetics*, vol. 30, no. 11, pp. 1513–1518, 2013.

[14] T. Janevic, L. G. Kahn, P. Landsbergis et al., "Effects of work and life stress on semen quality," *Fertility and Sterility*, vol. 102, no. 2, pp. 530–538, 2014.

[15] H. Yang, Q. Chen, N. Zhou et al., "Lifestyles associated with human semen quality: results from MARHCS cohort study in Chongqing, China," *Medicine (Baltimore)*, vol. 94, no. 28, 2015.

[16] J. Jurewicz, M. Radwan, W. Sobala et al., "Lifestyle and semen quality: role of modifiable risk factors," *Systems Biology in Reproductive Medicine*, vol. 60, no. 1, pp. 43–51, 2014.

[17] R. Z. Liu, J. C. Gao, H. G. Zhang, R. X. Wang, Z. H. Zhang, and X. Y. Liu, "Seminal plasma zinc level may be associated with the effect of cigarette smoking on sperm parameters," *Journal of International Medical Research*, vol. 38, no. 3, pp. 923–928, 2010.

[18] M. F. Hamad, N. Shelko, S. Kartarius, M. Montenarh, and M. E. Hammadeh, "Impact of cigarette smoking on histone

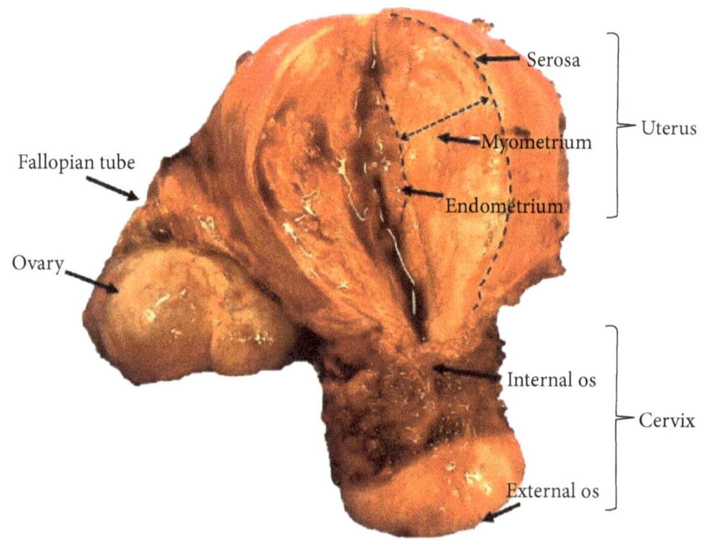

Figure 1: Human uterus and cervix removed at hysterectomy, with a vertical incision on the anterior aspect, representing macroscopic uterine anatomy.

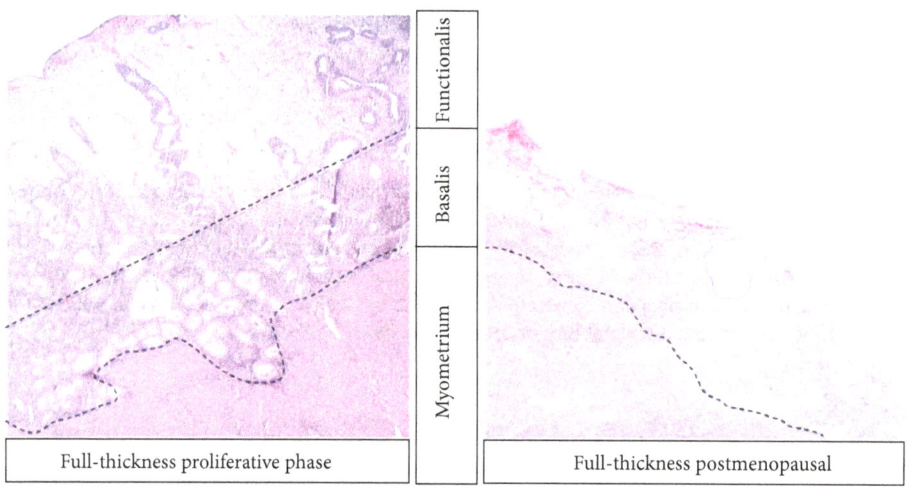

Figure 2: Representative micrograph (4x) of full-thickness human uterine biopsies taken from pre- and postmenopausal women, containing both endometrium and subendometrial myometrium stained with haematoxylin and eosin.

biopsy methods, either using suction (pipelle) curettes (Figure 3) or scraping with metal curettes. However, the deeper basalis is not usually accessible in a preserved intact premenopausal uterus, and with pipelle or even more extensive curette biopsies, the amount of functionalis obtained depends hugely on the optimal sampling technique and on the cycle phase. For example, pipelle biopsies obtained at the time of spontaneous (menstrual phase) or iatrogenic (traumatic) bleeding may contain mostly blood without much endometrial tissue. Some of these problems can be overcome by adapting special techniques in an intact uterus, such as resection of the endometrium under direct vision with hysteroscopy to obtain a full-thickness endometrial sample containing basalis. However, this is usually an additional and a more invasive procedure, which may not be routinely performed, therefore will require further ethical considerations, necessitating additional time, counselling regarding specific-risks, and thus resources [6]. The premenopausal basalis can also be harvested as a wedge biopsy from a hysterectomy specimen, where a full-thickness endometrial sample can be obtained containing the functionalis, the basalis, and the underlying myometrium [7] (Figure 3). It is important to note, however, that the indication for hysterectomy is usually an underlying uterine pathology, such as heavy menstrual bleeding, endometriosis, or malignancy [8]; therefore, the samples may not be representative of a normal healthy endometrium. Furthermore, most women undergo hysterectomy for benign conditions when medical therapy fails, thus will be routinely still on hormonal treatment, such as the Mirena intrauterine device or gonadotropin-releasing hormone (GnRH) analogue treatments. Such exogenous hormones will alter endometrial phenotype and function, and therefore, a wash out period after hormone exposure is indicated when examining the normal endometrium (of at least 3 months after being on any hormonal therapy) to avoid exogenous hormonal influence. Some authors have harvested placental bed biopsies at the time of

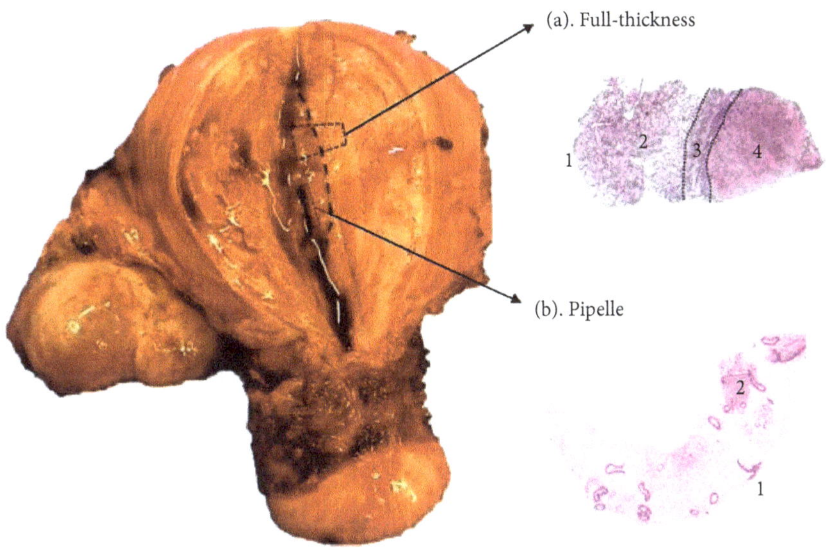

FIGURE 3: Image of a human uterus with representative micrographs of (a) full-thickness endometrial biopsy (100x) from a hysterectomy specimen and (b) pipelle endometrial biopsy (4x), depicting the distinct anatomical areas included in each of them when the human uterus is sampled with different methods. (1) Luminal epithelium, (2) functionalis, (3) basalis, and (4) myometrium.

delivery of a baby, where decidual tissue with some superficial myometrial tissue is obtained [9].

Contrastingly, in postmenopausal women and premenopausal women on hormonal preparations that preclude the influence of cyclical ovarian hormones on the endometrium, (e.g. GnRH analogues), there is no endometrial functionalis layer. Therefore, when the endometrium is sampled, the harvested biopsies will only contain the stem cell-rich basalis layer of the endometrium [10, 11]. Furthermore, full-thickness biopsies taken from this thin endometrium in a hysterectomy sample (and even possibly from a curettage) invariably contain the underlying myometrium; thus, the studies examining the expression of endometrial-specific genes may be affected by the myometrial expression levels that are included in the whole biopsy. In endometrial cancer research, it is challenging, and not usually possible, to obtain a full-thickness uterine biopsy for snap freezing or RNA studies, as the specimen must be initially preserved whole for pathologists' scrutiny and staging purposes [3]. Hence, curettes or pipelle biopsies are the only available sampling methods for most studies. Depending on the size and the nature of the cancer, a superficial endometrial biopsy may contain a malignant or benign endometrium, or a combination. The actual proportion of cancer cells included in a whole frozen or freshly collected tissue biopsy may affect the data obtained but is not easy to determine. Haematoxylin and eosin (H&E) staining and morphological assessment of the frozen tissue sections may be suitable in some instances. Furthermore, others have also explored the possibility of examining the uterine fluid that represents the cytokine or metabolic milieu of the endometrium related to a particular pathology [12].

There are significant changes in the endometrial cell phenotype and function during different phases of the menstrual cycle [1, 13], including proliferation, decidualisation, and changes in hormone responsiveness. The cellular composition also changes significantly across the menstrual cycle. For example, a sample containing secretory-phase functionalis layer will contain leucocytes accounting for up to 30% stromal cells due to the massive leucocyte infiltration that occurs at the end of the cycle [14]. These changes in cellular proliferation and composition are mainly limited to the functionalis layer, which is relevant to fertility and premenopausal gynaecological conditions, such as heavy menstrual bleeding [15, 16]. Therefore, fertility researchers focus mainly on this layer for the obvious reasons, and they often take biopsies that only contain the functionalis layer from women who wish to preserve their uterus and thus their fertility [17, 18]. In contrast, stem cell biologists focus more on the basalis layer since it has been postulated to harbour endometrial stem cells [5, 10].

Since the endometrium is the primary target organ for ovarian hormones, the endometrial biopsy should naturally be examined in the context of the menstrual cycle phase and thus with relevance to the distinct ovarian hormonal influence of that phase [1]. Frequently, cell type-specific gene expression or protein quantitative studies process whole endometrial samples without necessarily considering the differing cell types included in each sample [19–21]; therefore, cell type-specific changes maybe diluted or masked in the results obtained by analysing the whole biopsy. Unless normalisation using a specific marker is performed, such as marking epithelial cells with cytokeratin to assess the proportion of the particular cell type present in the biopsy, the final results will be prejudiced by the heterogeneity of the cell types included [11, 22, 23].

The cell-cell interaction between the different cell types of the endometrium is also important, with evidence suggesting that cross-talk between the epithelial and stromal cells plays an important role in hormonal regulation, for example, in the context of steroid hormone receptor expression [1, 2]. Methods which do not disturb the tissue architecture but directly assess the gene or protein expression at a cellular level, such as *in situ* hybridisation [11], immunohistochemistry [21], or immunofluorescence [23], will remove this bias. Isolating cells directly can also be achieved with antibody-based fluorescence-activated cell sorting (FACS) [10] or magnetic bead sorting [23] which will also allow extended functional studies in the isolated, viable cells employing either in vitro or in vivo models. Techniques such as laser capture microdissection [24, 25] can also be employed to extract a particular cell type from a frozen tissue section. This method will allow direct comparison and further in-depth analysis of endometrial epithelial and stromal cells from the different endometrial compartments. Furthermore, the novel technique imaging mass cytometry (Fluidigm) has recently been optimised for the first time in the endometrium, broadening our ability to study the endometrium in detail [26]. Techniques like this provide a remarkable platform for highly detailed functional and phenotypic analysis of endometrial tissue, in this case employing metal-labelled antibodies, rather than the fluorochromes that are used in traditional flow cytometry or in immunofluorescence studies. Therefore, it allows simultaneous analysis of a greater number of markers in a single endometrial tissue section. Although cell type-specific spatial expression of genes or gene products can be observed with aforementioned methods, the quantification still poses a challenge. The use of a variety of semiquantitative scoring systems[2] and computer-based image analysis methods [14] has attempted to reduce observer bias; but none have removed the problem completely. The use of these new techniques and further studies on optimising the analytic methods used will continue to increase our understanding of the human endometrial architecture and cell-specific functions.

In order to avoid common pitfalls, researchers examining endometrial biopsies should follow the already published, elaborative, and standard operating procedures that are available for specific pathologies [7, 27]. These were designed to harmonise the data generated using human endometrial samples and to improve the quality, reproducibility, and clinical translatability of the research.

2.1. Solutions for Common Problems with Endometrial Sampling

2.1.1. Pipelle Endometrial Biopsy/Endometrial Curettings. The main problems encountered with these biopsies are (1) the inclusion of insufficient endometrial material and (2) sampling of endometrial functionalis only, unless in certain patients (e.g. postmenopausal women or those on particular hormonal preparations such as gonadotrophin-releasing hormone analogues/progestogens, which curtail the effects of dynamic and cyclical ovarian hormones to produce an endometrial functionalis). To rectify or account for these issues, careful histological evaluation of the biopsy content should be undertaken by a trained histopathologist and reported in the publication accordingly [2, 4, 10, 11, 17].

2.1.2. Harvesting the Endometrium from Hysterectomy Samples. Studies collecting the endometrium from hysterectomy samples should, from the outset, clarify if they intend to collect either full-thickness samples (which requires opening of the uterine cavity) or other scraping or suction methods that would access mostly the endometrial functionalis. When the full-thickness endometrium is collected, the methodology should include details on the exact location in the uterine cavity (e.g., fundal, anterior, or posterior wall) where the biopsy is taken. If the study compared data generated using samples of the endometrium from women who have only a basalis layer (e.g., postmenopausal), with the endometrium of premenopausal women who have a thicker endometrium with obvious basalis and functionalis regions, it is essential to clarify the exact layer that is compared to provide robust and reproducible results [2]. Inclusion of myometrium cells in the whole "endometrial" sample in a full-thickness sample can affect some data. For example, if myometrial cells have a distinct gene expression pattern that may erroneously be interpreted as relevant to the endometrium. The use of specific techniques such as laser capture microdissection would allow accurate isolation of a particular cell type in this instance. If the endometrium is obtained from the hysterectomy specimen using suction or scraping without opening the uterus, the precautions mentioned in Section 2.1.1 above should be followed.

3. Harvesting the Myometrium

Myometrial samples are most commonly harvested during a caesarean section (CS), as the myometrium is easily accessible from the uterine incision [28]. The uterine incision at a routine CS is a transverse incision on the anterior aspect of the lower uterine segment. The lower segment of the uterus is typically developed at late gestation and in labour and lies between the physiological retraction ring and the obstetrical internal os [29]. It is a thinner, more fibrous part of the myometrium, which is also less active than the rest of the uterine corpus in a labouring uterus [30, 31]. A myometrial biopsy can be taken from the upper or the lower edge of the transverse uterine incision [28]. Myometrial functional studies as well as many molecular biological studies are often performed on these biopsies. However, the results can be affected by obesity, diabetes, gestation, the presence or absence of labour, singleton or twin pregnancy, and fibrosis from previous uterine surgery [32–35]. Furthermore, data should be interpreted in the context of these biopsies being obtained from a gravid uterus, which has undergone massive hypertrophy [36] and has been exposed to the pregnancy related hormonal milieu [37]. The location of the myometrial biopsy may also have implications for data analysis; for example, a biopsy taken from the upper uterine segment at a classical CS (where a vertical incision is made into the upper uterine segment) may have different properties to the myometrium obtained from a lower uterine segment [38]; however, in relation to contractility studies, current evidence suggests that there is no significant difference between myometrial biopsies obtained from upper and lower uterine segments [39].

The nonpregnant myometrium can be sampled at the time of gynaecological surgery, typically after hysterectomy

[40] or at myomectomy. Myomectomy samples may contain leiomyomatous tissue, but a sample obtained at hysterectomy can be taken from any part of the uterus, with or without commonly occurring pathological lesions such as leiomyomata or adenomyomas [16]. Interestingly, published functional studies commonly compare the nonpregnant and pregnant myometrium, for example assessing the contractility of muscle fibres, but do not necessarily consider the impact of comparing muscle fibres derived from different uterine areas [41, 42]. This may impact the quality of the data generated, for example, if the non-pregnant myometrial fibres were obtained from the uterine fundus, whilst pregnant myometrium was derived from the lower segment of the uterus [43]. This issue is further complicated by the fact that no discernible lower segment exists in a nonpregnant uterus; thus, we propose that attempts should be made to collect myometrial tissue from the anterior lower uterine body in nonpregnant uterus and from the upper edge of the transverse CS incision to strive to obtain similar tissue for comparative studies. Finally, since the myometrium contains distinct myometrial layers [43, 44], the exact layer muscle fibres are derived from may also confound the results.

4. Conclusion

In summary, uterine biopsies are a valuable source of human tissue, and studies using these biospecimens have contributed significantly to our current understanding of pregnancy, fertility, and many gynaecological disorders. When collecting and processing uterine biopsies for studies and biobanking, careful consideration is essential of the many pitfalls that can confound the results obtained from them, and strict adherence to published standard operative procedures is also imperative. This will enable researchers to utilise these important biospecimens to discover diagnostic and therapeutic targets for the benefit of millions of women suffering from obstetric and gynaecological conditions.

Authors' Contributions

D.K.H. conceived the manuscript. A.M., A.K., M.A., R.A., N.T., and D.K.H. prepared the first draft. A.M. and D.K.H. revised the manuscript critically and prepared the references. All authors revised and read the manuscript and approved the submitted final version.

Acknowledgments

The authors would like to thank the Liverpool Women's NHS Foundation Trust and the University of Liverpool, for their continued support. This work was supported by the Wellbeing of Women (grant numbers ELS706, RG1073, and RG2137), the National Institute of Health Research (ACF and ACL), and the Liverpool Women's Hospital cancer charity.

References

[1] D. K. Hapangama, A. M. Kamal, and J. N. Bulmer, "Estrogen receptor β: the guardian of the endometrium," *Human Reproduction Update*, vol. 21, no. 2, pp. 174–193, 2015.

[2] A. M. Kamal, J. N. Bulmer, S. B. DeCruze, H. F. Stringfellow, P. Martin-Hirsch, and D. K. Hapangama, "Androgen receptors are acquired by healthy postmenopausal endometrial epithelium and their subsequent loss in endometrial cancer is associated with poor survival," *British Journal of Cancer*, vol. 114, no. 6, pp. 688–696, 2016.

[3] R. A. A. Alnafakh, M. Adishesh, L. Button, G. Saretzki, and D. K. Hapangama, "Telomerase and telomeres in endometrial cancer," *Frontiers in Oncology*, vol. 9, p. 344, 2019.

[4] A. J. Valentijn, G. Saretzki, N. Tempest, H. O. Critchley, and D. K. Hapangama, "Human endometrial epithelial telomerase is important for epithelial proliferation and glandular formation with potential implications in endometriosis," *Human Reproduction*, vol. 30, no. 12, pp. 2816–2828, 2015.

[5] N. Tempest, A. Maclean, and D. K. Hapangama, "Endometrial stem cell markers: current concepts and unresolved questions," *International Journal of Molecular Sciences*, vol. 19, no. 10, p. 3240, 2018.

[6] N. Bourdel, P. Chauvet, E. Tognazza, B. Pereira, R. Botchorishvili, and M. Canis, "Sampling in atypical endometrial hyperplasia: which method results in the lowest underestimation of endometrial cancer? A systematic review and meta-analysis," *Journal of Minimally Invasive Gynecology*, vol. 23, no. 5, pp. 692–701, 2016.

[7] M. Adishesh, A. Fyson, S. B. DeCruze et al., "Harmonisation of biobanking standards in endometrial cancer research," *British Journal of Cancer*, vol. 117, no. 4, pp. 485–493, 2017.

[8] S. Sourial, N. Tempest, and D. K. Hapangama, "Theories on the pathogenesis of endometriosis," *International Journal of Reproductive Medicine*, vol. 2014, Article ID 179515, 9 pages, 2014.

[9] J. N. Bulmer, P. J. Williams, and G. E. Lash, "Immune cells in the placental bed," *The International Journal of Developmental Biology*, vol. 54, no. 2-3, pp. 281–294, 2010.

[10] A. J. Valentijn, K. Palial, H. al-lamee et al., "SSEA-1 isolates human endometrial basal glandular epithelial cells: phenotypic and functional characterization and implications in the pathogenesis of endometriosis," *Human Reproduction*, vol. 28, no. 10, pp. 2695–2708, 2013.

[11] N. Tempest, A. M. Baker, N. A. Wright, and D. K. Hapangama, "Does human endometrial LGR5 gene expression suggest the existence of another hormonally regulated epithelial stem cell niche?," *Human Reproduction*, vol. 33, no. 6, pp. 1052–1062, 2018.

[12] H. C. Fitzgerald, L. A. Salamonsen, L. J. Rombauts, B. J. Vollenhoven, and T. A. Edgell, "The proliferative phase underpins endometrial development: altered cytokine profiles in uterine lavage fluid of women with idiopathic infertility," *Cytokine*, vol. 88, pp. 12–19, 2016.

[13] A. Kamal, N. Tempest, C. Parkes et al., "Hormones and endometrial carcinogenesis," *Hormone Molecular Biology and Clinical Investigation*, vol. 25, no. 2, pp. 129–148, 2016.

[14] J. A. Drury, K. L. Parkin, L. Coyne, E. Giuliani, A. T. Fazleabas, and D. K. Hapangama, "The dynamic changes in the number of uterine natural killer cells are specific to the eutopic but not to the ectopic endometrium in women and in a baboon

model of endometriosis," *Reproductive Biology and Endocrinology*, vol. 16, no. 1, p. 67, 2018.

[15] S. Biswas Shivhare, J. N. Bulmer, B. A. Innes, D. K. Hapangama, and G. E. Lash, "Menstrual cycle distribution of uterine natural killer cells is altered in heavy menstrual bleeding," *Journal of Reproductive Immunology*, vol. 112, pp. 88–94, 2015.

[16] D. K. Hapangama and J. N. Bulmer, "Pathophysiology of heavy menstrual bleeding," *Women's Health*, vol. 12, no. 1, pp. 3–13, 2016.

[17] D. K. Hapangama, M. A. Turner, J. A. Drury et al., "Endometriosis is associated with aberrant endometrial expression of telomerase and increased telomere length," *Human Reproduction*, vol. 23, no. 7, pp. 1511–1519, 2008.

[18] C. D. Williams, J. F. Boggess, L. R. LaMarque et al., "A prospective, randomized study of endometrial telomerase during the menstrual cycle," *The Journal of Clinical Endocrinology and Metabolism*, vol. 86, no. 8, pp. 3912–3917, 2001.

[19] H. O. D. Critchley, K. A. Robertson, T. Forster, T. A. Henderson, A. R. W. Williams, and P. Ghazal, "Gene expression profiling of mid to late secretory phase endometrial biopsies from women with menstrual complaint," *American Journal of Obstetrics and Gynecology*, vol. 195, no. 2, pp. 406–414.e7, 2006.

[20] A. P. Ponnampalam, G. C. Weston, A. C. Trajstman, B. Susil, and P. A. Rogers, "Molecular classification of human endometrial cycle stages by transcriptional profiling," *Molecular Human Reproduction*, vol. 10, no. 12, pp. 879–893, 2004.

[21] D. Mathew, J. A. Drury, A. J. Valentijn, O. Vasieva, and D. K. Hapangama, "In silico, in vitro and in vivo analysis identifies a potential role for steroid hormone regulation of FOXD3 in endometriosis-associated genes," *Human Reproduction*, vol. 31, no. 2, pp. 345–354, 2016.

[22] A. Kamal, A. Valentijn, R. Barraclough et al., "High AGR2 protein is a feature of low grade endometrial cancer cells," *Oncotarget*, vol. 9, no. 59, pp. 31459–31472, 2018.

[23] D. K. Hapangama, J. Drury, L. da Silva et al., "Abnormally located SSEA1+/SOX9+ endometrial epithelial cells with a basalis-like phenotype in the eutopic functionalis layer may play a role in the pathogenesis of endometriosis," *Human Reproduction*, vol. 34, no. 1, pp. 56–68, 2019.

[24] A. Yanaihara, Y. Otsuka, S. Iwasaki, K. Koide, T. Aida, and T. Okai, "Comparison in gene expression of secretory human endometrium using laser microdissection," *Reproductive Biology and Endocrinology*, vol. 2, no. 1, p. 66, 2004.

[25] A. Maclean, J. Bhullar, S. Miwa et al., "Differential expression of hormone metabolising enzymes defines endometrial epithelial sub-populations," *BJOG-An International Journal of Obstetrics and Gynaecology*, vol. 126, pp. E134–E134, 2019.

[26] A. Maclean, J. Bhullar, S. Miwa et al., "Blair Bell Research Society: annual academic meeting abstracts," *BJOG: An International Journal of Obstetrics & Gynaecology*, vol. 126, no. 6, pp. e125–e141, 2019.

[27] A. F. Vitonis, K. Vincent, N. Rahmioglu et al., "World Endometriosis Research Foundation Endometriosis Phenome and Biobanking Harmonization Project: II. Clinical and covariate phenotype data collection in endometriosis research," *Fertility and Sterility*, vol. 102, no. 5, pp. 1223–1232, 2014.

[28] S. Arrowsmith, P. Keov, M. Muttenthaler, and C. W. Gruber, "Contractility measurements of human uterine smooth muscle to aid drug development," *Journal of Visualized Experiments*, no. 131, article e56639, 2018.

[29] C. P. Wendell-Smith, "The lower uterine segment," *The Journal of Obstetrics and Gynaecology of the British Empire*, vol. 61, no. 1, pp. 87–93, 1954.

[30] C. Sparey, S. C. Robson, J. Bailey, F. Lyall, and G. N. Europe-Finner, "The differential expression of myometrial connexin-43, cyclooxygenase-1 and -2, and Gs alpha proteins in the upper and lower segments of the human uterus during pregnancy and labor," *The Journal of Clinical Endocrinology and Metabolism*, vol. 84, no. 5, pp. 1705–1710, 1999.

[31] K. Wedenberg, G. Ronquist, A. Waldenstrom, and U. Ulmsten, "Regional differences in energy charge of the pregnant human uterus regardless of functional status in comparison with the non-pregnant uterus," *Biochimica et Biophysica Acta*, vol. 1058, no. 2, pp. 147–151, 1991.

[32] J. Zhang, L. Bricker, S. Wray, and S. Quenby, "Poor uterine contractility in obese women," *BJOG : An International Journal of Obstetrics and Gynaecology*, vol. 114, no. 3, pp. 343–348, 2007.

[33] S. Arrowsmith, A. Kendrick, J. A. Hanley, K. Noble, and S. Wray, "Myometrial physiology–time to translate?," *Experimental Physiology*, vol. 99, no. 3, pp. 495–502, 2014.

[34] P. Turton, S. Arrowsmith, J. Prescott et al., "A comparison of the contractile properties of myometrium from singleton and twin pregnancies," *PLoS One*, vol. 8, no. 5, article e63800, 2013.

[35] O. Santos Filho Ode, L. M. Nardozza, E. Araujo Junior, L. C. Rolo, L. Camano, and A. F. Moron, "Cesarean uterine scar evaluation by the grey-level histogram," *Revista da Associacao Medica Brasileira (1992)*, vol. 56, no. 1, pp. 99–102, 2010.

[36] O. Shynlova, R. Kwong, and S. J. Lye, "Mechanical stretch regulates hypertrophic phenotype of the myometrium during pregnancy," *Reproduction*, vol. 139, no. 1, pp. 247–253, 2010.

[37] S. Wray and C. Prendergast, "The myometrium: from excitation to contractions and labour," *Advances in Experimental Medicine and Biology*, vol. 1124, pp. 233–263, 2019.

[38] S. Astle, S. Thornton, and D. M. Slater, "Identification and localization of prostaglandin E2 receptors in upper and lower segment human myometrium during pregnancy," *Molecular Human Reproduction*, vol. 11, no. 4, pp. 279–287, 2005.

[39] M. J. Luckas and S. Wray, "A comparison of the contractile properties of human myometrium obtained from the upper and lower uterine segments," *BJOG : An International Journal of Obstetrics and Gynaecology*, vol. 107, no. 10, pp. 1309–1311, 2000.

[40] A. M. Darwish, A. M. Makhlouf, A. A. Youssof, and H. A. Gadalla, "Hysteroscopic myometrial biopsy in unexplained abnormal uterine bleeding," *European Journal of Obstetrics, Gynecology, and Reproductive Biology*, vol. 86, no. 2, pp. 139–143, 1999.

[41] M. J. Luckas, M. J. Taggart, and S. Wray, "Intracellular calcium stores and agonist-induced contractions in isolated human myometrium," *American Journal of Obstetrics and Gynecology*, vol. 181, no. 2, pp. 468–476, 1999.

[42] R. A. Word, J. T. Stull, M. L. Casey, and K. E. Kamm, "Contractile elements and myosin light chain phosphorylation in myometrial tissue from nonpregnant and pregnant women," *The Journal of Clinical Investigation*, vol. 92, no. 1, pp. 29–37, 1993.

[43] H. N. Aguilar and B. F. Mitchell, "Physiological pathways and molecular mechanisms regulating uterine contractility," *Human Reproduction Update*, vol. 16, no. 6, pp. 725–744, 2010.

[44] S. Weiss, T. Jaermann, P. Schmid et al., "Three-dimensional fiber architecture of the nonpregnant human uterus determined ex vivo using magnetic resonance diffusion tensor imaging," *The Anatomical Record. Part A, Discoveries in Molecular, Cellular, and Evolutionary Biology*, vol. 288A, no. 1, pp. 84–90, 2006.

6

Combined Intranasal Insulin/Saxagliptin/Metformin Therapies Ameliorate the Effect of Combined Oral Contraceptive- (COC-) Induced Metabolic Syndrome (MetS) with a Major Target on Glucose Metabolism in Adult Female Wistar Rats

Saheed Olanrewaju Afolabi, Joy Folahan, Olalekan Agede, and Olufunke Olorundare

Department of Pharmacology and Therapeutics, University of Ilorin, Ilorin, Nigeria

Correspondence should be addressed to Saheed Olanrewaju Afolabi; afolabi.so@unilorin.edu.ng

Academic Editor: Vikas Roy

Objective. To evaluate the effect of the chronic use of combined oral contraceptives (COCs: ethinyl estradiol and levonorgestrel) on the indices of metabolic syndrome in adult female Wistar rats and possible therapeutic management. *Materials and Methods.* 64 female Wistar rats received either distilled water, norethindrone (NOR), COC, intranasal insulin (INI), metformin (MET), saxagliptin (SAX), INI+MET, and INI+SAX. After 8 weeks of exposure to COC, the animals were sorted into the therapeutic groups. Several parameters were assayed for, such as body weight changes, fasting blood glucose (FBG) level, insulin levels, inflammatory cytokines, and glycated hemoglobin (Hb1Ac). *Results.* The levels of FBG, insulin, and Hb1Ac were increased consequent upon COC treatment. Treatment with INI+SAX and INI+MET reduced significantly the levels of FBG and Hb1Ac; in addition, the level of insulin was significantly increased in the INI+MET groups ($p \leq 0.05$). Serum lipid profile analysis showed a statistical reduction in high-density lipoprotein (HDL) level; this reduction was also significantly reversed in the INI+SAX group. Reduced catalase activity observed in the COC group was reversed in the INI+MET group ($p \leq 0.05$). A nonsignificant increase in the level of TNF-α as a result of COC treatment was reversed by INI and INI+MET treatment. Liver GLUT4 and G-6-phosphate levels were significantly increased by COC treatment, and this effect was reversed by INI+SAX in both assays, respectively ($p \leq 0.01$). *Conclusions.* The use of MET and SAX in combination with INI has been shown to reverse some indices of MetS. This study proposes a clinical phase to backup and ascertain these preclinical findings.

1. Introduction

Premenopausal women are active users of hormonal contraceptives. In the last decade, there has been an upsurge in this usage; scientific reports have estimated that over 150 million sexually active women subscribe to these pharmaceuticals globally [1–3]. Commercially available formulations consisting of a synthetic estrogen and progestin constitute the globally recognized combined oral contraceptives (COCs) [4, 5]. In addition to its contraceptive effects, constant administration of COC is also being explored as a therapeutic intervention against polycystic ovary syndrome (PCOS) and dysmenorrhea [6, 7]. However, the use of COC has been linked with disruption in body weight regulation, arterial blood pressure, glucose metabolism, and general homeostatic regulations in females [8, 9]. Endocrinologists and researchers in the field of reproductive health suggest that continuous prescription of COC should be revised with respect to these adverse effects [10, 11]. Ethinyl estradiol (EE), synthesized from 17β-estradiol (E2), is the most used synthetic estrogen in COC [7, 12, 13]; it is an estrogen receptor agonist. Over the years, ethinyl estradiol has been used for menopausal symptoms, gynecological disorders, and some forms of hormone-sensitive cancers [14–16]. Currently, EE is almost exclusively employed for the adjunctive role it plays in the COC, making it the most widely used estrogen [17]. Levonorgestrel (LEV) is a use-alone emergency contraceptive pill and is also formulated with estrogen in some COC [18]. It is a progestin that works principally by preventing ovulation and enhancing the closure of the cervix to prevent the entry of sperm, similar to the hormone progesterone [19, 20]. LEV is a synthetic steroid (17α-ethynyl-18-methyl-19-nortestosterone) derived from testosterone [21].

The combination of these hormones has been studied for their therapeutic efficacy in women who have PCOS, a pathological condition characterized by dysregulation in and carbohydrate metabolism in women [22, 23]. Generally, COCs from its inception have been linked with dysregulation of glucose homeostasis. The COCs containing norethindrone and EE have reportedly increased glycemia levels in premenopausal women [24]; this effect was in tandem with COC containing levonorgestrel and EE [25].

Glycemic regulation is under the control of the hormone, insulin. When glucose level in the extracellular fluid increases, it is transported to the pancreatic β-cells and its consequent metabolism raises the intracellular ATP/ADP ratio. This closes the ATP-sensitive/K+ channels (KATP), causing depolarization of the β-cell membranes and activation of Ca^{2+}-activated voltage channels; the Ca^{2+} influx then activates the release of insulin granules via exocytosis [26, 27]. Insulin resistance (IR) is a metabolic disorder that features a decreased response to both exogenous and endogenous insulin in cells, specific adipose tissues, skeletal muscles, and the whole body. IR is one of the major indicators and pathological driver of metabolic syndrome, a disease condition caused by a myriad of metabolic mishaps which features IR, hyperinsulinemia, glucose intolerance, and dyslipidemia [28, 29]. Metabolic syndrome is suggested to be the most important medical problem of the 21st century. Insulin resistance is a known risk factor for type 2 diabetes [30, 31]. Metformin is an oral hypoglycemic agent belonging to the biguanide class of antidiabetic agents. It is often used as first-line treatment of diabetes [32, 33]. It improves hyperglycemia primarily through its suppression of hepatic glucose production, increases insulin sensitivity, enhances peripheral glucose uptake, upregulates oxidation of fatty acid [34], and downregulates glucose absorption from the gastrointestinal tract. A member of the dipeptidyl peptidase-4 (DPP-4) inhibitor group of oral hypoglycemics, saxagliptin is approved by the US Food and Drug Administration and the European Medicines Agency. DPP-4 inhibitors are believed to be therapeutically effective in the management of IR and thus could prevent metabolic syndrome [35].

Here, we set out to investigate the effect of combined oral contraceptives (ethinyl estradiol and levonorgestrel) and minipill (norethindrone) on adult female albino rats; and the possible ameliorative effect of single/combined administration of saxagliptin, intranasal insulin and metformin on the metabolic syndrome status.

2. Materials and Methods

2.1. Experimental Groups. Adult female Wistar rats (64) were obtained from an animal house facility in Ogbomosho, Oyo state, Nigeria, and housed in groups of eight and allowed to acclimatize for 7 days in the animal housing facility of the Faculty of Basic Medical Sciences, University of Ilorin, Nigeria. Housing conditions were temperature of 25°C and a 12 : 12 light : dark cycle with light on by 07 : 00 and off at 1900. The animals were housed in metabolic cages with wood shavings as beddings replaced fortnightly. Animals had unrestricted access to rat pelletized feed from Top Feed Nigeria Ltd. (consisting of maize, soybean, GNC, corn brown, wheat offal, palm kernel cake, and bone) and water ad libitum. Animals were monitored and cleaned up daily. All eight groups received distilled water/NOR/COC for 8 weeks; then, each group received various therapeutic regimen for 7 days as outlined below. All protocols involving the use of experimental animals were duly approved by the University Ethical Committee with the approval number UERC/ASN/2020/2028. The international guide to handle and use of experimental animals by the National Research Council [36] and Committee for the Update of the Guide for the Care and Use of Laboratory Animals [37] was strictly adhered to during the animal handling phase of this study.

The animal experimental groupings are underlisted.

Group 1. Control

Group 2. Norethindrone (NOR), 1.4 mg/kg/day

Group 3. Combined oral contraceptives (EE and LEV; COC), 7.6 mg/kg/day

Group 4. COC+intranasal insulin (INI: 2 IU, 1 IU/10 μl and 10 μl/nostril)

Group 5. COC+metformin (MET: 150 mg/kg/day)

Group 6. COC+saxagliptin (SAX: 10 mg/kg/day)

Group 7. COC+INI+MET

Group 8. COC+INI+SAX

2.2. Drugs. Recombinant human insulin (actrapid, 100 IU/ml) was purchased from Novo Nordisk, combined oral contraceptives (ethinyl estradiol and levonorgestrel) were from Bayer USA, and metformin, norethindrone (minipill), and saxagliptin were purchased from MedPlus pharmacy Ilorin. All biochemical reagents including ELISA kits for rat insulin, glucose-6-phosphate, lipids, and glucokinase were purchased from Elabscience (US). All other chemicals were of analytical grade and commercially available. Accu-Chek glucometer and glucose strips were purchased from Roche Diagnostic, USA (Micropipette P-10, Eppendorf).

2.3. Intranasal Insulin Administration. According to the method described by Njan et al. [38], rats were anesthetized by placing them in tightly sealed transparent glass jars containing isoflurane (5%) obtained from Southern Anesthesia & Surgical, (West Columbia, US) for brief periods (<30 s), removed, and restrained in the supine position. A total of 2 IU (1 IU/10 μl and 10 μl/nostril) of rapid acting insulin or vehicle (0.9% Sodium Chloride, NaCl) was rapidly dispensed intranasally using a micropipette (P-10, Eppendorf). This procedure lasted for about 15 s. Animals became conscious in another 15–20 s and were observed physically before returning to the metabolic cages.

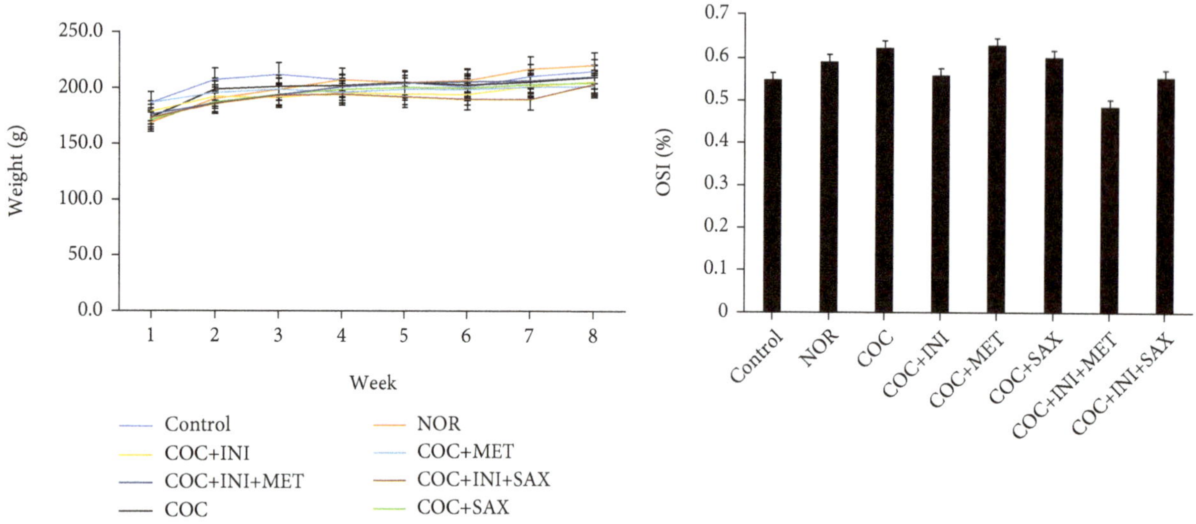

(a) (b)

FIGURE 1: (a) The effect of treatment groups on weekly body weight monitoring. There was no statistically significant alteration in the weight of the treatment groups when compared with the control at $p \leq 0.05$; mean ± SEM, $n = 8$. (b) The organosomatic index (OSI) carried out on the pancreas showed no statistical difference in the weight of the organ in the treatment group when compared with the control $p \leq 0.05$; mean ± SEM, $n = 8$.

2.4. Measurement of Body Weight, Organosomatic Index, Fasting Blood Glucose, and Glucose Tolerance Test. Body weights of control and experimental rats were analyzed weekly throughout the experimental phase. At the end of the experimental period, the animals were sacrificed, the pancreas was harvested, and the organosomatic index was calculated (i.e., weight of the pancreas as a percentage of the animal body weight). Fasting blood glucose levels were analyzed using a glucometer (Accu-Chek Performa, Roche Diagnostic, USA). An oral glucose tolerance test (OGTT) was performed using an oral dose of glucose (2 g/kg) for 2 h after 8 consecutive weeks of treatment. Prior to the OGTT procedure, animals were fasted overnight and given only water to drink throughout the time. The blood samples were collected from each group just before glucose administration (0 min) and at 30, 60, and 120 min after glucose administration.

2.5. Plasma and Serum Biochemical Assays. Albino rats were sacrificed using isoflurane (5% W) anesthesia, and blood was collected by cardiac puncture. Serum was isolated by centrifugation (LABCENT 5000) at 3000 rpm 15 min as per standard protocols. Serum insulin, C-peptide, C-reactive protein (CRP), and Adenosine Deaminase (ADA) levels were assayed by the solid-phase enzyme-linked immunosorbent assay (ELISA) (Millipore; Billerica, USA, cat. no.: EZRMI-13K). Method described by Wilson and Spiger [39] was used to determine the lipid profile. Lipoproteins were fractionated by a dual precipitation technique of and high-density lipoprotein (HDL) and low-density lipoprotein (LDL) [40]. Total cholesterol (TC) and triglycerides (TGs) were measured using commercially available kits (Abcam, UK) following the manufacturer's protocol. Glycosylated hemoglobin (HbA1C) levels were estimated by the method described by Rao and Pattabiraman [41].

2.6. Pancreatic and Liver Homogenate Assays. Liver and pancreas homogenates, 10% (w/v), were prepared in a potassium phosphate buffer 0.05 M, pH 7.4. Elvehjem homogenizer (Dominique Dutscher, Issy-les-Moulineaux, France) was used. The homogenates were centrifuged for 10 min at 3000 × g at 4°C, and the supernatant aliquots were saved and stored at -20°C. The homogenate protein content was measured according to the method described by Lowry et al. [42]. Superoxide dismutase (SOD) activity was measured by rate of inhibition of pyrogallol autooxidation on a spectrophotometer at 470 nm according to the method of Marklund and Marklund [43]. SOD activity was expressed as units per milligram protein. The method described by Rotruck et al. was used to determine the glutathione peroxidase (GPx) level. It was calculated by the rate of NADPH oxidization spectrophotometrically at 340 nm [44]. GPx activity was presented as micrograms (μg) of reduced glutathione (GSH) expended/min/mg protein. The method described by Sinha was used to quantify the catalase (CAT) activity as estimated by monitoring the decomposition of H_2O_2 spectrophotometrically at 240 nm [45]. Levels of tumor necrosis factor-alpha (TNF-α; cat. no.: CSB-E04741m), interleukin-1 beta (IL-1β; cat. no.: CSB-E04621m). and interleukin-6 (IL-6; cat. no.: CSB-E04627m) were assessed in the pancreas supernatant by ELISA using anti-mouse antibody (CUSABIO Life Sciences, Wuhan, China) based on the manufacturer's instructions.

Liver xanthine oxidase level was determined using methods described by Mohamed et al. [46]; membrane GLUT4 transporters were quantified using ELISA kit procured from Life Science Inc. (USA) following the manufacturer's

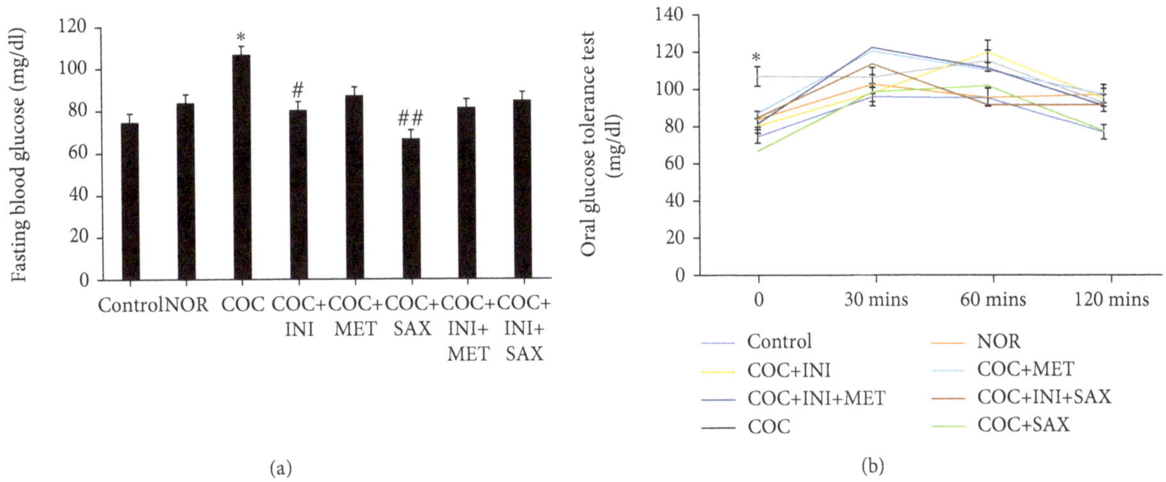

FIGURE 2: (a) COC caused a significant increase in the fasting blood glucose level when compared with control ($^*p \leq 0.05$); this increase was significantly reversed by administration of SAX ($^{\#\#}p \leq 0.01$). INI administration also reduced the FBG significantly ($^{\#}p \leq 0.05$); mean ± SEM, $n = 8$. (b) The oral glucose tolerance test showed an initial increase in the blood glucose. However, there was no significant effect on the tolerance test among the tested group in the course of the 120 mins tolerance test; mean ± SEM, $n = 6$.

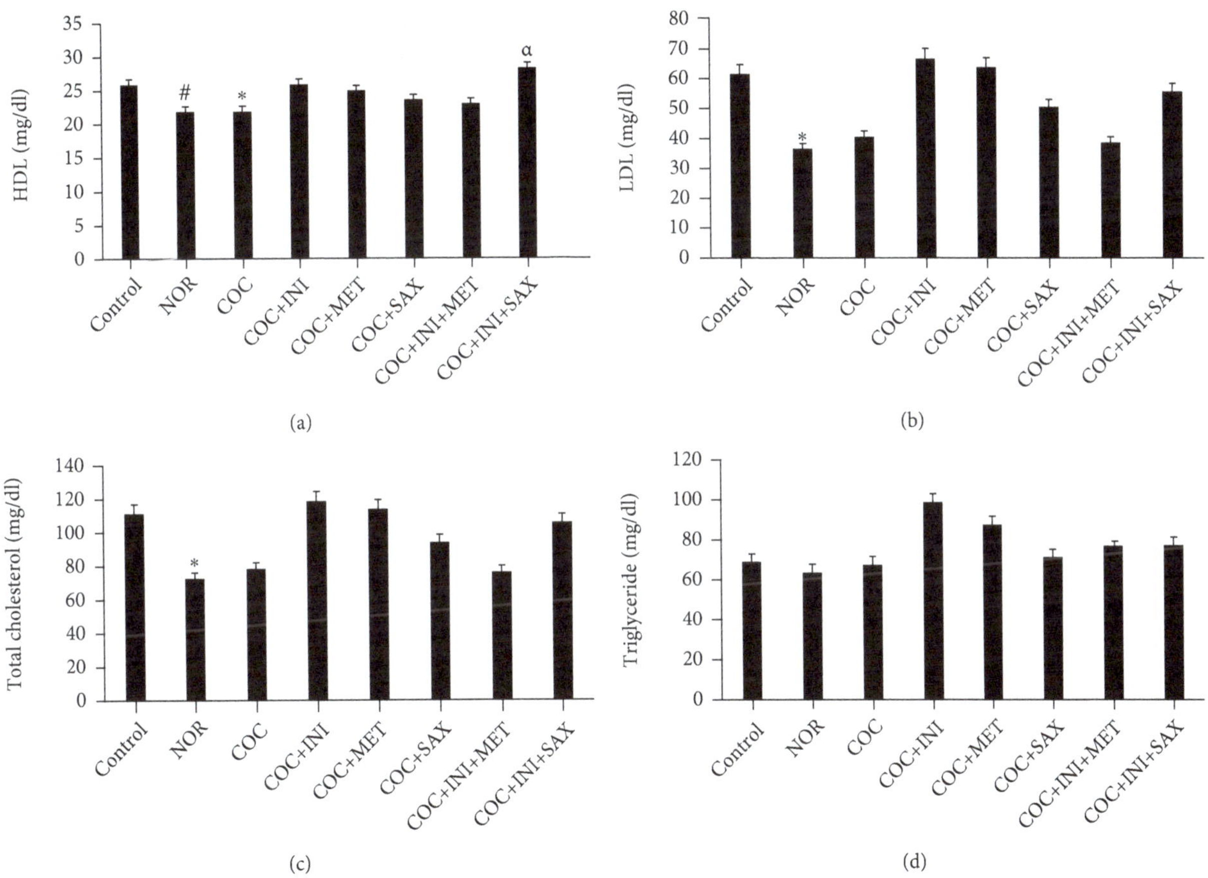

FIGURE 3: (a) COC caused a significant decrease in HDL level when compared with control ($^*p \leq 0.05$); this was also observed in the NOR group ($^{\#}p \leq 0.05$). INI+SAX significantly ($^{\alpha}\ p \leq 0.05$) increased the HDL level when compared with the COC group. (b, c) A significant reduction in the LDL and total cholesterol levels of the NOR-treated group, respectively ($^*p \leq 0.05$) (mean ± SEM, $n = 8$).

instructions [47]; glucokinase (GCK) level was quantified using the ELISA method in accordance with the instructions of the GCK ELISA kit (provided by Beijing Lvyuan Bode Biotechnology Co., Ltd.)

2.7. Statistical Analysis. Results are presented as means ± SEM, one-way ANOVA, parametric (unpaired Student's *t*-test), or nonparametric (Mann-Whitney *U*-test) unpaired tests also using GraphPad Prism® version 6.00 for Windows

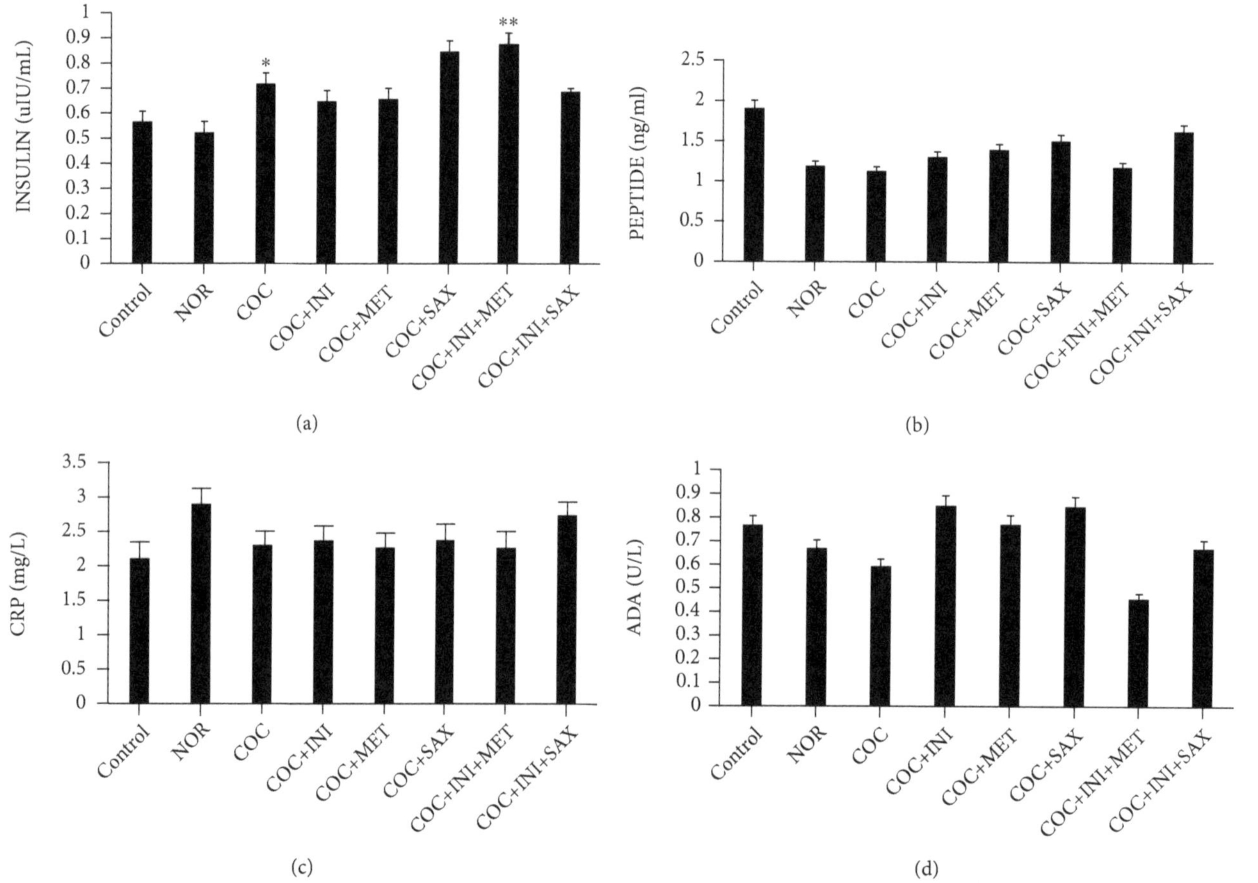

FIGURE 4: (a) COC caused a significant increase in insulin level when compared with control (*$p \leq 0.05$); this was also observed in the INI+MET group (**$p \leq 0.01$) when compared with the COC group. (b, c) No significant difference across the groups for C-peptide and CRP, respectively (mean ± SEM, $n = 8$).

(San Diego, CA, USA). The level of significance was set at $p < 0.05$.

3. Results

3.1. Body Weight and Pancreatic Organosomatic Index Evaluation. The 9-week study featured a weekly monitoring of the animal weight per group ($n = 8$). There was no statistically significant difference across the treatment group (Figure 1(a)). This trend was similar in the organosomatic index, which also showed no significant alteration in this index across the experimental groups (Figure 1(b)).

3.2. Fasting Blood Glucose Level and Oral Glucose Tolerance Test. There was a significant increase in the fasting blood glucose level of the COC group ($p \leq 0.05$); this alteration was however reversed in the INI group ($p \leq 0.05$) and the SAX group ($p \leq 0.01$) (Figure 2(a)). The OGTT showed no significant effect across the treatment groups except for the initial spike in glucose level observed at the 0 min timepoint (Figure 2(b)).

3.3. Serum Lipid Profile Analysis. HDL levels were significantly reduced in both COC ($p \leq 0.05$) and NOR ($p \leq 0.05$) groups. This reduction was reversed in the INI+SAX group ($p \leq 0.05$) (Figure 3(a)). The NOR group showed a significant reduction in both LDL and total cholesterol levels ($p \leq 0.05$) (Figures 3(b) and 3(c), respectively). There was no significant alteration in the triglyceride level across the experimental groups.

3.4. Evaluation of Insulin, C-Peptide, C-Reactive Protein, and ADA Levels. Insulin level was significantly increased in the COC group ($p \leq 0.05$) when compared with the control; this level was further increased in the INI+MET group ($p \leq 0.01$) (Figure 4(a)). The C-peptide, C-reactive protein, and ADA levels were not significantly different across the experimental groups (Figures 4(b)–4(d), respectively).

3.5. Assessment of Antioxidant Parameters on Pancreas Homogenate. Catalase level was significantly reduced in the COC group when compared with the control ($p \leq 0.05$); this reduction was reversed in the INI+MET group ($p \leq 0.01$). SOD, GPx, and GSH levels were not significantly affected across the experimental groups (Figures 5(b)–5(d)); total protein and MDA levels were not also significantly affected across the experimental groups (Figures 6(a) and 6(b)).

3.6. Assessment of TNF-α, IL-6, and IL-1β Levels in Pancreas Homogenate. Figures 7(a)–7(c) show that levels of TNF-α,

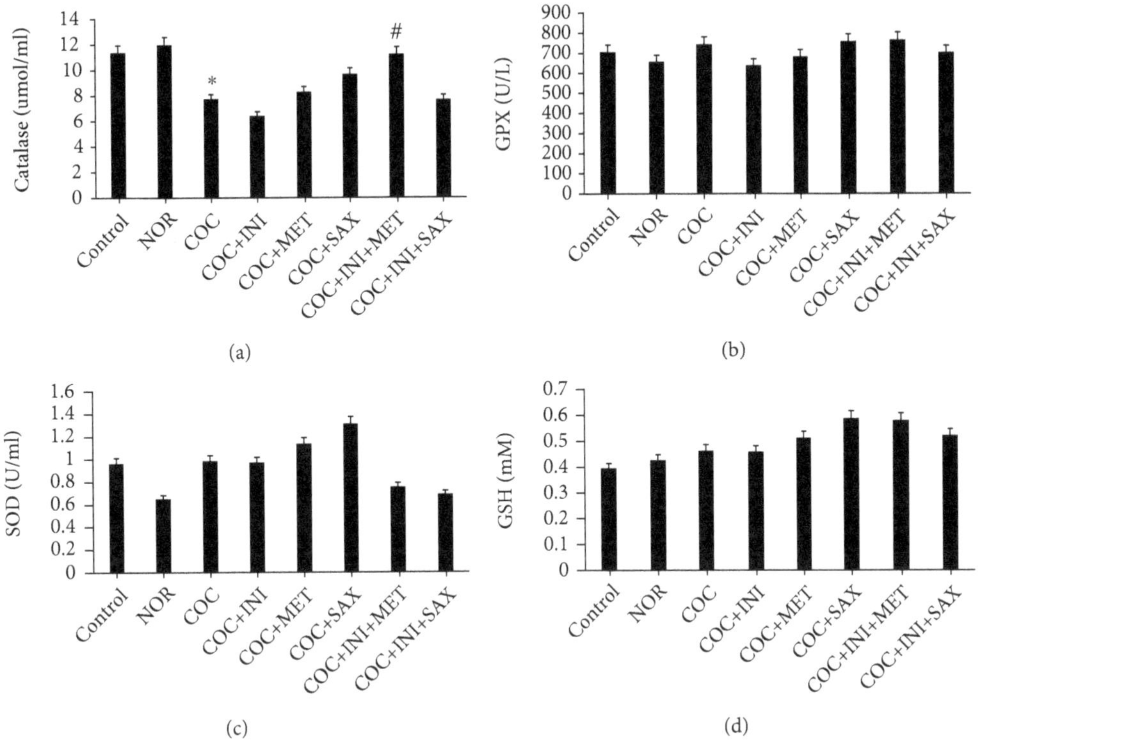

FIGURE 5: (a) COC caused a significant decrease in catalase level when compared with control ($^{*}p \leq 0.05$); this decrease was reversed in the INI+MET group ($^{\#}p \leq 0.01$) when compared with the COC group. (b, c) No significant difference across the groups for SOD and GPX, respectively (mean ± SEM, $n = 6$).

IL-6, and IL-1β were not significantly different statistically in comparison with the control. However, nonstatistical compares suggest an increase in the TNF-α levels in the COC group and a subsequent reduction in the MET and INI+ MET groups.

3.7. Evaluation of Glucokinase, G6P, and GLUT4 Levels in Liver Homogenate. COC caused a significant decrease in glucokinase level when compared with control ($^{**}p \leq 0.01$); this decrease was not reversed by any of the treatment group when compared with the COC group (Figure 8(a)). COC increased the G6P level ($^{**}p \leq 0.01$). This effect was reversed significantly by the INI+SAX group ($^{\#\#}p \leq 0.01$) (Figure 8(b)). COC increased the GLUT4 levels significantly ($^{**}p \leq 0.01$); this effect was reversed in INI+MET ($^{*}p \leq 0.05$) and INI+SAX ($^{\#\#}p \leq 0.01$) (Figure 8(c)).

3.8. Evaluation of Plasma HbA1c and Liver Xanthine Oxidase Levels. Glycated hemoglobin (HbA1c) levels assayed for in the plasma showed a significant increase in the COC group ($^{*}p \leq 0.05$); this effect was reversed significantly in the MET, SAX, and INI+MET groups ($^{**}p \leq 0.01$) (Figure 9(a)). Xanthine oxidase levels were not significantly different across the experimental groups (Figure 9(b)).

4. Discussion

A constellation of metabolic abnormalities which features hyperglycemia, hyperinsulinemia, and hyperlipidemia among other disorders was initially termed as "Insulin resistance syndrome" [48]. These metabolic abnormalities, generally now referred to as metabolic syndrome (MetS), are increasing at an alarming rate, becoming a major public and clinical problem worldwide [49]. MetS has been linked to cardiovascular dysfunction and a major risk factor in the development of type 2 diabetes mellitus [50, 51]. This present study sets out to unravel the effect of combined oral contraceptives (COCs) on specific elements of MetS and the possible benefits of intranasal insulin (INI), metformin (MET), and saxagliptin (SAX) in various combination regimens in the management of this syndrome. It is expected that the results from this study shed light on the underlying therapeutic intervention for this disorder occasioned by a chronic administration of COC in adult female albino Wistar rats.

Body weight changes and particularly body mass index (BMI) have been linked directly to metabolic syndrome status in humans [52], with a particular interest in the relationship between MetS and waist circumference [53, 54]. Weekly monitoring of the experimental groups showed that the chronic exposure to combined oral contraceptives did not affect the animal body weight during the study. In their study, Ghezzi et al. postulated that weight loss or distortion takes place in the early developmental stages of the animals, and this study attributed the unlikelihood of weight gain at maturity to a physiological decline in the development of the animals at adulthood [55]. This phenomenon is in tandem with our findings, since adult female Wistar rats were used. Organosomatic index of the pancreas was also in line with the body weight changes, and this is expected due to the fact that insulin resistance may not be a sign of toxicity

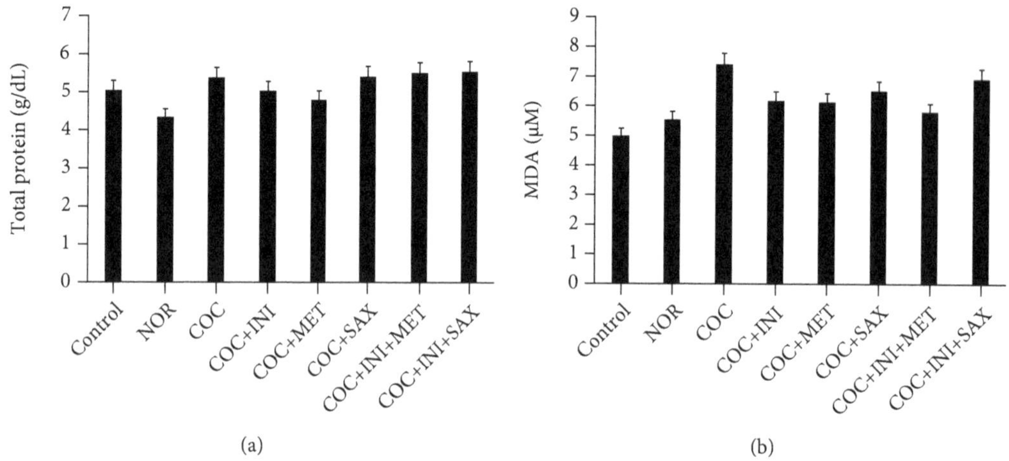

FIGURE 6: (a, b) No significant alterations across the test groups for total protein and MDA levels, respectively; $p \leq 0.05$; mean ± SEM, $n = 6$.

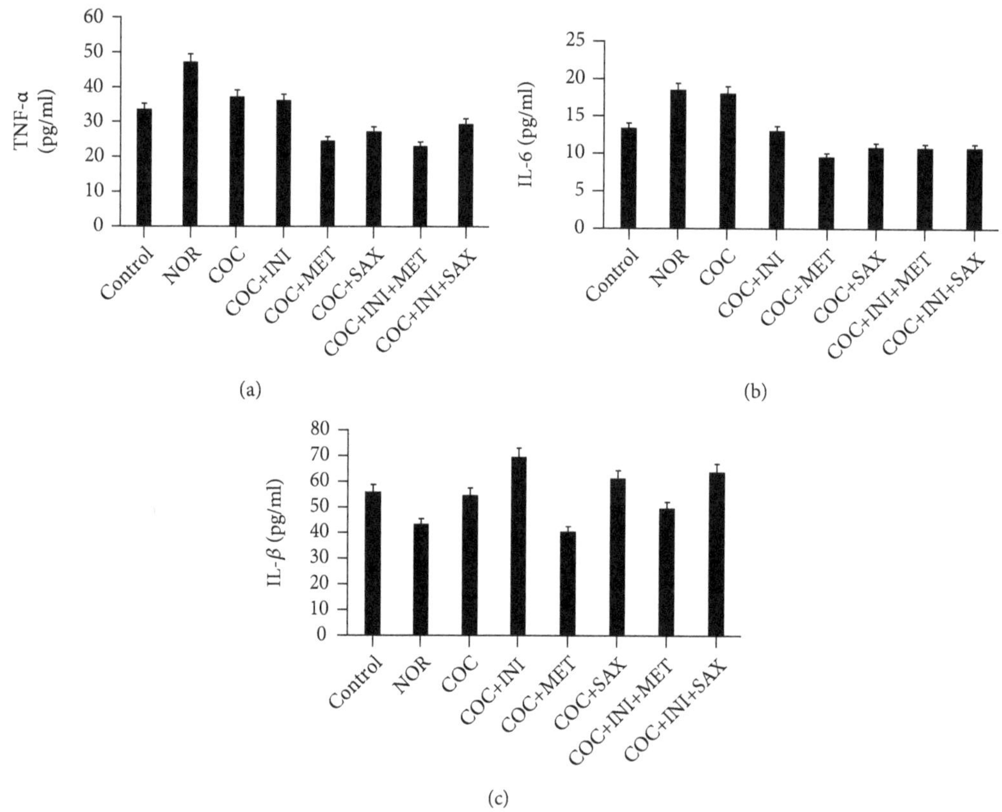

FIGURE 7: (a–c) No statistically significant alterations across the test groups for the inflammatory mediators: TNF-α, IL-6, and IL-1β, respectively. However, there is a nonstatistical increase in the level of TNF-α and IL-6 in the COC group and a subsequent reduction in the MET and INI+MET groups for both mediators, $p \leq 0.05$; mean ± SEM, $n = 6$.

to the pancreas, since this is not insulin insufficiency as seen in the etiology of type 1 diabetes mellitus [56]. Organosomatic index is a more definitive examination of organ weight which shows the proportional sizes of organs and depicts the status of organ systems. Organ sizes relative to body weight may change faster than organism weight and are an important indicator of organ toxicity. Organosomatic indices have been globally accepted as a pointer of organ-system integrity of animals [57].

High blood glucose (hyperglycemia) and hyperinsulinemia are major features of metabolic syndrome and particular risk factors in type 2 diabetes mellitus [50]. Use of combined oral contraceptive induces significant increases in both fasting blood glucose and insulin levels; this establishes the fact that the continuous use of this contraceptive predisposes to type 2 diabetes mellitus and cardiovascular dysfunctions. Treatment with saxagliptin markedly reduced the fasting blood glucose levels, and a reduction in glycemic

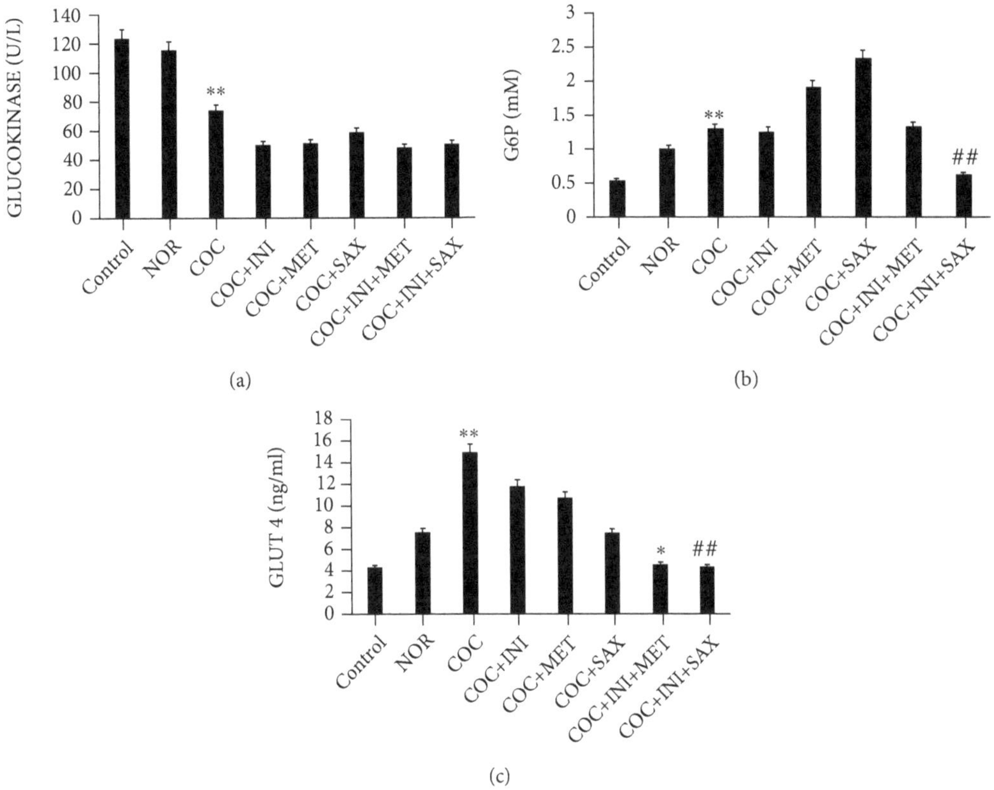

FIGURE 8: (a) COC caused a significant decrease in glucokinase level when compared with control ($^{**}p \leq 0.01$); this decrease was not reversed by any of the treatment group ($p \leq 0.01$) when compared with the COC group. (b) COC increased the G6P level ($^{**}p \leq 0.01$); this effect was reversed significantly by the INI+SAX group ($^{\#\#}p \leq 0.01$). (c) COC increased the GLUT4 levels significantly ($^{**}p \leq 0.01$); this effect was reversed in INI+MET ($^{*}p \leq 0.05$) and INI+SAX ($^{\#\#}p \leq 0.01$) (mean ± SEM, $n = 6$).

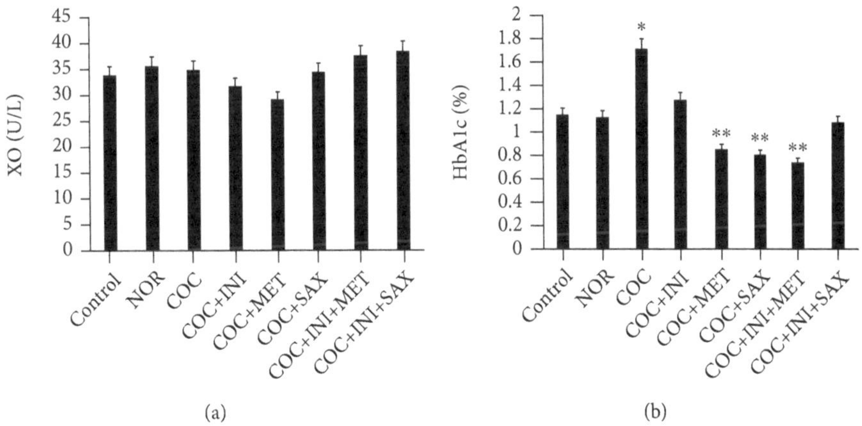

FIGURE 9: (a) No significant alterations across the test groups for xanthine oxidase (XO), $p \leq 0.05$; (b) COC increased significantly the level of HBA1c when compared with the control ($^{*}p \leq 0.05$); this effect was reversed significantly in the MET, SAX, and INI+MET groups ($^{**}p \leq 0.01$); mean ± SEM, $n = 6$; $n = 8$.

level was also observed in the intranasal insulin group. Insulin resistance depicted by hyperinsulinemia can dysregulate glucose metabolism generating chronic hyperglycemia, leading to the onset of cardiac related abnormalities [58]. A proper management of the elements of MetS in women of reproductive age can prevent the development of cardiovascular diseases, which is the global leading cause of death [59]. C-reactive peptide, C-peptide, and ADA levels were not significantly affected; also, the oral glucose tolerance test was not affected by the combined oral contraceptives.

Lipid profile analysis, with particular focus on the HDL, LDL, and triglyceride level, has been specifically linked to metabolic syndrome [60]. Combined oral contraceptive use reduced the level of HDL; this reduction was reversed by intranasal insulin and saxagliptin combined therapy; LDL and total cholesterol levels were reduced by the administration of norethindrone; however, triglyceride levels were not affected by the combined contraceptives. Insulin resistance alters systemic lipid metabolism leading to the development of dyslipidemia [61]; the 3 popular lipid-related aberrations are as follows: (1) upregulated levels of plasma triglycerides, (2) low levels of high-density lipoprotein, and (3) the presence of low-density lipoproteins. These features, in combination with dysfunction of the endothelial, which can also be caused by disrupted insulin signaling, are important underlying factors to formation of atherosclerotic plaques [58].

The association between oxidative stress and insulin resistance has been reported to be a predisposing link to cardiovascular diseases [62]. Pancreatic homogenate antioxidant assay showed that the level of catalase enzyme was significantly reduced consequent upon exposure to combined oral contraceptives; this reduction was reversed by treatment with intranasal insulin and metformin combination therapy. Catalase is an antioxidant enzyme which catalyzes the breakdown of hydrogen peroxide to water and oxygen. It is crucial for the protection of cells from oxidative damage by reactive oxygen species (ROS) [63]. Deficiency or malfunction of catalase is postulated to be related to the pathogenesis of many age-associated degenerative diseases like diabetes mellitus, hypertension, anemia, and vitiligo [64]. Other antioxidant parameters such as SOD, GSH, GPx, and MDA levels were not affected significantly by treatment with the combined oral contraceptive in this study.

Glycated hemoglobin (HbA1c) levels have been used as a diagnostic parameter for profiling insulin resistance in patients and a probe for type 2 diabetes mellitus [65]. We checked for the effect of combined oral contraceptive treatment on HbA1c and discovered a significantly high level ($p \leq 0.05$); this effect was reversed in the MET, SAX, and INI+SAX groups ($p \leq 0.01$), suggesting their efficacy in the management of MetS caused by the use of combined oral contraceptive which could subsequently lead to the prevention of type 2 DM and cardiotoxicity. The formation of the sugar-hemoglobin linkage indicates the presence of excessive sugar in the bloodstream, often indicative of diabetes [66]. HbA1C is of particular interest because it is easy to detect. Liver GLUT4 level was upregulated in the COC group and subsequently reversed in the INI+MET and INI+SAX groups. However, we suggest this could be as a result of the length of the study; we expected a reduction in the level of GLUT4 activity. During the normal physiology of glucose-stimulated secretion of insulin, beta-cells release insulin into circulation, activating GLUT4-dependent glucose uptake into peripheral tissue. Glucokinase level was significantly reduced in the COC group; glucose-6-phosphate levels were increased in the same group but subsequently reduced in the INI+SAX group. Glucokinase converts glucose to glucose-6-phosphate which may be converted to glycogen for storage [67]. Inflammatory cytokines such as TNF-α, IL-6, and IL-1β play significant roles in the etiology of metabolic syndrome. Scientific evidence suggests that obesity, in particular chronic visceral adiposity, is associated with inflammatory markers including interleukin-6 (IL-6) and tumor necrosis factor-alpha (TNF-α) [68]. Studies have shown that IL-6 and TNF-α are secreted from infiltrated macrophages into adipose tissue and have critical roles in MetS, insulin resistance, nonalcoholic fatty liver disease, and atherogenesis [69]. Our study showed that these cytokines (TNF-α and IL-6) were affected without statistical significance. Nonstatistically significant increase in TNF-α and in COC-treated group was reversed by administration of MET and combined INI+MET. These suggest an early stage or development of MetS can be arrested with these therapeutic regimens.

5. Conclusion

Findings from this study show that chronic combined oral contraceptive treatment predisposes female albino rats to metabolic syndrome which features hyperglycemia, dyslipidemia, hyperinsulinemia, etc., all of which were featured in this present study. The use combination therapies particularly involving saxagliptin and metformin corrected some of these metabolic abnormalities that have a direct link to glucose metabolism. Thus, the metabolic syndrome status of combined oral contraceptive users should be closely monitored, and therapeutic interventions should be employed to prevent development of type 2 DM and other cardiovascular pathologies. A clinical study should be engaged in order to establish the translational relevance of these findings in women of reproductive age.

Authors' Contributions

All authors made significant contributions to conception and design, acquisition of the data, or analysis and development of the manuscript. SOA and OO conceptualized the work and worked extensively on the development of the manuscript. SOA, FJ, and OA carried out the laboratory work including providing expertise in the methods used and the overall inference from the findings of the research work. All authors read and approved the final manuscript.

Acknowledgments

We thank Pharmacist Chloe Fatigun and Mr. Benjamin Ejimkonye for their technical support during the research.

References

[1] K. Daniels and J. C. Abma, *Current Contraceptive Status among Women Aged 15-49: United States, 2015-2017*, National Center for Health Statistics, 2018, https://www.cdc.gov/nchs/products/databriefs/db388.html.

[2] L. S. Mørch, C. W. Skovlund, P. C. Hannaford, L. Iversen, S. Fielding, and Ø. Lidegaard, "Contemporary hormonal contraception and the risk of breast cancer," *The New England Journal of Medicine*, vol. 377, no. 23, pp. 2228–2239, 2017.

[3] R. Sitruk-Ware and A. Nath, "Metabolic effects of contraceptive steroids," *Reviews in Endocrine & Metabolic Disorders*, vol. 12, no. 2, pp. 63–75, 2011.

[4] D. B. Cooper and H. Mahdy, *Oral Contraceptive Pills*, StatPearls, 2020.

[5] K. M. Curtis, N. K. Tepper, T. C. Jatlaoui et al., "US medical eligibility criteria for contraceptive use, 2016," *Morbidity and Mortality Weekly Report*, vol. 65, no. 3, pp. 1–3, 2016.

[6] J. Y. Jeong, M. K. Kim, I. Lee et al., "Polycystic ovarian morphology is associated with primary dysmenorrhea in young Korean women," *Obstetrics & Gynecology Science*, vol. 62, no. 5, p. 329, 2019.

[7] V. de Leo, M. C. Musacchio, V. Cappelli, P. Piomboni, and G. Morgante, "Hormonal contraceptives: pharmacology tailored to women's health," *Human Reproduction Update*, vol. 22, no. 5, pp. 634–646, 2016.

[8] S. Manzoor, M. A. Ganie, S. Majid et al., "Analysis of intrinsic and extrinsic coagulation pathway factors in OCP treated PCOS women," *Indian Journal of Clinical Biochemistry*, vol. 17, pp. 1–10, 2020.

[9] Q. Wang, P. Würtz, K. Auro et al., "Effects of hormonal contraception on systemic metabolism: cross-sectional and longitudinal evidence," *International Journal of Epidemiology*, vol. 45, no. 5, pp. 1445–1457, 2016.

[10] S. Panicker, S. Mann, J. Shawe, and J. Stephenson, "Evolution of extended use of the combined oral contraceptive pill," *The Journal of Family Planning and Reproductive Health Care*, vol. 40, no. 2, pp. 133–141, 2014.

[11] A. Edelman, M. F. Gallo, M. D. Nichols, J. T. Jensen, K. F. Schulz, and D. A. Grimes, "Continuous versus cyclic use of combined oral contraceptives for contraception: systematic Cochrane review of randomized controlled trials," *Human Reproduction*, vol. 21, no. 3, pp. 573–578, 2006.

[12] F. de Castro Coelho and C. Barros, "The potential of hormonal contraception to influence female sexuality," *The Journal of Reproductive Medicine*, vol. 2019, article 9701384, pp. 1–9, 2019.

[13] F. Z. Stanczyk, D. F. Archer, and B. R. Bhavnani, "Ethinyl estradiol and 17β-estradiol in combined oral contraceptives: pharmacokinetics, pharmacodynamics and risk assessment," *Contraception*, vol. 87, no. 6, pp. 706–727, 2013.

[14] S. Christin-Maitre, "Use of hormone replacement in females with endocrine disorders," *Hormone Research in Pædiatrics*, vol. 87, no. 4, pp. 215–223, 2017.

[15] N. Santoro, R. Worsley, K. K. Miller, S. J. Parish, and S. R. Davis, "Role of estrogens and estrogen-like compounds in female sexual function and dysfunction," *The Journal of Sexual Medicine*, vol. 13, no. 3, pp. 305–316, 2016.

[16] H. Kuhl, "Pharmacology of estrogens and progestogens: influence of different routes of administration," *Climacteric*, vol. 8, Suppplement 1, pp. 3–63, 2005.

[17] G. Evans and E. L. Sutton, "Oral contraception," *Medicina Clínica*, vol. 99, no. 3, pp. 479–503, 2015.

[18] K. K. Scarsi, K. M. Darin, S. Nakalema et al., "Unintended pregnancies observed with combined use of the levonorgestrel contraceptive implant and efavirenz-based antiretroviral therapy: a three-arm pharmacokinetic evaluation over 48 weeks," *Clinical Infectious Diseases*, vol. 62, no. 6, pp. 675–682, 2016.

[19] R. Peck, W. Rella, J. Tudela, J. Aznar, and B. Mozzanega, "Does levonorgestrel emergency contraceptive have a post-fertilization effect? A review of its mechanism of action," *The Linacre Quarterly*, vol. 83, no. 1, pp. 35–51, 2016.

[20] C. Kahlenborn, R. Peck, and W. B. Severs, "Mechanism of action of levonorgestrel emergency contraception," *The Linacre Quarterly*, vol. 82, no. 1, pp. 18–33, 2015.

[21] J. Elks, Ed., *The Dictionary of Drugs: Chemical Data: Chemical Data, Structures and Bibliographies*, Springer, 2014.

[22] L. Li, R. Zhang, J. Zeng et al., "Effectiveness and safety assessment of drospirenone/ethinyl estradiol tablet in treatment of PCOS patients: a single center, prospective, observational study," *BMC Women's Health*, vol. 20, no. 1, pp. 1–7, 2020.

[23] A. S. De Melo, R. Reis, R. A. Ferriani, and C. Vieira, "Hormonal contraception in women with polycystic ovary syndrome: choices, challenges, and non-contraceptive benefits," *Open Access Journal of Contraception*, vol. Volume 8, pp. 13–23, 2017.

[24] I. J. Halperin, S. Sujana Kumar, D. F. Stroup, and S. E. Laredo, "The association between the combined oral contraceptive pill and insulin resistance, dysglycemia and dyslipidemia in women with polycystic ovary syndrome: a systematic review and meta-analysis of observational studies," *Human Reproduction*, vol. 26, no. 1, pp. 191–201, 2011.

[25] O. A. Adeyanju, O. A. Soetan, A. O. Soladoye, and L. A. Olatunji, "Oral hormonal therapy with ethinylestradiol–levonorgestrel improves insulin resistance, obesity, and glycogen synthase kinase-3 independent of circulating mineralocorticoid in estrogen-deficient rats," *Canadian Journal of Physiology and Pharmacology*, vol. 96, no. 6, pp. 577–586, 2018.

[26] P. Rorsman and M. O. Huising, "The somatostatin-secreting pancreatic δ-cell in health and disease," *Nature Reviews. Endocrinology*, vol. 14, no. 7, pp. 404–414, 2018.

[27] P. V. Röder, B. Wu, Y. Liu, and W. Han, "Pancreatic regulation of glucose homeostasis," *Experimental & Molecular Medicine*, vol. 48, no. 3, article e219, 2016.

[28] J. Myers, P. Kokkinos, and E. Nyelin, "Physical activity, cardiorespiratory fitness, and the metabolic syndrome," *Nutrients*, vol. 11, no. 7, p. 1652, 2019.

[29] K. D. Bruce and F. R. Cagampang, "Epigenetic priming of the metabolic syndrome," *Toxicology Mechanisms and Methods*, vol. 21, no. 4, pp. 353–361, 2011.

[30] G. Ricci, I. Pirillo, D. Tomassoni, A. Sirignano, and I. Grappasonni, "Metabolic syndrome, hypertension, and nervous system injury: epidemiological correlates," *Clinical and Experimental Hypertension*, vol. 39, no. 1, pp. 8–16, 2017.

[31] M. D. DeBoer, M. J. Gurka, S. H. Golden et al., "Independent associations between metabolic syndrome severity and future coronary heart disease by sex and race," *Journal of the American College of Cardiology*, vol. 69, no. 9, pp. 1204-1205, 2017.

[32] K. Ganesan and S. Sultan, *Oral Hypoglycemic Medications*, StatPearls, 2019.

[33] J. Grisouard, K. Timper, T. M. Radimerski et al., "Mechanisms of metformin action on glucose transport and metabolism in human adipocytes," *Biochemical Pharmacology*, vol. 80, no. 11, pp. 1736–1745, 2010.

[34] S. Correia, C. Carvalho, M. S. Santos et al., "Metformin protects the brain against the oxidative imbalance promoted by type 2 diabetes," *Medicinal Chemistry*, vol. 4, no. 4, pp. 358–364, 2008.

[35] P. Sa-nguanmoo, P. Tanajak, S. Kerdphoo et al., "SGLT2-inhibitor and DPP-4 inhibitor improve brain function via attenuating mitochondrial dysfunction, insulin resistance, inflammation, and apoptosis in HFD-induced obese rats," *Toxicology and Applied Pharmacology*, vol. 333, pp. 43–50, 2017.

[36] National Research Council, *Sustainability and the US EPA*, National Academies Press, 2011.

[37] U. Albus, "Guide for the care and use of laboratory animals (8th edn)," *Laboratory Animals*, vol. 46, no. 3, pp. 267-268, 2012.

[38] A. A. Njan, C. O. Fatigun, A. M. Alli-Oluwafuyi et al., "Effect of intranasal insulin on peripheral glucose profile in dexamethasone-induced insulin resistance in Wistar rats," *Beni-Suef University Journal of Basic and Applied Sciences*, vol. 7, no. 4, pp. 516–524, 2018.

[39] D. E. Wilson and M. J. Spiger, "A dual precipitation method for quantitative plasma lipoprotein measurement without ultracentrifugation," *The Journal of Laboratory and Clinical Medicine*, vol. 82, no. 3, pp. 473–582, 1973.

[40] A. Hafiane and J. Genest, "High density lipoproteins: measurement techniques and potential biomarkers of cardiovascular risk," *BBA Clinical*, vol. 3, pp. 175–188, 2015.

[41] P. Rao and T. N. Pattabiraman, "Further studies on the mechanism of phenol-sulfuric acid reaction with furaldehyde derivatives," *Analytical Biochemistry*, vol. 189, no. 2, pp. 178–181, 1990.

[42] O. H. Lowry, N. J. Rosebrough, A. L. Farr, and R. J. Randall, "Protein measurement with the Folin phenol reagent," *The Journal of Biological Chemistry*, vol. 193, no. 1, pp. 265–275, 1951.

[43] S. Marklund and G. Marklund, "Involvement of the superoxide anion radical in the autoxidation of pyrogallol and a convenient assay for superoxide dismutase," *European Journal of Biochemistry*, vol. 47, no. 3, pp. 469–474, 1974.

[44] J. T. Rotruck, A. L. Pope, H. E. Ganther, A. B. Swanson, D. G. Hafeman, and W. G. Hoekstra, "Selenium: biochemical role as a component of glutathione peroxidase," *Science*, vol. 179, no. 4073, pp. 588–590, 1973.

[45] A. K. Sinha, "Colorimetric assay of catalase," *Analytical Biochemistry*, vol. 47, no. 2, pp. 389–394, 1972.

[46] S. S. Mohamed Isa, A. Ablat, and J. Mohamad, "The antioxidant and xanthine oxidase inhibitory activity of Plumeria rubra flowers," *Molecules*, vol. 23, no. 2, p. 400, 2018.

[47] A. U. Kabir, M. B. Samad, A. Ahmed et al., "Aqueous fraction of Beta vulgaris ameliorates hyperglycemia in diabetic mice due to enhanced glucose stimulated insulin secretion, mediated by acetylcholine and GLP-1, and elevated glucose uptake via increased membrane bound GLUT4 transporters," *PLoS One*, vol. 10, no. 2, article e0116546, 2015.

[48] D. E. Moller and K. D. Kaufman, "Metabolic syndrome: a clinical and molecular perspective," *Annual Review of Medicine*, vol. 56, no. 1, pp. 45–62, 2005.

[49] M. G. Saklayen, "The global epidemic of the metabolic syndrome," *Current Hypertension Reports*, vol. 20, no. 2, p. 12, 2018.

[50] M. K. Lee, K. Han, M. K. Kim et al., "Changes in metabolic syndrome and its components and the risk of type 2 diabetes: a nationwide cohort study," *Scientific Reports*, vol. 10, no. 1, p. 2313, 2020.

[51] S. C. Marott, B. G. Nordestgaard, A. Tybjærg-Hansen, and M. Benn, "Components of the metabolic syndrome and risk of type 2 diabetes," *The Journal of Clinical Endocrinology and Metabolism*, vol. 101, no. 8, pp. 3212–3221, 2016.

[52] M. B. Schulze, "Metabolic health in normal-weight and obese individuals," *Diabetologia*, vol. 62, no. 4, pp. 558–566, 2019.

[53] M. Gao, J. Lv, C. Yu et al., "Metabolically healthy obesity, transition to unhealthy metabolic status, and vascular disease in Chinese adults: a cohort study," *PLoS Medicine*, vol. 17, no. 10, article e1003351, 2020.

[54] A. Lukács, E. Horváth, Z. Máté et al., "Abdominal obesity increases metabolic risk factors in non-obese adults: a Hungarian cross-sectional study," *BMC Public Health*, vol. 19, no. 1, 2019.

[55] A. C. Ghezzi, L. T. Cambri, J. D. Botezelli, C. Ribeiro, R. A. Dalia, and M. A. de Mello, "Metabolic syndrome markers in Wistar rats of different ages," *Diabetology and Metabolic Syndrome*, vol. 4, no. 1, p. 16, 2012.

[56] M. Wolosowicz, B. Lukaszuk, and A. Chabowski, "The causes of insulin resistance in type 1 diabetes mellitus: is there a place for quaternary prevention?," *International Journal of Environmental Research and Public Health*, vol. 17, no. 22, p. 8651, 2020.

[57] N. Gupta, D. K. Gupta, and P. K. Sharma, "Condition factor and organosomatic indices of parasitized Rattus rattus as indicators of host health," *Journal of Parasitic Diseases*, vol. 41, no. 1, pp. 21–28, 2017.

[58] V. Ormazabal, S. Nair, O. Elfeky, C. Aguayo, C. Salomon, and F. A. Zuñiga, "Association between insulin resistance and the development of cardiovascular disease," *Cardiovascular Diabetology*, vol. 17, no. 1, pp. 1–4, 2018.

[59] L. Kazlauskienė, J. Butnorienė, and A. Norkus, "Metabolic syndrome related to cardiovascular events in a 10-year prospective study," *Diabetology and Metabolic Syndrome*, vol. 7, no. 1, p. 102, 2015.

[60] A. Tahir, P. J. Martinez, F. Ahmad et al., "An evaluation of lipid profile and pro-inflammatory cytokines as determinants of cardiovascular disease in those with diabetes: a study on a Mexican American cohort," *Scientific Reports*, vol. 11, no. 1, p. 2435, 2021.

[61] D. M. Erion, H. J. Park, and H. Y. Lee, "The role of lipids in the pathogenesis and treatment of type 2 diabetes and associated co-morbidities," *BMB Reports*, vol. 49, no. 3, pp. 139–148, 2016.

[62] S. Dzięgielewska-Gęsiak, D. Stołtny, A. Brożek, M. Muc-Wierzgoń, and E. Wysocka, "Are insulin-resistance and oxidative stress cause or consequence of aging," *Experimental Biology and Medicine*, vol. 245, no. 14, pp. 1260–1267, 2020.

[63] P. Chelikani, I. Fita, and P. C. Loewen, "Diversity of structures and properties among catalases," *Cellular and Molecular Life Sciences*, vol. 61, no. 2, pp. 192–208, 2004.

[64] A. Nandi, L. J. Yan, C. K. Jana, and N. Das, "Role of Catalase in Oxidative Stress- and Age-Associated Degenerative Diseases," *Oxidative Medicine and Cellular Longevity*, vol. 2019, Article ID 9613090, 19 pages, 2019.

[65] G. Saravia, F. Civeira, Y. Hurtado-Roca et al., "Glycated hemoglobin, fasting insulin and the metabolic syndrome in males. Cross-sectional analyses of the Aragon workers health study baseline," *PLoS One*, vol. 10, no. 8, article e0132244, 2015.

[66] S. I. Sherwani, H. A. Khan, A. Ekhzaimy, A. Masood, and M. K. Sakharkar, "Significance of HbA1c test in diagnosis and prognosis of diabetic patients," *Biomarker Insights*, vol. 11, pp. BMI.S38440–BMI.S38104, 2016.

[67] N. B. Whitticar and C. S. Nunemaker, "Reducing glucokinase activity to enhance insulin secretion: a counterintuitive theory to preserve cellular function and glucose homeostasis," *Frontiers in Endocrinology*, vol. 11, p. 378, 2020.

[68] M. Mohammadi, M. H. Gozashti, M. Aghadavood, M. R. Mehdizadeh, and M. M. Hayatbakhsh, "Clinical significance of serum IL-6 and TNF-α levels in patients with metabolic syndrome," *Reports of Biochemistry & Molecular Biology*, vol. 6, no. 1, pp. 74–79, 2017.

7

Determinants of Skilled Birth Attendant Utilization at Chelia District, West Ethiopia

Adugna Dufera,[1] Elias Teferi Bala,[2] Habtamu Oljira Desta,[2] and Kefyalew Taye[2]

[1]*Department of General Public Health, College of Medicine and Health Science, Ambo University, Ambo, West Shoa, Ethiopia*
[2]*Department of Public Health College of Medicine and Health Science, Ambo University, Ambo, Ethiopia P.O. Box 19*

Correspondence should be addressed to Habtamu Oljira Desta; oljirah@gmail.com

Academic Editor: Hind A. Beydoun

Background. An estimated 303,000 maternal deaths occurred globally in 2015 from which sub-Saharan Africa alone accounted for 201,000 (66%) of the maternal deaths, and most of these are attributed to complications of pregnancy and childbirth due to the absence of institutional delivery by skilled attendants. *Objective.* The aim of this study was to assess institutional delivery utilization and associated factors among mothers who gave birth in the last one year in Chelia District. *Methodology.* A community-based cross-sectional study design supplemented by a qualitative method was employed from March 15 to 30, 2018. A multistage sampling technique was used to select 475 study participants. Quantitative data were collected using structured questionnaires, and focus group discussions were employed to get qualitative data. The data were entered to EpiData version 3.1 and exported to the statistical package version 21 for analysis. Descriptive statistics and bivariate and multivariate logistic regression analysis were computed to measure the strength of association between dependent and independent variables at a p value of <0.05. *Results.* Among the respondents, 216 (46.2%) utilized institutional delivery service. Monthly income (AOR = 4.465, 95%CI = 1.729, 11.527), antenatal care attendance (AOR = 0.077, 95%CI = 0.008, 0.73), knowledge of mothers about their expected date of delivery (AOR = 0.297, 95%CI = 0.179, 4.93), intended pregnancy (AOR = 0.326, 95%CI = 0.162 , 0.654), discussion with health extension workers about the place of delivery at home visit (AOR = 0.11, 95%CI = 0.023, 0.523), knowledge of mothers about the existence of the waiting area in health facilities (AOR = 0.14, 95%CI = 0.023, 0.84), and number of children (AOR = 0.119, 95%CI = 0.029, 0.485) had a significant association with institutional delivery utilization. *Conclusion.* Utilization of institutional delivery was low and far away from the expected country target in the district. The health sector should strive to increase proportion of institutional delivery by reaching pregnant mothers with timely antenatal care service provision and enhancing family planning provision.

1. Introduction

The majority of maternal health complications and deaths occurred in low- and middle-income countries (LMIC) where three quarters of the deaths are due to direct obstetric complication [1, 2]. Although maternal deaths worldwide have decreased by 45% since 1990, 800 women still die each day from largely preventable causes before, during, and after the time of giving birth. Ninety-nine percent of the preventable maternal deaths occur in low- and middle-income countries [3].

An estimated 295,000 maternal deaths occurred globally in 2017, making an overall MMR of 211 maternal deaths per 100,000 live births. Out of this, least developed countries account for a maternal mortality rate of 415 per 100,000 live births, with sub-Saharan Africa being the only region with very high MMR 542 per 100,000 live births and Ethiopia accounting for 14,000 maternal deaths [4, 5].

It is indicated that the risk of dying from a maternal cause for a woman in developing countries especially in Africa is around 23 times higher than that for a woman living in developed countries and the maternal mortality ratios are 495 and 12 per 100,000 women in Africa and in developed regions, respectively [6, 7].

From the recent Ethiopian Demographic and Health Survey report, the estimate of the maternal mortality ratio was 412 deaths per 100,000 live births, which could be prevented through skilled personnel intervention for all maternal services particularly before, during, and after childbirth [8].

Appropriate delivery care is crucial for both maternal and prenatal health, and increasing skilled attendants at birth is the central goal of the safe motherhood and child survival movements. In addition to professional attention, it is important that mothers deliver their babies in an appropriate setting where lifesaving equipment and hygienic conditions can also help reduce the risk of complications that may cause death or illness to mother and child [4, 9].

When a woman dies in childbirth, her infant and any other children's survival is threatened. Infants without a mother are more likely to die within two years. Children up to 10 years whose mothers die are 3 to 10 times more likely to die within two years than children living with mothers [10, 11].

Literatures recommend that the best way to assure a safe and successful delivery outcome remains to be ensuring the presence of a skilled birth attendant in every childbirth [12, 13]. This can be realized by increasing proportions of institutional deliveries [14].

Home delivery is common in many developing countries including Ethiopia. A high rate of home delivery was reported from Malawi, Nepal, Zaria (Northern Nigeria), and Pakistan [2, 7, 15], and many studies in Ethiopia, such as in Tigray, Arsi, and Dodota districts, indicated low utilization of institutional delivery. Similarly, the 2016 EDHS report revealed that the majority of births were being attended by traditional birth attendants at home [8, 15–17].

Different studies have indicated that institutional delivery service utilization is determined by complex interacting factors such as level of need, distance, economic factors, awareness and satisfaction, sociodemographic characteristics, and administrative arrangements [12, 13, 18].

Beside importance of institutional delivery, there was very limited evidence regarding the raised issues. Therefore, this study was aimed at investigating the level of institutional delivery service utilization and factors associated with it in Chelia District, western part of Ethiopia. The findings may be of immediate benefit to the West Shoa Zone health department in the implementation of future conducive strategies aimed at modifying factors in the health system in the community as agents of change to enhance institutional delivery.

2. Methods and Materials

2.1. Study Area and Design. The study was conducted in Chelia District West Shoa Zone, Oromiya regional state, Ethiopia. The district has 18 rural and 2 urban kebeles (kebele refers to the lowest administrative unit in Ethiopia). The total population of the district is 108,886 out of which women of childbearing age and expected pregnancies were 24,096 and 3,778, respectively. On the other hand, in the district, there were one general hospital, four health centers, eighteen health posts, and nine private clinics. The study was conducted starting from March 15 to 30, 2018. A community-based cross-sectional study design supplemented by a qualitative study was utilized.

2.2. Study Populations and Sample Size. All women of the reproductive age group were the source population for this study. Randomly selected women who gave birth in the last 12 months were included in the study. The following assumptions were considered while calculating the sample size. Ninety-five percent confidence level (95% CI) of obtaining mothers who gave birth at the health institutions from the population within 5% margin of error and using $p = 16.9\%$ institutional delivery prevalence of Gonji Kolela District of Amhara Region, Ethiopia [12].

$$n = \frac{(Z\alpha/2)^2 (P)\,(1-p)}{d^2} = \frac{(1.96)^2 (0.169)\,(1-0.169)}{0.05^2} = 216. \tag{1}$$

Considering the design effect of 2 and 10% nonresponse rate, the final sample size was 475.

2.3. Sampling Technique. The multistage sampling technique was used to select the study participants. Six kebeles (one urban and five rural) which account for 30% of the total kebeles were selected from each stratum using a lottery method, and 475 study participants were selected from each selected kebele proportionally using systematic sampling methods. The first HH was sampled using the lottery method by going at the health post of the kebele, and the sampling interval was calculated as $K = (N/n) = 1179/475{\sim}3$. Thus, households were selected by using a systematic sampling procedure in an interval of every 3rd households in each kebele. Since mothers in the specific kebeles were expected to be homogenous in many ways, convenient sampling was employed for FGD to select easily accessible mothers for the discussion. Five FGDs having 6 to 8 participants were employed.

2.4. Data Collection Tool

2.4.1. Quantitative Data. A structured questionnaire which included sociodemographic and health service utilization factors was prepared based on the objectives of the study after reviewing different literatures. Then, the questionnaire was translated to the local language to facilitate the data collection process.

2.4.2. Qualitative Data. To have an in-depth insight into the factors related to the place of delivery, qualitative data was collected. Five focus group discussions were held in the district. Three groups consisted of mothers, and the remaining two groups were husbands. Each FGD had 6 to 8 participants. Each session took a time span of one to one and half hour. The groups were made homogeneous in terms of sex and social classes. Settings for the discussions were arranged with privacy for participants, comfortable situation (location), lesser noise (by avoiding noisy areas), nonthreatening environment, and easily accessible location. The recruited supervisors were used as the facilitator and note taker while the principal investigator has modulated the discussion.

2.5. Data Processing and Analysis

2.5.1. Quantitative Data. Data was coded and entered to Epi-Data version 3.1 and exported to SPSS version 21 for analyses. Frequency, mean, and standard deviations from descriptive statistics and analytic statistics such as bivariate and multivariable logistic regression analyses were computed to determine the association of various factors on the outcome variable. Variables having a p value less than or equal to 0.05 on binary logistic regression were the candidate for multiple logistic regressions. Statistical significance was declared at $p < 0.05$. The strength of association between independent and dependent variables was assessed using the adjusted odds ratio with 95% confidence interval.

2.5.2. Qualitative Data. Data was transcribed into Afaan Oromo text by the principal investigator from replaying the recorded discussions and using the written note from ideas raised during the sessions and translated into the English language for analysis. Different ideas in the text were merged in their respective thematic areas and analyzed thematically. Then, the result was presented in narration by triangulating with the quantitative findings.

2.6. Ethical Consideration. Ethical clearance was received from the Ethical Review Committee of College of Medicine and Health Science of Ambo University on February 28, 2018, with reference no. CMHS-ERC: 28/2010. Verbal consent was obtained from the study subjects after they had been informed about the objectives and procedures of the study including their right to withdraw themselves from participation any time they want.

3. Results

3.1. Sociodemographic Characteristics. A total of 468 mothers who gave birth in the last twelve months were interviewed making a response rate of 98.5%. Out of the interviewed mothers, 396 (84.6%) were rural dwellers and 161 (34.4%) were in the age category of 25-29 years. The mean age of the respondents was 28.85 years with the standard deviation (SD) of 5.58. Most of the respondents 302 (64.53%) were Protestant in religion whereas majority of them 427 (91.24%) were Oromo in ethnicity. The mean monthly income of the respondents was 1221.18 ETB with a standard deviation of 1632.94 (Table 1).

3.2. Obstetric Characteristics of the Respondents. During the last pregnancy, 395 (84.4%) of the mothers had attended ANC visit. Among the mothers who attended ANC, more than half 237 (60%) visited health facilities less than four times. About 164 (35%) of the respondents faced more than five pregnancies including the current (Table 2).

3.3. Institutional Delivery Service Utilization. Among the study participants, only 216 (46.2%) gave births at health institutions and the rest delivered at home. Mothers who gave birth at health facilities justified what made them go to health institution to give birth. The points raised as reasons for their institutional delivery were as follows: previous better outcome with delivering at health facility, need better services, I was told to deliver at health facility, and health facility was near to me (Figure 1).

3.4. Factors Affecting Institutional Delivery Service Utilization. Multivariate analysis showed that monthly income, ANC attendance during the last pregnancy, EDD information, intended pregnancy, discussion with HEWs about the place of delivery, knowledge of mothers about the existence of the waiting area in health facilities, and number of children had a significant statistical association with the utilization of institutional delivery service (see Table 3).

Mothers who have six or more children were about 88.1% ($AOR = 0.119$, $95\%CI = 0.029, 0.485$) less likely to utilize institutional delivery as compared to those who have three or less children. In addition, mothers who did not get discussion with HEWs about the place of delivery were 89% ($AOR = 0.11$, $95\%CI = 0.023, 0.523$) less likely to utilize institutional delivery than those who got the discussion. Similarly, mothers who become pregnant without their need were 67.4% ($AOR = 0.326$, $95\%CI = 0.162, 0.654$) less likely to utilize institutional delivery as compared to those who got intended pregnancy. Furthermore, mothers who did not attend ANC during the last pregnancy were 92.3% less likely to give birth at health institutions than those who attended ANC ($AOR = 0.077$, $95\%CI = 0.008, 0.73$). Finally, this study also showed that having knowledge of EDD increases the likelihood of giving birth at health institutions. Mothers who did not know their EDD during pregnancy were 70.3% less likely to utilize institutional delivery than those who knew it ($AOR = 0.297$, $95\%CI = 0.179, 4.93$) (Table 3).

Qualitative data from FGD also showed that income affects institutional delivery service utilization. A FGD participant spoke that "…there is difference between poor and riches in utilizing institutional delivery; even in the absence of ambulance, using local ambulance was challenge in that no one carries pregnant of poor family. In the presence of money sky is a way" (a 47-year-old participant's husband who has 8 children).

A 36-year-old rural dweller mother of 6 children said "… Giving normal birth is not in the hand of peoples; it is just from God. I believe that God is with me at where ever I go; so, no need of going here and there."

A mother aged 34 years added that "...let ears of pregnant do not hear this; I know many mothers who died in Hospitals, no one died at home to give birth. What God determined for us could not be left at everywhere."

4. Discussion

The results of this study showed that mothers who utilized institutional delivery service were 46.2% (95% CI: 41.8, 50.9) in the district and more than half of the mothers (53.8%) gave birth at home. This magnitude of institutional delivery was low when compared with the health sector development plan of the country. However, it is higher than

Table 1: Sociodemographic characteristics of mothers who gave birth in the last one year in Chelia District, western Ethiopia (March 2018) ($N = 468$).

Variables	Categories	Frequency	Percent
Age of the respondents	≤20	37	7.9
	20-24	60	12.8
	25-29	161	34.4
	30-34	126	26.9
	>35	84	18
Religion of the respondents	Orthodox	149	31.84
	Muslim	3	0.64
	Wakefata	14	2.99
	Protestant	302	64.53
Ethnicity of the respondents	Oromo	427	91.24
	Amhara	22	4.70
	Tigre	1	0.21
	Gurage	18	3.85
Marital status of the respondents	Single	20	4.27
	Married	428	91.45
	Divorced	14	3
	Widowed	6	1.28
Educational status of the husbands	Unable to read and write	113	26.40
	Primary school	161	37.62
	Secondary school	96	22.43
	College and above	58	13.55
Educational status of the respondents	Unable to read and write	176	37.6
	Primary school	179	38.2
	Secondary school	70	15
	College and above	43	9.2
Occupation of the respondents	Government or NGO employee	42	8.97
	Merchant	33	7.05
	Housewife	51	10.90
	Daily labor	28	5.98
	Private employee	65	13.89
	Farmer	244	52.14
	Unemployed	5	1.07
Residence of the respondents	Rural	396	84.6
	Urban	72	15.4
Access to information sources like radio or television	Yes	168	35.9
	No	300	64.1
Average monthly income of the respondents	≤500	154	32.91
	501-1000	178	38.03
	1001-1500	53	11.32
	>1500	83	17.74

those in studies conducted in Gonji Kolela District of Amhara Region, Ethiopia; Dodota District of Oromiya, Ethiopia; and Sekela District of Amhara, Ethiopia, which were 16.9%, 18.2%, and 12.1%, respectively [6, 10, 12, 13]. Similarly, this finding was higher than that of the 2016 EDHS report of the national and Oromiya region which were 26% and 18.8%, respectively [12, 19, 20]. The difference may be due to the study period, geography of the health facility,

TABLE 2: Obstetric characteristics of mothers who gave birth in the last one year in Chelia District, western Ethiopia (March 2018) ($n = 468$).

Variables	Alternatives	Frequency	Percent
Number of children	≤3	234	50.0
	4-5	137	29.3
	≥6	97	20.7
Gravidity	≤2	134	28.6
	3-4	154	32.9
	≥5	180	38.5
Parity	≤2	151	32.3
	3-4	153	32.7
	≥5	164	35.0
Status of the new born	Alive	454	97.0
	Other*	14	3
Home delivery assistant	Family/neighbors/friends	153	61
	Health extension workers	25	10
	TBAs	56	22
	None	18	7
Knowledge of pregnancy danger signs	Yes	199	42.5
	No	269	57.5
ANC attendance	Yes	395	84.4
	No	73	15.6
ANC started time in gestational weeks	≤12 weeks	126	31.9
	13-24	241	61.01
	>24	28	7.09
Number of ANC visits	One	7	1.77
	Two	73	18.48
	Three	157	39.75
	Four	95	24.05
	Beyond 4	63	15.95
Knowledge about EDD	Yes	189	47.85
	No	206	52.15
Delivery site	Home	252	53.8
	Health facility	216	46.2

* indicates still birth or death within seven days.

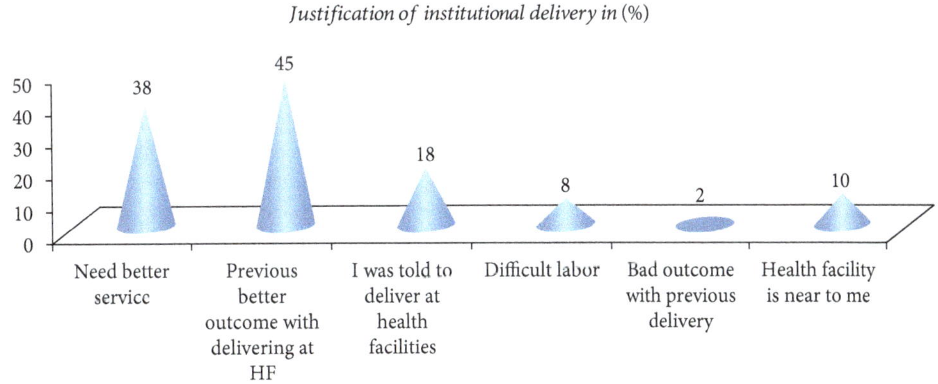

FIGURE 1: Justifications given by mothers who utilized institutional delivery in Chelia District (March 2018).

Table 3: Factors associated with institutional delivery service utilization of mothers who gave birth in the last one year in Chelia District, western Ethiopia (March 2018) ($n = 468$).

Variables	Alternatives	Delivery sites HF	Delivery sites Home	COR (95% CI)	AOR (95% CI)
Monthly income	≤500	41	113	1	1
	501-1000	82	96	2.35 (1.48, 3.74)**	3.64 (1.63, 8.15)**
	1001-1500	28	25	3.087 (1.61, 5.89)**	3.01 (1.106, 8.152)*
	>1500	65	18	9.95 (5.28, 18.73)**	4.46 (1.72, 11.52)**
Number of children	≤3	130	104	1	
	4-5	54	83	0.52 (0.33, 0.79)**	0.39 (0.142, 1.09)
	≥6	32	65	0.39 (0.24, 0.646)**	0.119 (0.029, 0.48)**
Residence of the respondents	Rural	162	234	0.23 (0.131, 0.40)**	5.74 (0.9, 36.59)
	Urban	54	18	1	1
HEWs ever visit home	Yes	78	72	1	1
	No	138	180	0.708 (0.47, 1.04)	
Discussion with HEWs about the delivery place	Yes	72	56	1	1
	No	6	16	0.29 (0.107, 0.79)*	0.11 (0.02, 0.52)**
ANC attendance	Yes	211	184	1	1
	No	5	68	0.06 (0.025, 0.16)**	0.07 (0.008, 0.73)*
Knowledge about EDD	Yes	138	51	1	1
	No	73	133	0.20 (0.132, 0.31)**	0.29 (0.179, 4.93)**
Intended pregnancy	Yes	195	172	1	1
	No	21	80	0.23 (0.137, 0.39)**	0.32 (0.162, 0.65)**
Knowledge about the existence of waiting areas in public HF	Yes	182	161	1	1
	No	34	91	0.33 (0.21, 0.517)**	0.14 (0.02, 0.84)*

*p value < 0.05, **p value < 0.01. HF = health facilities.

and existence of free ambulance service. For instance, if free ambulance service is given, pregnant mothers will reach health institutions without transport expense. On the other hand, the finding of this study was lower than those of studies conducted in Dejen District, Ethiopia, and Bench Maji Zone, southern Ethiopia, which were 71.7% and 78.3%, respectively [13, 14]. These differences may be due to the study period and area in which health facilities could be easily accessible and sustainable ambulance services might be in place.

The result of this study revealed that income had a significant association with institutional delivery service utilization. Mothers who earn beyond 1,500 Ethiopian birr were 4.46 times more likely to give birth at health facility as compared to those who earn less than 500 Ethiopian birr. This finding was consistent with other research findings reported in northern Karnataka of India and Gonji Kolela District of Amhara [9, 13, 21]. The possible explanation for this consistency could be the importance of money in life facilitation for human beings regardless of the residence area.

ANC attendance during the last pregnancy was also another determinant factor of institutional delivery. Mothers who did not attend ANC during the last pregnancy were 92.3% less likely to utilize institutional delivery service as compared to those who attended ANC. This finding was similar to the findings from studies conducted in Goba District of Oromiya of Ethiopia and Tigray of Ethiopia [22, 23]. ANC service is a contact point for health workers with pregnant mothers to promote an institutional delivery and provide information for mothers on the status of their pregnancy which in turn alerts them to decide where to give birth. This finding was supported also by qualitative data.

A mother who completed grade 12 participated in FGD and also raised that "giving birth in Health facility is important. It was God who gave this wisdom for health professionals. Utilizing the services is not sin. Many mothers start services during pregnancy, but some do this only to know sex of the unborn. I and my neighbor attended the service and we got advice about our place of delivery from health professionals during the visits. Finally, both of us gave birth at the facility."

The results of this study showed also that institutional delivery service utilization was significantly influenced by the number of children the respondents have. Women who possess more than five children were about 88.1% less likely to deliver at health facilities than those who possess three or less children. This may be due to the fact that their previously experienced home delivery may make them confident enough to be riskless for the next childbirth among those who have more children.

In the presence of a home visit program by HEWs, the existence of discussion about the place of delivery with pregnant women was significantly associated with institutional delivery service utilization. Mothers who have not discussed with HEWs regarding the delivery place were 89% less likely to utilize institutional delivery service as compared to those who had the discussion. This may be because of awareness gained when family-based discussion with HEWs takes place during home visit.

Qualitative finding also showed that information from health extension workers is crucial for the health of the community. A 47-year-old FGD discussant father of 8 children said that "formerly health extension workers visit our home and give health information for our women, but currently they simply earn salary; they do not know us, we do not know them."

Not only is ANC service during pregnancy important for medical checkup and risk assessment but it also exposes the pregnant mothers to useful health information like eating habit, their EDD, and delivery preparation. This study found that EDD information is another significant factor for institutional delivery service utilization. Mothers who had not been informed about their EDD during pregnancy were 70.3% less likely to utilize institutional delivery service than those who knew their EDD. If delivery appointment is approximately predicted and known, mothers may prepare themselves accordingly by making some necessary arrangements for the delivery. This may keep the mothers alert and help them utilize institutional delivery service.

One of the institutional delivery service-promoting factors that recently started in public health facilities of our country is a waiting area with home-like environment for laboring mothers. This factor was significantly associated with institutional delivery service utilization in this study. Mothers who did not know that a home-like waiting area was available in health facilities were 86% less likely to utilize institutional delivery service as compared to those who knew it. Promoting this waiting area encompasses some food services such as porridge and coffee which were considered common food for mothers who gave birth. This may attract mothers to be in health facilities before and after birth just as their home. Qualitative findings also revealed significance of this factor.

As qualitative data indicated, hospitality and sympathy of health care providers determine the health-seeking behavior of clients. A 27-year-old FGD discussant mother of 2 children stated that "I have delivered in health facility; before that I went there with my aunt. We faced a compassionate and respectful attendant; she approached us as our sister and helped our aunt to give normal birth. There was coffee ceremony during that night. This makes me give birth at Health facility."

The study revealed also that intent of mothers about pregnancy was also significantly associated with the institutional delivery service utilization. Mothers who got accidental pregnancy were 67.4% less likely to utilize institutional delivery service as compared to those who got pregnant intentionally. Intended pregnancy makes the family eagerly ready for birth of the new born, and this may create conducive conditions for the mothers to deliver at health facilities.

5. Conclusion and Recommendation

This study revealed that proportion of women utilizing institutional delivery service in the study area was still low as compared to national and regional target of the country. Antenatal care attendance, family income, number of children, expected date of delivery information, intended pregnancy, existence of the delivery place related to the discussion between HEWs and mothers during home visit, and knowledge of the existence of home-like environment in public health facilities were factors affecting institutional delivery utilization of women in the district.

Since institutional delivery is vital for the well-being of both mothers and newborns, it is recommended to be enhanced throughout the district. Health extension workers should strengthen home visits focusing on households with pregnant mothers to expose them to health information and antenatal care services. Antenatal care service providers also should tell each pregnant mother about their expected date of delivery and the existence of respective caregivers with full-package waiting areas in the facility. Unintended pregnancy and a high number of children should be minimized through family planning service provision since they in turn affect institutional delivery service utilization. Pregnant mothers should visit health institutions as early as possible so as to get necessary services and health information prior to their delivery time.

The District Health Office should strive to enhance a pregnant registration system in the community, promoting conference of pregnant mothers with midwives or health extension workers and antenatal care service provision strategies for all eligible mothers through strong and continued monitoring of the work of health extension workers throughout the district so that institutional delivery utilization will be improved. The District Health Office should also have a discussion forum with traditional birth attendants and other home delivery assistants so that they should promote institutional delivery by skilled attendants rather than assisting at home.

Abbreviations

ANC: Antenatal care
EDD: Expected date of delivery
EDHS: Ethiopian Demographic and Health Survey
EPMM: Ending preventable maternal mortality
FGDs: Focus group discussions
HEWs: Health extension workers
HF: Health facility
SDGs: Sustainable development goals
HSTP: Health sector transformational plan
TBAs: Traditional birth attendants
SBAs: Skilled birth attendants.

Authors' Contributions

AD conceptualized the paper, searched the literature, trained field researchers for data collection, and wrote the results and discussion sections. ET and HO contributed to the design of the study and provided advice regarding methods and data interpretation and took part in qualitative data analysis. KT has critically reviewed the result and prepared the manuscript for publication. Finally, all authors have proofread the final manuscript.

Acknowledgments

It gives us great honor to thank all study participants for their cooperation in providing the necessary information. Our gratitude is great to research assistants who participated in data collection and supervision in this study. Finally, we greatly thank Mr. Guta Dufera for his financial support and Chelia District Health Office staffs for their contribution during data collection.

References

[1] P. C. Chi, *Impact of armed conflict on maternal and reproductive health in sub-Saharan Africa*, 2016.

[2] S. Dhakal, E. van Teijlingen, E. A. Raja, and K. B. Dhakal, "Skilled care at birth among rural women in Nepal: practice and challenges," *Journal of Health, Population, and Nutrition*, vol. 29, no. 4, pp. 371–378, 2011.

[3] J. B. de Mesquita and E. Kismödi, "Maternal mortality and human rights: landmark decision by United Nations human rights body," *Bulletin of the World Health Organization*, vol. 90, no. 2, 2012.

[4] S. R. Bhalotra, D. Clarke, J. Gomes, and A. Venkataramani, *Maternal mortality and women's political participation*, 2018.

[5] World Health Organization, *Trends in maternal mortality 2000 to 2017*, estimates by WHO, UNICEF, UNFPA, World Bank Group and the United Nations Population Division, 2019.

[6] World Health Organization, *Trends in Maternal Mortality: 1990 to 2013: Estimates by WHO, UNICEF, UNFPA, The World Bank and the United Nations Population Division*, WHO, Geneva, Switzerland, 2014.

[7] S. Agha, "Impact of a maternal health voucher scheme on institutional delivery among low income women in Pakistan," *Reproductive Health*, vol. 8, no. 1, 2011.

[8] E. Demographic, *Health survey 2011 central statistical agency Addis Ababa*, Ethiopia ICF International Calverton, Maryland, USA, 2012.

[9] A. J. Kesterton, J. Cleland, A. Sloggett, and C. Ronsmans, "Institutional delivery in rural India: the relative importance of accessibility and economic status," *BMC Pregnancy and Childbirth*, vol. 10, no. 1, 2010.

[10] L. Alkema, D. Chou, D. Hogan et al., "Global, regional, and national levels and trends in maternal mortality between 1990 and 2015, with scenario-based projections to 2030: a systematic analysis by the UN Maternal Mortality Estimation Inter-agency Group," *The Lancet*, vol. 387, no. 10017, pp. 462–474, 2016.

[11] Y. T. Assfaw and M. S. Sebastian, *Determinants of antenatal care, Institutional delivery and skilled birth attendant utilization in Samre Saharti District, Tigray, Ethiopia*, Doctoral dissertation, Umeå International School of Public Health, 2010.

[12] H. Bayu, M. Adefris, A. Amano, and M. Abuhay, "Pregnant women's preference and factors associated with institutional delivery service utilization in Debra Markos Town, North West Ethiopia: a community based follow up study," *BMC Pregnancy and Childbirth*, vol. 15, no. 1, 2015.

[13] A. S. Teferra, F. M. Alemu, and S. M. Woldeyohannes, "Institutional delivery service utilization and associated factors among mothers who gave birth in the last 12 months in Sekela District, North West of Ethiopia: a community-based cross sectional study," *BMC Pregnancy and Childbirth*, vol. 12, no. 1, 2012.

[14] World Health Organization, *Strategies Towards Ending Preventable Maternal Mortality (EPMM)*, WHO, Geneva, Switzerland, 2015.

[15] M. Palamuleni, "Determinants of non-institutional deliveries in Malawi," *Malawi Medical Journal*, vol. 23, no. 4, pp. 104–108, 2011.

[16] A. A. Fikre and M. Demissie, "Prevalence of institutional delivery and associated factors in Dodota Woreda (district), Oromia regional state, Ethiopia," *Reproductive Health*, vol. 9, no. 1, 2012.

[17] M. Abera and T. Belachew, "Predictors of safe delivery service utilization in Arsi Zone, South-East Ethiopia," *Ethiopian Journal of Health Sciences*, vol. 21, no. 3, 2011.

[18] N. K. Beam, *Women and men's preferences for delivery services in rural Ethiopia*, Doctoral dissertation, UCSF, 2016.

[19] CSA, *Ethiopian Demographic and Health Survey 2016*, Central Statistical Agency Addis Ababa, Ethiopia, 2017.

[20] Y. Tsegay, T. Gebrehiwot, I. Goicolea, K. Edin, H. Lemma, and M. Sebastian, "Determinants of antenatal and delivery care utilization in Tigray region, Ethiopia: a cross-sectional study," *International Journal for Equity in Health*, vol. 12, no. 1, p. 30, 2013.

[21] World Health Organization, *Country cooperation strategy for WHO and Morocco: 2008-2013*, No. WHO-EM/ARD/031/E, 2010.

[22] W. Van Lerberghe, Z. Matthews, E. Achadi et al., "Country experience with strengthening of health systems and deployment of midwives in countries with high maternal mortality," *The Lancet*, vol. 384, no. 9949, pp. 1215–1225, 2014.

[23] D. Odo and D. Shifti, "Institutional delivery service utilization and associated factors among child bearing age women in Goba Woreda, Ethiopia," *Journal of Gynecology and Obstetrics*, vol. 2, no. 4, pp. 63–70, 2014.

8

Barriers to Maternal and Child Health Care Service Uptake in Assosa Zone, Benishangul Gumuz Region, Ethiopia: A Qualitative Study

Mulatu Agajie,[1] Solen Abera,[1] Eshetu Yimer,[2] Gizachew Yaregal,[2] Amir Muhidin,[3] Wagari Kelbessa,[1] Dula Ayana,[1] and Debebe Shaweno[4]

[1]*Assosa University, College of Health Science, Department of Public Health, Ethiopia*
[2]*Benishangul Gumuz Regional Health Bureau, Ethiopia*
[3]*Assosa General Hospital, Ethiopia*
[4]*School of Health and Related Research, University of Sheffield, Sheffield, England, UK*

Correspondence should be addressed to Mulatu Agajie; agajiemulatu@gmail.com

Academic Editor: Vikas Roy

Background. Ethiopia has reduced maternal mortality from 871 to 412 per 100,000 live births between 2000 and 2016. In 2019, under-5 mortality rates in Ethiopia were 55 deaths per 1,000 live births. Benishangul Gumuz was the second-largest region in the under-5 mortality rate (98/1,000 live births) in the country. Maternal and child health care service uptake is an important indicator of health outcomes. This study is aimed at exploring major barriers to maternal and child health care uptake in Assosa Zone. *Methods.* This study was conducted in the Bambasi, Menge, and Sherkole districts of the Assosa Zone from July 17 to August 31/2019. The study explored the life experience of study participants about MCH services. The sampling technique was purposive, and data collection methods were focus group discussions, key informant interviews, and in-depth interviews. Data were analyzed thematically. *Result.* The main barriers to child health care services were financial problems, lack of knowledge, preference of traditional medicines for a sick child, women having no time to care for their sick child, poor roads. poor health facility readiness, the poor economy of families, lack of ambulance, cultural and traditional beliefs, providers being male, and unprofessional behaviors which were the major barriers hindering the uptake of maternal health service utilization. *Conclusion.* Poor health facility readiness, indirect costs, inaccessibility to health facilities, and cultural and traditional practices were among the major barriers to service uptake identified by this research in the study area.

1. Introduction

The global maternal mortality ratio has decreased by 44% between 1990 and 2015 [1]. But, still, now, hundreds of thousands of mothers are dying from easily preventable causes [2]. Globally, the underfive mortality rate dropped to 41 deaths per 1,000 live births in 2016 from 93 in 1990, a 56 percent decline [3]. Maternal and child healthcarc service uptake is an important indicator of the health outcomes of mothers and children [4]. Ethiopia has also reduced maternal death from 871 to 412 between 2000 and 2016 [5]. Between 2005 and 2019, Ethiopia has reduced the underfive mortality rate from 123 to 55 deaths per 1,000 live births, the infant mortality rate from 77 to 43 deaths per 1,000 live births, and neonatal mortality rate from 39 to 30 deaths per 1,000 live births [6]. Ethiopia has to do much more to reach the goal of reducing the global maternal mortality ratio to less than 70 per 100,000 live births, neonatal mortality rate to less than 12 per 1,000 live births, and underfive mortality rate to less than 25 per 1,000 live births [7]. The reduction of maternal, neonatal, infant, and underfive mortality rates is by large attributable to the utilization of promotive, preventive, and curative primary health care interventions [8]. According to Ethiopian mini DHS 2019, coverage of ANC 4+ visit was 43%, skilled delivery was 50%, PNC in the first two days after delivery was 34%, and modern contraceptive use was 41%, which indicates even though maternal health services are available free of charge, women are not motivated to use the services. There is much variability between regions of Ethiopia; Benishangul Gumuz Region is the second highest in underfive mortality which is 98 deaths per 1,000 live births [5]. Barriers to health care services have many impacts on maternal and child health and survival, particularly in rural settings where there is inadequate access or poor utilization of health services. Therefore, exploring major barriers to maternal and child health care uptake in the study area could inform program managers about where to focus interventions that can reduce maternal and newborn mortality and improve their health outcomes.

2. Materials and Methods

2.1. Study Area and Period. A qualitative study was conducted in rural kebeles of the Bambasi, Menge, and Sherkole districts of the Assosa Zone in the Benishangul Gumuz Region between July 17 and August 31/2019. The study population was women development army members, (clan, religious, and kebele) leaders, and health extension workers, health workers working in underfive clinics, and mothers of children with chronic and acute illnesses. The FGDs were held separately for both sexes.

2.2. Study Population. The Sampling technique was purposive, and data collection methods were focus group discussions (FGD), key informant interviews (KII), and in-depth interviews (IDI). A total of 15 FGDs, 8 KII, and 9 IDI were conducted. One hundred sixty-seven participants have participated in the study. Data were analyzed using a thematic analysis approach. Focus group discussions were held among members of the women's development army, clan, kebele, and religious leaders. Key informant interviews were held with health extension workers and among health care workers in health centers and in-depth interviews with women whose children had chronic illnesses. Idea saturation for our study was reached after interviewing 150 FGD participants, 8 key informant interviewees, and 9 in-depth interview participants.

2.3. Research Instruments and Data Collection. FGD was held separately for both sexes using the guideline. In-depth interviews and KII were also conducted using interview guides to collect the data. During focus group discussions, one person facilitated the discussion whereas the other took important notes and tape-recorded them.

2.4. Data Quality and Analysis. Data collectors were selected based on their experience in qualitative research and training in the data collection process. At the end of every day, a debriefing session between data collectors was done. The interviews were conducted in the participant's local language and translated to English; the researcher was fluent in both languages. All interview records were transcribed verbatim. The guides for interviews and FGD were pretested on 5 percent of the total samples outside the actual data collection sites before actual data collection, and amendment was done accordingly. The objective of the research was clearly described to respondents before taking the interviews. The audio voice was recorded from the respondents and finally transcribed. Mixed methods (FGD, IDI, KII, and observation) among different participants for data collection were used to cross-verify the collected data. Supervision meetings and discussions were also conducted to authenticate collected data. Health facility readiness assessment tools with the parameters, facility staffing, infrastructure, availability of transportation for emergencies, communication, power supply, source of water, infection prevention, processing equipment for use, waste disposal system, supervision, general services, and structure and availability of basic supplies were assessed using standard checklists to determine whether the facilities had fulfilled the minimum standard requirements. One hundred thirty study participants have claimed that superstitions are responsible for not availing the available health care facility. Themes were identified after reading and rereading the data, and finally, the analysis was performed thematically.

2.5. Ethical Considerations. Ethical clearance was obtained from the ethical review committee of Assosa University. Participants were informed about the objective of the study and the right to refuse or withdraw from the study at any time. Audio recordings and transcripts were kept confidential and codes were used instead of names. Before the interview, informed and verbal consent was obtained from the participants.

3. Results

A total of fifteen focus group discussants, eight key informant interviewees, and nine in-depth interviewees have participated in the study. The age of study participants has ranged from 24 to 63 years.

When asked what actions they take when children get sick; the majority of FGD participants said that despite many barriers they are facing at the health facilities, they still go to health facilities for treatment. Almost all participants across all districts indicated timely care-seeking for a sick child in their community which was reported to be a big challenge because of financial problems, remoteness of health facility, preference of traditional medicine over modern medicine, and women's workload, the traditional belief that the illness is due to evil eyes, and unavailability of basic medical supplies. The participants also agreed low utilization of child health care services because of the knowledge gap in the community about the importance of preventive child health care.

When asked whether childhood and newborn illness treatment was available at the community level, almost all participants from FGD and IDI revealed that there is no treatment for sick children and newborns in their communities.

"The health care providers are not responsible and not respecting us, even when we request an ambulance, they always reply no fuel." (Woman, FGD, 35 years).

Another FGD participant said that *"Few mothers do not want to take their sick child to a health facility because diseases like malnutrition are due to evil eyes and health care providers do nothing for them and they believe taking them to traditional healer would be better. This is why malnutrition in children in our community became a huge problem. They do not accept the advice we give them."* (Woman, FGD, 40 years).

"I was dissatisfied with the care given to my sick child in the nearest health center because; there is no drug, no diagnostic materials, and no committed health workers and long waiting time." (Woman, IDI, 26 years).

"....within the last five years, death due to malnutrition has occurred, mostly the community considers malnutrition as a punishment of sin from the Lord and believed to be due to evil eyes and they do not take malnourished children to a health facility for treatment. The other reason that makes malnutrition common is that most mothers are passing their time on gold mining leaving their children at home meanwhile no one cares and no food for these children." (Menge, KII, HEW).

All FGD participants across the three districts agreed on the importance of antenatal care for mother and child health; however, the timing to make the first visit was usually taken as a norm to be after five months of pregnancy and missing the appointments.

As reported by one of the KII:

"Almost all farming and gold mining in our community are undertaken by women; farmland and mining sites are far away from home, they go in the morning and get back home in the evening and they miss their appointment days. The other challenge is that villages are far from the health center and the roads are not good, especially during the rainy seasons it is not functional. In addition, most of them do not have money to pay for transportation." (Menge, HEW, KII, 29 years).

Almost all FGD participants and KII reflected the importance of skilled delivery and prefer to deliver at a health facility. In contrast to this, most births occur at home because of different barriers: remoteness of the villages from the health facility, disrespect and uncaring providers, and unavailability of foods and drinks at health facilities for delivered mothers.

One of the FGD participants said

"The reason for the very poor quality of services is that delivery attendants have no skills and knowledge and when they are asked for help they usually humiliate us. Some are not disciplined, they are making women's critical situations as a point of discussion and enjoyment which is unacceptable and discouraging. When women hear this information, they do not want to go to a health facility for delivery; they prefer to deliver at home where they are being respected." (Sherkole woreda, clan leader, FGD, 45 years).

Another FGD participant stated *"....Delivering at a health facility is very good but the most barriers for mothers are that many women who come from remote and stay longer do not get food and drinks at health facilities especially "Muk" which is important for mothers immediately after delivery; why not the government provide foods and drinks for laboring mother at a health facility?* (Bambasi, woman, FGD, 42 years).

Another key informant said

"Mostly women complain that the health centers have no waiting rooms, where women stay if they come to health center during labor time. The reasons for the absence of waiting room for delivery are lack of budget and attention to this problems. Another reason why women deliver at home is that women fear to be attended by male midwives." (Sherkole health center, KII).

Another key informant said

[1] "....lack of transport, lack of support from husband, economic problems, lack of ambulance service; midwives being male were the major reasons for very low institutional delivery. Women are encouraged by the elders to deliver at home. Elders convince them as if they safely deliver at home than at health facility." (Sherkole HEW).

Regarding postnatal care service uptakes, participants of FGD and KII across the three districts agreed that postnatal care is the less utilized MCH service in all communities and considered it not important. Women are not allowed to go outside the home 45 days after delivery, because culturally, it is believed that women face great health problem and she may bleed if she moves outside and may die.

"...our communities culturally do not allow women to move outside the home 45 days *after delivery. And we health care providers also do not provide PNC services at home because usually, the health center did not assign providers for it."* (Menge, KII, HW).

All FGDs and KIIs participants reported that family planning is also a less utilized maternal health service in their respective communities. Culturally, women are not allowed to use family planning because of strong male dominance and opposition and taken to be as opposing to what Allah says to humans. Usually, children are seen as an asset in the community. One key informant said that

"Family planning is less utilized services, because of husband opposition and it is forbidden to take family planning, visible implant. Women who took implants are not allowed to enter in mosques." (Sherkole, HEW).

In all communities, poverty was reported to be the primary barrier to timely seek treatment for children. Participants indicated that the decision-making power of MCH services is dominantly made by husbands. Money is controlled exclusively by husbands.

One member of the participants said

"When at home; we abuse our wife's right using family planning but at the meeting, we do not tell the fact, we mostly describe as if we allow our wife to use family planning."

(Menge, clan leader, FGD, 45 years).

Another member of the participants said that

".......our husbands are supporting us in many ways, except opposing family planning use. Women do not take any family planning without the willingness of their husbands, even it is difficult to request about it." (Menge, woman, FGD, 46 years).

All participants reported remoteness to the health facilities, unavailability of an ambulance, lack of basic supplies, poor compassion, caring, and respectful providers, and long waiting time at health facilities which were the major barriers that affect service utilization of mothers and their children.

4. Discussion

This study was aimed at exploring barriers to maternal and child health care service utilization in three districts of Assosa Zone, Benishangul Gumuz Region, Ethiopia. Health care service uptake during pregnancy, delivery, and postpartum period has significant importance for the survival and health of both mother and child. Despite these services are being provided free, the majority of women are not using them. Study participants have identified various barriers to maternal and child health care service uptake.

In the current study, child's health care service uptake from public health facilities was hindered by poor health-facility basic supplies, dependence on traditional medicine, traditional beliefs, inadequate public transport, and poor roads, low economic status of families, women's workload, and poor ICCM and CBNC implementation at the community level. The traditional belief at the community level was identified as an important barrier to timely accessing health care service uptake in the current study. Child health care services are poorly utilized if it has financial expenses such as buying drugs from private clinics and transportation costs and might delay or prevent poor families to seek care and can increase the risk of dying and severity of the disease. Similar findings were reported in Burkina Faso [9] and Ghana [10]. Another barrier was elders were perceived to be unsupportive to seek treatment for sick children from health facilities. The ICCM/CBNC services at the community level were also not fully functional, and the participants knew little about the services. These findings are consistent with previous studies in low- and middle-income countries [11], Malawi [12], and Wolkayit [13].

In this study, the knowledge about the importance of ANC was reported to be good, but the importance of making the first ANC early and visiting all ANC appointments is inadequate. Distant health facilities, women's heavy workload, the long waiting time to receive care, and limited transport availability appeared as a reason for late and missed ANC utilization. In line with these findings, studies conducted in Nepal [14] and South Sudan [10, 15] showed women often did not have enough time to visit a health facility due to their workloads. Another study conducted in Sierra Leone [16] revealed ANC was not timely due to lack of transport, distant health facilities, and social norms to delay care seeking until pregnancy is visible. Other similar findings were reported from Ghana [17], rural Tanzania [18], Malawi [19], and Senegal [20].

The Ethiopian government has subsidized MCH services to make them affordable, acceptable, and available. Despite these initiatives, our findings showed that the quality of services, providers being male, unavailability of foods and drinks, lack of ambulance, inconvenient waiting rooms, long-distance from health facilities, and unprofessional behaviors were among many barriers that limited women's access to skilled delivery services. The health care providers should respect the reproductive rights of laboring mothers such as keeping their confidentiality, providing care with respect and dignity, and the service should be mother-friendly services. Similar findings were reported from Sidama Zone [21], selected towns in Ethiopia [22], and Ethiopia [23]. Physical abuse including slapping at the delivery bed was also reported in Nigeria [24]. A study from Eastern Nepal [25] reported as laboring mothers were not comfortable exposing their body parts to male providers. Most pregnant women have taken home as a natural place of delivery where they could get adequate foods and drinks, where they are being emotionally supported by family members and being respected. This finding is consistent with a study in rural areas of Nepal [14], preference of home delivery for the wish to be cared for by family members, greater freedom of movement at home, and the possibility to obtain appropriate "hot" foods.

Currently, in Ethiopia, only 50% of women get assistance from skilled providers, whereas half have no access to skilled care, which increases the risk of morbidity and mortality to mothers [26].

The Ethiopian government has taken encouraging measures in availing ambulances for laboring mothers to move them timely to health facilities; however, participants in this particular study reported very limited availability of ambulances for laboring women. This finding revealed the demand for skilled delivery at a health facility, but unavailability of an ambulance and/or fuel and lack of alternative transportation means during labor and emergency could delay or prevent from going to the health facility. This finding is supported by a study done in rural Ghana [17] that demonstrated that distant health facilities and lack of ambulances play a significant role in reduced skilled delivery service utilization.

PNC was reported to be the less utilized maternal health service. Even though there was a difference among districts, PNC was reported to have no advantages unless mothers face health problems. This study also revealed that culturally, women were not allowed to move outside the home 45 days after delivery which was perceived to expose mothers to bleeding. Thus, most participants had poorly understood about complications of mothers and newborns after delivery. To reduce neonatal mortality, health extension workers were expected to provide postnatal care services after delivery through home visiting. Despite the importance of PNC visits, all women were not receiving PNC at home or health facilities because of HEW availability and performance. This finding is also supported by the study conducted in the Wolkaiye Tigray region [13], rural areas of Nepal [25], selected towns of Ethiopia [22], and Sierra Leone [16].

The main barriers to family planning service uptake reported by the participants were a strong cultural desire for large family size (perception of children as an asset), male opposition and domination, and religious restriction. Our findings are consistent with studies conducted in Burundi and Northern Uganda [27], Bale [28], and Rwanda [26], which have identified a lack of decision-making powers of women or husband domination and opposition and desire for a larger family as the reasons for not using family planning. This study showed an association between religious beliefs and family planning; it is forbidden to have implants and enter into the mosque. Consistent with our study in rural Tanzania [29] and South Africa [30], it showed religious and cultural norms as a barrier to family planning utilization.

5. Conclusion and Recommendations

The barriers identified gave us a clue why reducing maternal and newborn death in the region is a serious challenge for the government. Poor health facility readiness, indirect costs, inaccessibility to health facilities, and cultural and traditional practices were among the major barriers to service uptake identified by this research in the study area. Health facility readiness must be given due attention to improving the quality of maternal and newborn care. The practical solution must be considered for practical barriers to maternal and child health service utilization in the region. The government should address geographic access problems and transportation barriers. Different partners and stakeholders should do strong awareness creation and community mobilization programs about women empowerment through involving religious and clan leaders, traditional healers, and other relevant bodies to increase the uptake of MCH services in the region.

Abbreviations

CBNC: Community-Based Newborn Care
FGD: Focus group discussion
HEW: Health extension workers
HW: Health worker
ICCM: Integrated community case management
IDI: In-depth interview
KII: Key informant interview
KOICA: Korea International Cooperation Agency
MCH: Maternal and child health.

Authors' Contributions

All authors made substantial contributions in raising research ideas, designing the study, supervising the data collection process, result writing and analysis, and drafting the manuscript. We authors agreed and approved the manuscript for publication.

Acknowledgments

KOICA (Korea International Cooperation Agency) has supported the Benishangul Gumuz Regional Health Bureau financially, and the bureau has funded the research as part of the employment of the authors. Staffs from the funder bureau were involved in the manuscript writing editing approval and decided to publish the manuscript. The authors wish to thank KOICA for funding this research. We are also grateful to UNICEF, Emory University, Benishangul Gumuz regional, Health Bureau, and Assosa University for administrative support. In addition, we would like to thank community leaders, health workers, and women who generously shared their time, thoughts, and experiences. Data collectors also deserve our acknowledgment.

References

[1] J. Bongaarts, *WHO, UNICEF, UNFPA, World Bank Group, and United Nations population division trends in maternal mortality: 1990 to 2015 Geneva: World Health Organization, 2015*, Wiley Subscription Services, Inc, 2016.

[2] WHO, *World Health Statistics 2018: Monitoring Health for the SDGs Sustainable Development Goals*, World Health Organization, Geneva, 2018.

[3] UNICEF, *Levels & trends in child mortality: Report 2017. UNICEF, WHO, the World Bank, United Nations Population Division New York: UNICEF on behalf of the UN Inter-agency Group for Child Mortality Estimation*, UNICEF, 2017.

[4] WHO, *World health statistics 2016: monitoring health for the SDGs sustainable development goals*, World Health Organization, 2016.

[5] CSA, *Ethiopia Demographic and Health Survey 2016: key indicators report*, CSA and ICF, Addis Ababa, Ethiopia, and Rockville, Maryland, USA, 2016.

[6] EPHI, *Ethiopia mini demographic and health survey 2019: key indicators*, Central Statistical Agency, 2019.

[7] UN, *Transforming our world: the 2030 agenda for sustainable development*, Resolution adopted by the UN General Assembly, 2015.

[8] FMOH, *Health sector transformation plan (2015/16–2019/20)*, Ethiopia, Federal Ministry of Health Addis Ababa, 2015.

[9] L. R. Østergaard, P. J. Bjertrup, and H. Samuelsen, ""Children get sick all the time": a qualitative study of socio-cultural and health system factors contributing to recurrent child illnesses in rural Burkina Faso," *BMC Public Health*, vol. 16, no. 1, pp. 1–9, 2016.

[10] J. K. Ganle, B. Obeng, A. Y. Segbefia, V. Mwinyuri, J. Y. Yeboah, and L. Baatiema, "How intra-familial decision-making affects women's access to, and use of maternal health-care services in Ghana: a qualitative study," *BMC Pregnancy and Childbirth*, vol. 15, no. 1, p. 173, 2015.

[11] J. Sumankuuro, J. Crockett, and S. Wang, "Perceived barriers to maternal and newborn health services delivery: a qualitative study of health workers and community members in low and middle-income settings," *BMJ open*, vol. 8, no. 11, article e021223, 2018.

[12] E. A. Lungu, R. Biesma, M. Chirwa, and C. Darker, "Health-care seeking practices and barriers to accessing under-five child health services in urban slums in Malawi: a qualitative study," *BMC Health Services Research*, vol. 16, no. 1, pp. 1–11, 2016.

[13] A. M. Abraha, A. Myléus, P. Byass, A. Kahsay, and J. Kinsman, "Social determinants of under-5 child health: a qualitative study in Wolkayit Woreda, Tigray Region, Ethiopia," *PLoS One*, vol. 14, no. 6, article e0218101, 2019.

[14] R. Shah, E. A. Rehfuess, D. Paudel, M. K. Maskey, and M. Delius, "Barriers and facilitators to institutional delivery in rural areas of Chitwan district, Nepal: a qualitative study," *Reproductive Health*, vol. 15, no. 1, pp. 1–13, 2018.

[15] C. Wilunda, C. Scanagatta, G. Putoto et al., "Barriers to utilisation of antenatal care services in South Sudan: a qualitative study in Rumbek North County," *Reproductive Health*, vol. 14, no. 1, pp. 1–10, 2017.

[16] A. Sharkey, A. Yansaneh, P. S. Bangura et al., "Maternal and newborn care practices in Sierra Leone: a mixed methods study of four underserved districts," *Health Policy and Planning*, vol. 32, no. 2, pp. 151–162, 2017.

[17] J. K. Ganle, M. Parker, R. Fitzpatrick, and E. Otupiri, "A qualitative study of health system barriers to accessibility and utilization of maternal and newborn healthcare services in Ghana after user-fee abolition," *BMC Pregnancy and Childbirth*, vol. 14, no. 1, p. 425, 2014.

[18] F. August, A. B. Pembe, E. Kayombo, C. Mbekenga, P. Axemo, and E. Darj, "Birth preparedness and complication readiness–a qualitative study among community members in rural Tanzania," *Global Health Action*, vol. 8, no. 1, article 26922, 2015.

[19] C. S. Chimatiro, P. Hajison, E. Chipeta, and A. S. Muula, "Understanding barriers preventing pregnant women from starting antenatal clinic in the first trimester of pregnancy in Ntcheu District-Malawi," *Reproductive Health*, vol. 15, no. 1, p. 158, 2018.

[20] K. H. Kim, J. W. Choi, J. Oh, J. Moon, S. You, and Y. Woo, "What are the barriers to antenatal care utilization in rufisque district, Senegal?: a bottleneck analysis," *Journal of Korean Medical Science*, vol. 34, no. 7, 2019.

[21] A. Z. Kea, O. Tulloch, D. G. Datiko, S. Theobald, and M. C. Kok, "Exploring barriers to the use of formal maternal health services and priority areas for action in Sidama zone, southern Ethiopia," *BMC Pregnancy and Childbirth*, vol. 18, no. 1, p. 96, 2018.

[22] M. Kaba, G. Taye, M. Gizaw, and I. Mitiku, "Maternal health service utilization in urban slums of selected towns in Ethiopia: qualitative study," *Ethiopian Journal of Health Development*, vol. 31, no. 2, pp. 96–102, 2017.

[23] C. Fikru, M. Getinet, and T. Shaweno, "Proximate determinants of under-five mortality in Ethiopia: using 2016 nationwide survey data," *Pediatric Health, Medicine and Therapeutics*, vol. 10, pp. 169–176, 2019.

[24] M. A. Bohren, J. P. Vogel, Ö. Tunçalp et al., "Mistreatment of women during childbirth in Abuja, Nigeria: a qualitative study on perceptions and experiences of women and healthcare providers," *Reproductive Health*, vol. 14, no. 1, pp. 1–13, 2017.

[25] S. Lama and A. K. I. Krishna, "Barriers in utilization of maternal health care services: perceptions of rural women in eastern Nepal," *Kathmandu University Medical Journal*, vol. 12, no. 4, pp. 253–258, 2015.

[26] D. B. Farmer, L. Berman, G. Ryan et al., "Motivations and constraints to family planning: a qualitative study in Rwanda's southern Kayonza District," *Global Health: Science and Practice*, vol. 3, no. 2, pp. 242–254, 2015.

[27] P. C. Chi, P. Bulage, H. Urdal, and J. Sundby, "A qualitative study exploring the determinants of maternal health service uptake in post-conflict Burundi and northern Uganda," *BMC Pregnancy and Childbirth*, vol. 15, no. 1, 2015.

[28] A. Gonie, A. Wudneh, D. Nigatu, and Z. Dendir, "Determinants of family planning use among married women in bale eco-region, Southeast Ethiopia: a community based study," *BMC Women's Health*, vol. 18, no. 1, pp. 1–10, 2018.

[29] J. Baraka, A. Rusibamayila, A. Kalolella, and C. Baynes, "Challenges addressing unmet need for contraception: voices of family planning service providers in rural Tanzania," *African Journal of Reproductive Health*, vol. 19, no. 4, pp. 23–30, 2015.

[30] Y. M. Kriel, C. Milford, J. Cordero et al., "Male partner influence on family planning and contraceptive use: perspectives from community members and healthcare providers in KwaZulu-Natal, South Africa," *Reproductive Health*, vol. 16, no. 1, pp. 1–15, 2019.

9

Community-Based Essential Newborn Care Practices and Associated Factors among Women of Enderta, Tigray, Ethiopia, 2018

Gebrehiwot Gebremariam Weldeargeawi,[1] **Zenawi Negash,**[2] **Alemayehu Bayray Kahsay,**[3] **Yemane Gebremariam,**[4] **and Kidanemaryam Berhe Tekola**[5]

[1]*Department of Public Health, College of Medicine and Health Science, Adigrat University, Ethiopia*
[2]*JSI/Research and Training Institute, Inc., Tigray, Ethiopia*
[3]*School of Public Health, Mekelle University, Ethiopia*
[4]*School of Public Health, Mekelle University, Tigray, Ethiopia*
[5]*Department of Nutrition, School of Public Health, Mekelle University, Ethiopia*

Correspondence should be addressed to Gebrehiwot Gebremariam Weldeargeawi; gebrihet@gmail.com

Academic Editor: Hind A. Beydoun

Introduction. Neonatal mortality contributes a higher percentage of infant mortality, especially in developing countries including Ethiopia where the rate of institutional delivery is low. In Ethiopia, scientific evidences on the level of community-based essential newborn care practice were scanty and inconclusive. *Objectives.* The aim of the study was to assess community-based essential newborn care practices and associated factors among women who have infant < 12 months. *Methods.* A community-based cross-sectional study was employed among 634 randomly selected women who have infant < 12 months from June 23, 2017, to August 29, 2017, at Enderta district. Data was collected by a face-to-face interview through structured questionnaires, and it was coded, entered, and cleaned using EpiData version 3.1. Then, the data was exported to SPSS version 21 for analysis. Odds ratios and p value were computed to know the association between the independent variables with the dependent variable. Finally, a variable at p values of $p < 0.05$ was considered statistically significant with the outcome variable. *Result.* The overall community-based essential newborn care practice was found 40.7%. Educational status (AOR = 6.6, 95% CI, 2.49-11.97), previous ANC follow-up (AOR = 1.7, 95% CI, 1.2-3.80), weight of the child during birth (AOR = 1.3, 95% CI, 1.12-2.98), and place of delivery (AOR = 2.1, 95% CI, 1.50-4.63) were found to be significantly associated with community-based essential newborn care. Even though overall newborn practice was found to be good, the cord care practices were found to be poor that indicated there is a need to rise community awareness.

1. Background

Despite the observed declining in the proportion of deaths among children less than five years, neonatal mortality remains high. Globally, every year, nearly 46% of all deaths in children under five were among newborn infants. According to 2013 report, there were an estimated 2.9 million neonatal deaths annually within the first 4 weeks of their life. Almost 99% of these neonatal deaths occurred in the low- and middle-income countries with the highest rates (38%) in sub-Saharan African accounts globally [1].

Neonatal mortality forms almost two-thirds (1/5 million) of the 8 million annual deaths of children under one and almost 40% of all deaths of children under 5 years [2]. Three major causes, namely, complications of prematurity, intrapartum-related neonatal deaths, and neonatal infections, account for more than 85% of newborn deaths. Complications of prematurity are currently the second leading cause of death of children less than five years [1].

Cognizant of the magnitude of the problem, the World Health Organization has come up evidence-based cost-effective measures to improve neonatal outcomes to be used by all stakeholders who engaged with the neonate care, but the neonatal death still remains very high as compared with the overall child mortality rate [3]. In Ethiopia, the current neonatal mortality was 29 deaths per 1000 live births, which makes the highest of the recent infant mortality rates (IMR) which accounts about 63% [4]. Lack of knowledge on the primary caregiver and coupled with strong cultural beliefs influence neonatal survival because newborn care practices by the primary caregiver immediately after birth are important in determining neonatal mortality and morbidity rate [5].

Study conducted in Gulomekeda, Ethiopia, revealed that about 80.4% of mothers had good knowledge on essential newborn care, but 60% of mothers applied butter or oil on the cord stump [6]. Similarly, Ethiopia is one of the ten countries with the highest number of neonatal deaths globally, with an estimated 122,000 newborn deaths per year [7]. Another report from the country revealed that three quarters of newborns had clean cord cutting and tying of the umbilical cord, but only 12% of the mothers had a postnatal checkup within two days, and the quality of the health services they provided was very poor [8]. To alleviate this problem, the government of Ethiopia put efforts to implement the health policy and commitment to achieve the SDG by focusing mother and child health as its top priority [9]. Accordingly, the Federal Ministry of Health (FMOH) introduced prenatal and postnatal home visits by health extension workers (HEWs) in all parts of the country [9, 10] because majority of the neonatal deaths that occurred were preventable because the death is strongly associated with inadequate health care that the mother receives before and during pregnancy, childbirth, and the postnatal period [11–13] due to unavailability of the services, inadequate number of skilled personnel, geographical inaccessibility and poor quality of care, financial constraints, cultural practices, mothers awareness/knowledge about newborn care, maternal health and sociodemographic characteristics, and educational status of mothers [14, 15]. Thus, to decrease this neonatal morbidity and mortality rate, primary caregivers should have the appropriate knowledge and practices on essential neonatal care, but the available literature in Ethiopia did not provide much information about mothers' knowledge and associated factors on essential newborn care. Thus, in order to generate information on essential newborn care practice, this study has been conducted among those women who have an infant of less than 12 months, and it contributes for a careful design of initiative that was targeted to address this group of population through promoting community-based strategies.

2. Methods

2.1. Study Area and Design. The study was conducted in Enderta district, Tigray, Ethiopia, from December 2017 to March 2018. The district is found in the southern east of Tigray regional state, North Ethiopia. A community-based cross-sectional study design was employed among 634 women who had infants < 12 months. Women who had infants < 12 months were considered the as source population of the study, and randomly selected women who had infants < 12 months during the data collection period were considered the sample population. All women who had infants < 12 months prior to the data collection period of the study and who live in the study area for at least 6 months were included.

2.2. Sample Size and Techniques. The sample size was calculated using a single population proportion formula. According to the Ethiopian Demographic Health Survey 2011, the prevalence of initiated breastfeeding within one hour after delivery (one of the contributing factor) was 52% [4]. Consideration at 95% CI, 5% margin of error, and 10% nonresponse rate, the total sample size was 634 women. A multistage sample technique was employed to recruited participants. Five rural kebeles and two semiurban kebeles were selected by a lottery method first, and then, the total sample size was distributed randomly proportional to the size of the population in each selected kebeles. In Ethiopia, the health extension workers who are providing services for the local communities registered every mother who delivered an infant. These women who had infants < 12 months were selected through systematic random sampling from a list of women in each kebeles' delivered mothers registration book.

2.3. Data Collection Tools and Procedures. Data was collected through a face-to-face interview using pretested structured questionnaires. 10 diploma nurses and three degree midwifery professionals were recruited as data collectors and supervisors, respectively. Two-day training on the purpose of how to collect data and related issues was given for data collectors and supervisors by principal investigators before the actual data collection period. Daily basis checkup for complete filling of the questionnaires was also conducted by supervisors and principal investigators, and completed questionnaires were kept, whereas unfilled and partially filled questionnaires were excluded before analysis.

2.4. Data Analysis. Data was coded, entered, and cleaned using EpiData version 3.1 and exported to SPSS version 21 for analysis. Descriptive statistics such as frequencies and percent were computed. Bivariate and multivariable logistic regression analyses were employed. A variable that was significant in the bivariate logistic regression analysis (at p value < 0.2) was transferred to multivariable logistic regression analysis. Adjusted odds ratio was computed at 95% confidence interval (CI) to determine the effect of the independent variable to the outcome variable. Finally, a variable with p value less than 0.05 was declared statistically significant.

2.5. Ethical Approval. Ethical clearance was obtained from the institutional review board of the College of Health Sciences Mekelle University. An official letter of cooperation and support letter were obtained from Tigray Regional Health Bureau; a written letter was also obtained from the district health office of Enderta. Finally, written consent was secured from each participant. The participants were told about the aim of the study, and they were also informed that the information they provided will be kept confidential as the data will be used only for the purpose of generating new information before signing the prepared consent. They were also told they have the right to refuse the interview even in the midterm of the interview if they are incontinent.

3. Result

3.1. Sociodemographic and Economic Characteristics of the Participants. A total of 634 women who had infant less than 12 months were included in the study. About 202 (31.9%) belong to the age group of 25-29 years with a median age of 28 years. Majority, 517 (91.3%), were married, and two hundred fifty-four (40.1%) were also housewives. Regarding their educational status, 255 (40.2%) study subjects were not able to read and write. Majority, 278 (43.8), of the participants were farmer by their occupation with limited (2.4%) which were students (Table 1).

3.2. Obstetrics and Maternal Health Service History of the Participants. Study participants were asked their place of birth for the current infant, and out of the total study participants, 571 (91.1%) gave birth at a health institution. Five hundred fifty-seven (87.9%) had made ANC visit at least once for their recent infant, and 574 (90.5%) reported that they prepared necessary materials for the recent birth. Considering the ANC services, 81.5% of the participants have got counseling services on the advantage of ANC for their recent pregnancy, and 67.4% of them were also vaccinated for TT during ANC visits. Regarding on the post natal services 41.5% were not made post natal services for their recent preganancy.

Among the respondents, 515 (81.2%) heard information about immediate newborn care practice, of which 492 (77.6%) heard from health workers, with small number of them (16.7%) heard from their relatives (Table 2).

3.3. Community-Based Essential Newborn Care Practice of Mothers. Participants were asked about the correct practices on cord cutting, cord tying, application on the cord stump, breastfeeding initiation, colostrum feeding, and timing of newborn bathing, immunization, and place of delivery. The overall prevalence of community-based essential newborn care of mother in this was found to be about 40.7%.

Five hundred seventy-three (90.4%) of the respondents have used a new blade as an instrument for cord cutting, but 9.6% used an instrument they had used before. Five hundred three (79.3%) replied that nothing was placed on the umbilical cord of their newborn; however, significant proportion of them (20.7%) did apply something on the umbilicus (butter (74.8%), Vaseline or lotion (19.1%), and caw dug (6.1%)) on the umbilical cord of their newborn. Regarding the materials used for the cord cutting of the newborn, 63 (9.9%) of the participants replied they have used previously used materials. Similarly, about 15% of the participants gave the first milk to the newborn after 24 hours of birth. In addition, 473 (74.6%) of the participants of the study washed their newborn before 24 hours which is very dangerous to the newborn and can cause hypothermia (Table 3).

Table 1: Sociodemographic characteristic among women who have a child < 12 months in the rural community of Enderta district, southeast zone, Tigray, Ethiopia, 2017.

Variables		Frequency
Age of the mother	15-19	79 (12.5)
	25-29	202 (31.9)
	30-34	131 (20.7)
	35-39	78 (12.3)
	25-29	202 (31.9)
Marital status	Single	24 (3.8)
	Married	579 (91.3)
	Divorce	31 (4.9)
Monthly income	≤300	91 (14.4)
	301-600	140 (22.1)
	601-1000	101 (15.9)
	>1001	302 (47.6)
Educational status	Unable to read and write	255 (40.2)
	Able to read and write	84 (13.2)
	Elementary 1-8	207 (32.6)
	Secondary and above	88 (13.9)
Religion	Orthodox	610 (96.2)
	Muslim	24 (3.8)
Occupation	Governmental employee	29 (4.6)
	Housewife	254 (40.1)
	Farmer	281 (44.2)
	Daily laborer	24 (3.8)
	Merchant	31 (4.9)
	Student	14 (2.4)

3.4. Factors Associated with Community-Based Essential Newborn Care Practices. In this study, ANC visit, place of delivery, and educational level of participants have been found significantly associated variables with "community-based practice of essential newborn care." Participants who were able to read and write were 6.6 times more likely practiced ENBC than those who were unable to read and write (AOR = 6.6, 95% CI: 2.49-11.97). ANC visit was also statistically significantly associated with community-based ENBC practice. We found that participants who had ANC visits for the recent pregnancy were 1.6 times more likely practiced than those did not have ANC follow-up (AOR = 1.68, 95% CI: 1.19, 3.80). Again, women who gave birth at a health institution were 2.4 times more likely to practice ENBC as compared with those women who delivered at their home (AOR = 2.14, 95% CI: 1.50, 4.63). Similarly, women who born a child with a birth weight of >2.5 kg were 1.3 times more likely practicing ENBC than those who born a child with a birth weight of ≤2.5 kg (AOR = 1.34, 95% CI: 1.12, 2.98) (Table 4).

TABLE 2: Obstetrics and maternal health service among women who have children < 12 months in the rural community of Enderta district, southeast zone, Tigray, Ethiopia, 2018.

Variable		Frequency (percentage)
No. of pregnancy	0-1	166 (26.2)
	2-4	353 (55.7)
	≥5	115 (18.1)
No. of birth	0-1	174 (27.4)
	2-4	353 (55.7)
	≥5	107 (16.9)
ANC visit	Yes	557 (87.9)
	No	77 (12.1)
ANC assistance	Physician	8 (1.3)
	Health officer	165 (26)
	Nurse/midwife	360 (56.8)
	HEWs	24 (3.8)
Counseling recent ANC	Yes	517 (81.5)
	No	40 (6.3)
TT vaccination	Yes	427 (67.4)
	No	137 (21.6)
Attending monthly pregnant meeting	Yes	304 (47.9)
	No	330 (52.1)
Preparedness for delivery	Yes	574 (90.5)
	No	60 (9.5)
Materials prepared for delivery	Food	528 (83.3)
	Cloth	544 (85.8)
	Money	384 (60.6)
	Transport	183 (28.9)
Planned birth place	Yes	567 (89.4)
	No	67 (10.6)
Place of delivery	Health institution	571 (91.1)
	Home	63 (9.9)
Delivery attendant	Health profession	571 (90.1)
	TBA	32 (5)
	Relative and friend	31 (4.9)
Mode of delivery	Spontaneous vaginal delivery	544 (85.8)
	Instrumental delivery	52 (8.2)
	C/S	38 (6)
PNC visit	Yes	371 (58.5)
	No	263 (41.5)
Heard about immediate newborn care	Yes	515 (81.2)
	No	119 (18.8)
Source of information	HEW	387 (61)
	Health profession	492 (77.6)
	Mass media	265 (41.8)

4. Discussion

The present study found that 90.4% of women practice safe cord cutting using a new blade; this was higher than findings from Nepal (70.7%) [16]. The difference might be explained by the awareness about ENBC which was raised through time since the studies were done at different periods. It could be also due to the sociocultural differences between Ethiopia and Nepal. However, the finding was slightly lower than a study done in Tanzania (95%) [17]. The difference might be due to the awareness of the mothers about transmitted diseases which was better in Tanzania, and it may also be due to the information dissemination in Tanzania which was better than Ethiopia through better health coverage.

The timely initiation of breastfeeding observed in this study also was found 72.2%. This finding was similar with a notational report of EDHS, 2016 (73.6%) [9]; however, it was higher than studies from Tigray, Ethiopia (63%), Goba Woreda, Ethiopia (52.4%), and Addis Ababa, Ethiopia (58.2%) [9, 17–19]. The discrepancies on the finding might be due to mothers which may have better awareness about the advantage of early initiation of breastfeeding, and it could also be due to cultural practices, study area, and study period difference among the study participants.

In our study, women who can read and write were about 6.6 times more likely to report having experiences of community-based essential newborn practice than those who were unable to read and write. This finding was supported by a study conducted in Jimma, Ethiopia [20]. This might be related to the fact that educated mother may have better understanding about the ENBC practices, and they had the chance of accessing information from their schools and by reading books related to community-based essential newborn care. Similarly, women who had a history of ANC visit for the recent baby were more likely practiced as compared to their counterparts. This finding was consistent with a study done in Nepal, Tanzania, and Jimma [15, 16, 20]. This could be explained by women who attended ANC which may get information about the components and the importance of newborn care practice from health care providers.

Again, women who gave birth at health facilities for their recent baby were 2 times more likely reported as they were practiced than those who gave birth at their home. This may be evidenced by mothers who gave birth at health facilities which may have the chance for counseling about the danger of inappropriate child care practices, and in fact, they may have better engagement with health professionals while the problems were faced. Similarly, though the Government of Ethiopia had set a strategy, all mothers who gave birth should be visited by the health extension workers immediately after birth; mothers who gave birth at home were found less likely practicing essential newborn care; this might be because these mothers did not get appropriate information about essential newborn care practices.

Our study revealed that mothers who gave birth a newborn with a birth weight of <2.5 kg were more likely practicing essential newborn care than those who delivered <2.5 kg. This might be explained according to the newborn management guideline of Ethiopia; a newborn with a birth weight

Table 3: Practice of women who have children less than 12 months on essential newborn care, at Enderta district, southeast Tigray, North Ethiopia, 2017.

Variables	Characteristics	Frequency (percentage)
Essential newborn care practice	Yes	258 (40.7)
	No	376 (59.3)
Where do you put immediately after birth	On the mothers chest	429 (67.7)
	Others	205 (32.3)
Cord cutting instrument	New or boiled razor blade	573 (90.4)
	Used razor blade	61 (9.6)
Material used to tie cord	New string	542 (85.5)
	Other	92 (14.5)
Time of initiation of breastfeeding	Within 1 hour	458 (72.2)
	After 1 hour	176 (27.8)
Frequency of breastfeeding practices per day	<8 times	69 (10.9)
	≥8 times	565 (89.1)
Time of wash for the first time for newborn	After 24 hours	473 (74.6)
	Within 24 hours	161 (25.4)
Time of drying and wrapping the newborn	After delivery of placenta	274 (43.2)
	Do not know	23 (3.6)
	Before delivery of placenta	337 (53.2)
Did your baby received eye ointment from health care provider immediately after birth	Yes	571 (90.1)
	No	63 (9.9)
Did they apply anything on the baby's eye except ordered medication	Yes	267 (42.1)
	No	367 (57.9)
Types of some thing applied on the eye's of new born except ordered medication by health provider	Kuheli	236 (88.3)
	Butter	31 (12.7)
Did you apply anything to the cord	Yes	131 (20.7)
	No	503 (79.3)
What did you do the first milk or colostrum	Gave to baby	603 (95.1)
	Withdraw	31(4.9)
Was your baby vaccinated immediately after birth for BCG on the right	Yes	398 (62.8)
	No	236 (37.2)
What material was used to cut the umbilical cord	New and boiled razor	571 (90.1)
	Previously used razor	63 (9.9)
What material was applied on the cord	Butter applied	98 (73.8)
	Vaseline	25 (19.1)
	Animal dug	8 (6.1%)
Placement of the baby	On the mother's chest/belly	429 (67.7)
	Beside the mother	151 (23.8)
	On newborn bed/table	46 (7.3)
	Do not know	8 (1.3)
Initiation of breastfeeding	Within one hour	518 (81.7)
	2-24 hours after birth	16 (2.5)
	After 24 hours	100 (15.8)
Do you know danger sign	Yes	563 (88.8)
	No	71 (11.2)

Table 4: Factors associated with the community-based essential newborn care practices of women who have children < 12 months at Enderta district, southeast Tigray, North Ethiopia, 2017.

Variables	Category	ENBC practice Good practice	ENBC practice Poor practice	COR (95% CI)	AOR (95% CI)
Educational status	Unable to read and write	116	139	1	1
	Able to read and write	22	62	2.352 (1.363, 4.057)*	6.695 (2.494, 11.973)*
	Elementary 1-8	84	123	1.222 (.843, 1.771)	.348 (.179, .678)
	Secondary and above	36	52	1.205 (.738, 1.970)	.746 (.264, 2.107)
Gravidity	1 time	66	100	.559 (.334, .937)	.589 (.220, .978)
	2-4 times	161	192	.440 (.277, .699)	.686 (.314, 1.503)
	≥5 times	31	84	1	1
ANC visit	Yes	238	321	1.838 (1.090, 3.098)	**1.68 (1.19, 3.80)***
	No	22	55	1	1
Place of delivery	Health institution	204	290	2.612 (1.529, 4.463)	**2.14 (1.50, 4.63)***
	Home	39	24	1	1
Wt. of child during delivery	<2.5 kg	30	68	1.678 (1.057, 2.664)	1.34 (1.62, 2.98)
	≥2.5	228	308	1	1

of <2.5 kg should be managed as inpatient so that the essential newborn care practices will be provided by health professionals at the health facilities not by the parents themselves.

5. Conclusion

In this study, the overall CBEN care was better than from most similar studies of the region; however, their delay for the first bathing was very poor. Educational status of the mother, ANC visit, and place of delivery were found to be significantly associated with essential newborn care (ENBC) practices. Hence, there is a need of improving women education; community mobilization on initiation of breastfeeding and the ANC service utilization should be encouraged.

Abbreviations

ANC: Antinatal care
AOR: Adjusted odds ratio
BSC: Bachelor of science
COR: Crud odd ratio
CI: Confidence interval
EDHS: Ethiopian Demographic Health Survey
ENBC: Essential newborn care
ENCP: Essential newborn care practice
FMOH: Federal Ministry of Health
HEWs: Health extension workers
MPH: Master of public health.

Additional Points

Limitation of the Study. As far as our study was done among mothers who had less than 12 months old children and cross-sectional design, it might be affected by recalled bias.

Consent

The participants and other relevant stockholder for this study were told that the information collected from each of them could be published in an international journal so as to obtain important information that can help for policy makers and program designed to improve the community-based essential newborn care. Hence, we authors obtained consent to publish our work from the participants of the study and other stockholders (Tigray regional health office, district health office, and University ethical review board).

Acknowledgments

First of all, we would like to acknowledge Mekelle University College of Health Science for giving us this chance. Secondly, we are greatly indebted to Enderta district health office and health facilities for giving us indispensable information. Lastly, our deepest gratitude also goes to the study participants for their time and participating fully.

References

[1] UNICEF and UN Inter-agency Group for Child Mortality Estimation (IGME),, *Levels and trends in child mortality: report*, 2013.

[2] W. Moss, G. L. Darmstadt, D. R. Marsh, R. E. Black, and M. Santosham, "Research priorities for the reduction of perinatal and neonatal morbidity and mortality in developing country communities," *Journal of Perinatology*, vol. 22, no. 6, pp. 484–495, 2002.

[3] World Health Organization, *Essential newborn care report of a technical working group Geneva*, 1994.

[4] *Ethiopia Demographic and Health Survey 2011 report*, Mandley Software, Addis Ababa, Ethiopia, 2011.

[5] S. Meharban, *Care of newborn. 6th edition of neonatal acre*, Mandley Software, New Delhi, 2004.

[6] H. G. Misgna, H. B. Gebru, and M. M. Birhanu, "Knowledge, practice and associated factors of essential newborn care at home among mothers in Gulomekada District, Eastern Tigray, Ethiopia, 2014," *BMC Pregnancy and Childbirth*, vol. 16, no. 1, p. 144, 2016.

[7] J. E. Lawn, M. V. Kinney, R. E. Black et al., "Newborn survival: a multi-country analysis of a decade of change," *Health Policy and Planning*, vol. 27, supplement 3, pp. iii6–iii28, 2012.

[8] Ministry of Health (MOH) Ethiopia, *Health Sector Development Programme IV, 2010/11-2014/15*, Ministry of Health, Addis Ababa, Ethiopia, 2010.

[9] E.'s. H. E. Program, *Pathfinder International Support 2003-2007*, 2008.

[10] Mendley, *Ethiopia Demographic and Health Survey 2005*, Central Statistical Agency and ICF International, Addis Ababa, Ethiopia and Calverton, Maryland, USA, 2006.

[11] G. L. Darmstadt, D. A. Oot, and J. E. Lawn, "Newborn survival, changing the trajectory over the next decade," *Health Policy and Planning*, vol. 27, supplement 3, pp. iii1–iii5, 2012.

[12] World Health Organization, *Integrating maternal, newborn and child health programmers: report 2005.*

[13] Save the Children Ethiopia, *SNL/Save the Children Ethiopia COMBINE (unpublished data).*

[14] Federal Democratic Republic of Ethiopia, Ministry Of Health, *National Reproductive Health. Strategy 2006 – 2015.*

[15] D. Paudel, I. B. Shrestha, M. Siebeck, and E. Rehfuess, "Impact of the community-based newborn care package in Nepal: a quasi-experimental evaluation," *BMJ Open*, vol. 7, no. 10, article e015285, 2017.

[16] S. Penfold, Z. Hill, M. Mrisho et al., "A Large Cross-Sectional Community-based study of newborn care practices in southern Tanzania," *Plos One*, vol. 5, no. 12, p. e15593, 2010.

[17] Federal Ministry of Health of Ethiopia, *EDHS, 2016 report.*

[18] M. Ekubay, A. Berhe, and E. Yisma, "Initiation of breastfeeding within one hour of birth among mothers with infants younger than or equal to 6 months of age attending public health institutions in Addis Ababa, Ethiopia," *International Breastfeeding Journal*, vol. 13, no. 1, p. 4, 2018.

[19] T. Kokebie, M. Aychiluhm, and G. D. Alamneh, "Community based essential new born care practices and associated factors among women in the rural community of Awabel District, East Gojjam Zone, Amhara, Ethiopia, 2013," *International Journal of Advances in Scientific Research*, vol. 1, no. 1, pp. 17–27, 2015.

[20] E. Ekirapa-Kiracho, D. Barger, C. Mayora et al., "Uganda Newborn Study (UNEST) trial: Community-based maternal and newborn care economic analysis," *Health Policy and Planning*, vol. 32, supplement 1, pp. i42–i52, 2017.

10

Pregnancy Rate after Myomectomy and Associated Factors among Reproductive Age Women Who Had Myomectomy at Saint Paul's Hospital Millennium Medical College, Addis Ababa: Retrospective Cross-Sectional Study

Meseret Jeldu,[1] **Tadios Asres**,[2] **Temesgen Arusi**,[1] **and Muluken Gunta Gutulo**[3]

[1]*Wolkite University, Ethiopia*
[2]*Saint Paul's Millennium Medical College, Ethiopia*
[3]*Wolaita sodo univesrsity, Ethiopia*

Correspondence should be addressed to Temesgen Arusi; tematantu405@gmail.com

Academic Editor: Julio Rosa e Silva

Introduction. Uterine myoma occurs in 20-50% of reproductive age women. Uterine myomas may be associated with 5-10% of cases of infertility, but it is the sole cause or factor in only 2-3% of all infertility cases. Myomectomy is surgery done to remove myoma regardless of the methods. *Objective.* To assess impact of myomectomy on pregnancy rate and associated factors among reproductive age women who had myomectomy at St. Paul's Hospital Millennium Medical College, in Addis Ababa. *Methodology.* Hospital-based retrospective cross-sectional study was conducted to determine pregnancy rate after myomectomy and its associated factors. Patients who had myomectomy in SPHMMC from September 2012 to September 2017 were enrolled. Information was retrieved from hospital records and phone interviews with the patients. The strength of statistical association was measured by adjusted odds ratios and 95% confidence intervals. Statistical significance was declared at p value < 0.05. *Result.* Among 180 females participated in this study, 52.2% got pregnant after myomectomy. The result showed that females with age > 35 years were 0.31 times less likely to get pregnant after surgery than those ages 20-25 years [AOR = 0.31 (95% CI: 0.29-0.54)]. People with no infertility before surgery were 1.19 times more likely to be pregnant after surgery than those with unexplained infertility before the surgery [AOR = 1.19 (95% CI: 1.06-1.57)]. People with two uterine incisions were 0.06 times less likely [AOR = 0.06 (95% CI: 0.043-0.51)] while those with three or more than three incisions were 0.02 times less likely [AOR = 0.02 (95% CI: 0.002-0.22)] to get pregnant compared with those with one incision on uterine wall. *Conclusion.* Age, number of incision, and infertility before surgery were significantly associated with rate of pregnancy after myomectomy.

1. Introduction

Uterine myoma is a monoclonal, benign tumor arising from smooth muscles of the uterus. It occurs in 20-50% of reproductive age women and can be identified by ultrasound in approximately 80% of African-American and 70% of white American women by the time they reach menopause [1–3]. These tumors are classified based on their location and direction of growth: submucous, intramural, and subserous. Submucous myomas are proximate to the endometrium and grow toward and bulge into the endometrial cavity [1, 4–6].

The role of myomas as a causative factor in infertility remains controversial. It has been proposed that myomas interfere sperm transport, cause cervical and/or tubal blockage, distort endometrial cavity, or may cause inflammation to endometrium or secretion of vasoactive substances [2]. According to AFS guideline for practice, myomas may be associated with 5 to 10% of infertility but it is a sole factor in only 2 to 3% of all infertility cases. Even though myomectomy is the recommended treatment for symptomatic myomas among women wishing to preserve their fertility, the fertility performance of the women after this surgery is not thoroughly studied and detailed. It may also be associated with infertility due to extensive adhesion causing tubal blockage and intrauterine adhesions (IUAs) if endometrium is breached during surgery [1–3].

Myomectomy is found to significantly increase conception rate in women with myomas as a sole factor of infertility. The conception rate following myomectomy ranged from 25 to 77% in available retrospective studies [3]. In different retrospective study done at different hospitals and country showed improvement in fertility after myomectomy. Moreover, age of the women, presence of pelvic adhesion, and the presence of concomitant history of unexplained infertility have negative influence on chance of conception after myomectomy. There was no significant difference in pregnancy rate according to whether the uterine cavity is entered or not, preoperative size, location, and size of myoma(s) [2, 3, 7–9].

Many of the women with symptomatic myoma are in reproductive age group and need for future fertility [2, 7, 10–12]. There is shortage of data done in this area of interest as well as there is no research done on fertility performance after myomectomy in Ethiopia. For this reason and due to uncertainty of effect of myomectomy on pregnancy rate, physicians always face dilemma in counseling and management options of women with symptomatic myomas who need to conserve their fertility.

2. Materials and Methods

2.1. Study Area, Design, and Populations. Institution-based cross-sectional study was undertaken at St. Paul's Hospital Millennium Medical College, in Addis Ababa, the capital city of Ethiopia, from November 1, 2018, to December 30, 2018. It is the hospital with highest delivery rate and gives care to most of gynecologic patients in the city and other parts of the country. All women who had myomectomy at St. Paul's Hospital Millennium Medical College from September 2012 to September 2017 who are eligible were included under the study.

2.2. Sample Size Determination and Sampling Technique. All women who had abdominal myomectomy from September 2012 to September 2017 were included.

2.3. Inclusion and Exclusion Criteria

2.3.1. Inclusion Criteria. Women aged from 15 to 40 years of age at the time of surgery, those who had abdominal myomectomy from September 2012 to September 2017 and who volunteer to give information on phone interview.

2.3.2. Exclusion Criteria. Women with other significant infertility factor (i.e., tubal factor and abnormal SA of partner), those who are not wishing to conceive after myomectomy, those who had bilateral tubal ligation (BTL), those who have no phone number on patient medical record, and those who are not responding to phone call are unmatching identity between medical record name and phone responder.

2.4. Data Collection. The patient identification number of all cases of women who had abdominal myomectomy was taken from the hospital register of patient admission, operation room log book, and discharge log book from department of OBGYN. Their case files were retrieved from the medical record department of the hospital. A structured questionnaire written in English and customized for this study was used for data collection from each patient chart. The questionnaire includes sociodemographic, indication of myomectomy, intraoperative findings, and surgical techniques. Additionally, phone call was made to each patient for additional data that is not recorded in patient chart. Data collectors or interviewers were three trained OBGYN residents. The data collectors were trained for one day about the objectives of the study, techniques of collection, and how to fill the questionnaire. Every day, all of the collected data was reviewed and checked for completeness and relevance by the principal investigator. The collected data was cleaned and entered before analysis. The participants were informed that confidentiality of the information collected and the test result was insured.

2.5. Data Analysis. Data were checked for completeness and entered into Epi Info version 7.1 and then exported to SPSS version 23 for further data cleaning and analysis. Frequency distributions were obtained to check for data entry error (missing/unrecognized values and codes). Descriptive statistics, tables, graphs, means, and frequency distribution were used to present the information. The presence of an association between the independent and outcome variable was checked by the Pearson chi-square test. Additionally, each independent variable was fitted separately into bivariate logistic analysis to evaluate for the degree of association with the rate of pregnancy. Also, a further degree of association was assessed by multivariate logistic regression on variables with p values less than 0.25. The significance level was obtained with 95% CI and p value < 0.05 to evaluate the degree of association between factors and the rate of pregnancy.

2.5.1. Operation Definitions. Abortion is the process of pregnancy termination before the gestational age of viability (28 weeks/07months).

Spontaneous abortion is an abortion without medical or surgical intervention.

Abnormal uterine bleeding (AUB) is defined as menstrual bleeding that is not regular and cyclic and normal.

Infertility is one year unprotected sexual intercourse without conception.

Unexplained infertility is infertility in which there is no major causative factor in both partners.

Recurrent abortion refers to two or more consecutive spontaneous abortions.

3. Results

3.1. Socio Demographic Characteristics. A total of 180 women were included in this study. The mean (±SD) age of the women was 30 (±5.4 SD) and ranged from 20 to 40

Table 1: Sociodemographic characteristics of women who underwent myomectomy in SPHMMC, Addis Ababa, 2019.

Variable	Frequency
Age	
20-25	33
26-30	69
31-35	49
>35	29
Place of residence	
Urban	99
Rural	81
Education	
No formal education	68
Primary school	19
Secondary school	31
College	43
Unregistered	19
Occupation	
Housewife	62
Government employee	48
Merchant	21
Farmers	28
Private	21

years. The age distribution of the participant showed that large proportion 69 (38.3%) belongs to the age group of 26-30. The distribution of the respondent by educational status revealed that 68 (37.8%) of women had no formal education. The majority of the mothers were 62 (36.5%) housewives. More than half of the participant 99 (55.5%) of the women were urban residents (Table 1).

Table 2: Clinical characteristics before myomectomy of women who underwent myomectomy in SPHMMC, Addis Ababa, 2019.

Variable	Frequency
Primary indication for myomectomy	
AUB	80
Recurrent abortion	5
Unexplained infertility	36
Pelvic pain	42
Other	17
Infertility before surgery	
Yes	90
No	47
Unknown	43
Gravidity	
0	114
1	27
2	28
≥3	11
Parity	
0	120
1	31
2	23
≥3	6
Abortion before surgery	
Yes	27
No	153
Uterine size before surgery	
<12	19
≥12	161

3.2. Clinical Characteristics of Participants before Myomectomy. AUB was the primary indication for myomectomy for 80 (44.4%) of women, and for 42 (23.3%), pelvic pain was the primary indication for myomectomy. Unexplained infertility was the primary indication for myomectomy for 36 (20%) of the women. Half of the women 90 (50%) had infertility before surgery. One hundred fourteen (63.3%) of the women were nulligravid whereas 120 (66.7%) of the women were nulliparous. Regarding uterine size before surgery, 161 (89.4%) of the participants had ≥12 weeks uterine size (Table 2).

3.3. Intraoperative Finding of the Study Participants. Among females participated in this study, 75 (41.7%) of them had 1 to 3 myomas removed. For one hundred forty-seven (81.7%) of them, the largest size of myoma removed was >5 cm. Regarding location of the largest myoma removed, 136 (75.9%) of the participants belong to intramural type. In eighty-seven (48.3%) women, myomectomy was done through one incision on uterine wall. For 80 (44.4%) of the participants, location of incisions was on both posterior and anterior wall of the uterus. Fifty-six (31.1%) of the participant had endometrial cavity entered while undergoing the surgery (Table 3).

3.4. Pregnancy Rate after Myomectomy. Out of the 180 female who underwent myomectomy, 94 (52.2%) of them became pregnant after myomectomy while 86 (47.8%) of them did not get pregnant after myomectomy. Half of the participants were diagnosed with unexplained infertility before the surgery. The pregnancy rate was found to be 56.7% after myomectomy. Of thirty-six patients for whom myomectomy was done for unexplained infertility as a primary indication, 20 (55.6%) became pregnant (Figure 1).

3.5. Factors Associated with Pregnancy Rate after Myomectomy. Bivariate analysis was performed, and taking p value < 0.25 as a cut of point for determining significance, then multivariate analysis was conducted for those with p value $< 0.\ 25$. The seven covariates that were significantly associated (p value < 0.25) with fertility after myomectomy at the bivariate analysis were fitted into the backward stepwise multivariable logistic regression model to control for confounding. The final predictors of pregnancy rate after myomectomy were age, infertility before surgery, and number of incision (p value < 0.05). Age was significantly

Table 3: Intraoperative finding of women who underwent myomectomy, SPHMMC, Addis Ababa, 2019.

Variable	Frequency	Percentage
Number of myomas removed		
1-3	75	41.7
4-5	39	21.7
>5	60	33.3
Unspecified	6	3.3
Size of the largest myoma removed (cm)		
≤5	21	11.7
>5	147	81.7
Unspecified	12	6.7
Location of the largest myoma removed		
Submucous	24	13.4
Intramural	136	75.9
Subserous	13	7.3
Unspecified	6	3.4
Number of incision		
1	87	48.3
2	53	29.4
≥3	16	8.9
Unspecified	24	13.3
Location of incision(s) on the uterus		
Anterior wall	67	37.2
Posterior wall	21	11.6
Both anterior and posterior wall	80	44.4
Unspecified	12	6.7
Endometrial cavity entered		
Yes	56	31.1
No	124	68.9

associated with pregnancy rate after myomectomy. Participants aged >35 years were 0.31 times less likely to get pregnant after surgery than those aged 20-25 years [AOR = 0.31 (95% CI: 0.29-0.54)]. Infertility before surgery was the other predictor. People with no infertility before surgery were 1.19 times more likely to be pregnant after surgery than those with unexplained infertility before the surgery [AOR = 1.19 (95% CI: 1.06-1.57)]. Number of incision was also statistically significant in that people with two incisions were 0.06 times less likely while those with ≥3 incisions were 0.02 times less likely to get pregnant than those with one incision on the uterine wall [AOR = 0.06 (95% CI:0.05-0.51)] and [AOR = 0.02 (95% CI: 0.002-0.22)], respectively (Table 4).

4. Discussion

This is a health facility-based retrospective cross-sectional study aimed to assess the magnitude of pregnancy rate after myomectomy and associated factor(s) among women who underwent abdominal myomectomy surgery in SPHMMC from September 2012 to September 2017. The finding revealed that magnitude of fertility after myomectomy was

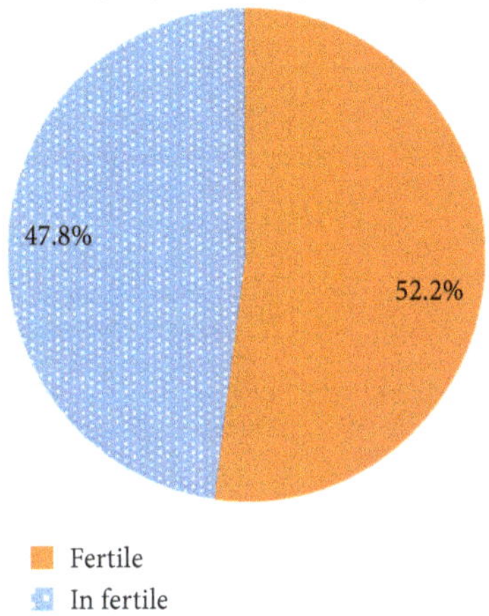

Figure 1: Pregnancy after myomectomy.

significantly associated with age, number of incisions, location of incision, and infertility before surgery.

Among female participated in this study 52.2% of the females got pregnant after myomectomy. This is almost similar to a study done in China which found that 50.3% of women after myomectomy were able to conceive [13]. The result of this study was higher than a study done in Hungary which stated that 40.4% of women got pregnant after myomectomy [14]. On the other hand, our study finding was lower than a study done in the UK which found that 57% pregnancy rate after myomectomy [3]; the finding from the USA found the same result as the UK finding which 57% pregnancy rate was after surgery [15]. Similar study done in New York also found 65.2% of pregnancy rate [16]. But in this study, there are 43 (23.9%) females whose history of infertility before surgery is unknown so that the overall prevalence of pregnancy after myomectomy may be affected negatively.

This study found that age was significantly associated with pregnancy rate after myomectomy. Participants aged >35 years were less likely to be pregnant than those age group 20-25 years. In a study done at Jessop Hospital, UK, women aged ≤35 had a significantly higher chance of conception (74%) than women ≥36 years (30%) [3]. Other study done in China also found that younger people have a higher pregnancy rate than older [13]. A study done in Senegal also support the result of this study; younger people get pregnant than those older people after myomectomy [17].

Number of incisions was also significantly associated with pregnancy rate after myomectomy. Participants who had both two and three and more than three incisions were less likely to get pregnant after myomectomy than those with only one incision. This can be explained by that as the number of incisions increases, the risk of adhesion possibly blocking fallopian tubes also increases [3, 7, 8]. Entry into endometrium cavity occurred on 56 females (45.16%) and has no association with the rate of pregnancy after the myomectomy. This finding is supported by other studies done in China and Hungary [13, 14].

Table 4: Bivariate and multivariate logistic regression analysis of factors associated with fertility after myomectomy, SPHMMC, Addis Ababa, 2019.

Variable	Fertility after myomectomy Yes, n (%)	No, n (%)	COR (95% CI)	AOR (95% CI)
Age				
20-25	13 (39.4)	20 (60.6)	1	
26-30	40 (57.9)	29 (42.0)	0.47 (0.20-1.09)	0.81 (0.27-2.46)
31-35	27 (55.1)	22 (44.9)	0.52 (0.21-1.29)	1.29 (0.35-4.69)
>35	14 (48.3)	15 (51.7)	0.69 (0.25-1.91)	0.31 (0.29-0.54)*
Primary indication for myomectomy				
AUB	42 (52.5)	38 (47.5)	1	
Recurrent abortion	4 (80.0)	1 (20.0)	0.28 (0.03-2.58)	0.21 (0.01-4.23)
Unexplained infertility	20 (55.6)	16 (44.4)	0.88 (0.40-1.94)	1.67 (0.50-5.48)
Pelvic pain	22 (52.4)	20 (47.6)	1.01 (0.47-2.12)	1.25 (0.45-3.46)
Other	6 (35.3)	11 (64.7)	2.02 (0.68-6.01)	1.65 (0.35-7.69)
Infertility before surgery				
Yes	51 (56.7)	39 (43.3)	0.41 (0.19-0.86)	0.30 (0.10-0.89)
No	28 (59.6)	19 (40.4)	1.36 (0.15-0.85)	1.19 (1.06-1.57)*
Unknown	15 (34.9)	28 (65.1)	1	
Uterine size before surgery				
<12	13 (68.4)	6 (31.6)	1	
≥12	81 (50.3)	80 (49.7)	2.13 (0.77-5.91)	1.51 (0.48-4.27)
No. of myomas removed				
1-3	36 (48.0)	39 (52.0)	1	
4-5	24 (61.5)	15 (38.5)	0.57 (0.26-1.27)	0.92 (0.33-2.57)
>5	33 (55.0)	27 (45.0)	0.75 (0.38-1.49)	1.34 (0.47-3.79)
Unspecified	—	4 (100.0)	—	—
No. of incision				
1	37 (42.5)	50 (57.5)	1	
2	33 (62.3)	20 (37.7)	0.45 (0.22-0.90)	0.06 (0.05-0.51)*
≥3	11 (68.8)	5 (31.3)	0.33 (0.10-1.05)	0.02 (0.002-0.22)*
Unspecified	13 (54.2)	11 (45.8)	0.62 (0.25-1.55)	0.08 (0.01-0.62)
Location of incision on the uterus				
Anterior wall	33 (49.3)	34 (50.7)	1	
Posterior wall	8 (38.1)	13 (61.9)	1.58 (0.58-4.29)	2.70 (0.73-9.95)
Both anterior and posterior wall	48 (60.0)	32 (40.0)	1.64 (0.33-1.94)	3.09 (0.98-51.04)
Unspecified	5 (41.7)	7 (58.3)	1.35 (0.39-4.71)	5.69 (0.57-11.64)

*p value < 0.05.

Infertility before surgery was also significantly associated with pregnancy rate after myomectomy. Participants who had a known infertility were less likely to get pregnant after myomectomy than those who did not complain failure to conceive before surgery. Infertility before myomectomy is a factor of poor prognosis for the subsequent pregnancy [17].

Although the overall pregnancy rate is relatively lower (52.2%) because of inclusion of patients whose fertility history before surgery was not known, Myomectomy improved pregnancy rate by 55.7% in patients with unexplained infertility. This figure is higher than the study done at Johns Hopkins University of school of medicine (51%) and lower than the one done at North Shore University Hospital (65.2%) [15, 16].

5. Limitation of the Study

Since this is retrospective study, we cannot reach to cause and effect associations. Additionally, this study was done in those patients for whom open laparotomy was done for myomectomy which is almost obsolete in other sites (endoscopic procedure) as result difficult to get data on myomectomy done with open laparotomy, because of lack of investigative modalities to properly put myoma as per FIGO classification, which is very important to correctly identify the location of myoma relative of endometrium and tubes.

6. Conclusion

Overall, half of the participants were able to get pregnant after myomectomy. Age, number of incisions, infertility before surgery, and location of incision were significantly associated with rate of pregnancy after myomectomy. Myomectomy improved pregnancy rate in those who had unexplained infertility before the index surgery.

Abbreviations

AFS: American Fertility Society
BS: Bilateral salpingectomy
BTL: Bilateral tubal ligation
HSG: Hysterosalpingography
IUA: Intrauterine adhesion
OBGYN: Obstetrics and Gynecology
RPL: Recurrent pregnancy loss
TAH: Tikur Anbessa Hospital
SA: Semen analysis
SPHMMC: Saint Paul's Hospital Millennium Medical College

Consent

Consent is not necessary.

Authors' Contributions

Dr. Meseret Olana is responsible for the proposal development, data collection, and data analysis; Dr. Tadios Mekonen and Mr. Muluken Gunta are responsible for the data collection and data analysis; and Dr. Temesgen Tantu is responsible for the data analysis, manuscript preparation, and correction.

Acknowledgments

The authors would like to acknowledge the Obstetrics and Gynecology Department of Saint Paul's Millennium Medical College. This work received support from the SPMMC, and it has no interest.

References

[1] J. S. Berek and H. PJA, *Berek & Novak, s gynecology 15th ed*, Artin teb, Tehran, 2012.

[2] M. Kasum, "Fertility following myomectomy," *Acta Clinica Croatica*, vol. 48, no. 2, pp. 137–143, 2009.

[3] T. Li, R. Mortimer, and I. Cooke, "Myomectomy: a retrospective study to examine reproductive performance before and after surgery," *Human Reproduction*, vol. 14, no. 7, pp. 1735–1740, 1999.

[4] C.-R. Garcia and R. W. Tureck, "Submucosal leiomyomas and infertility," *Fertility and Sterility*, vol. 42, no. 1, pp. 16–19, 1984.

[5] P. Vercellini, S. Maddalena, O. De Giorgi, A. Pesole, L. Ferrari, and P. G. Crosignani, "Determinants of reproductive outcome after abdominal myomectomy for infertility," *Fertility and Sterility*, vol. 72, no. 1, pp. 109–114, 1999.

[6] P. Seinera, C. Farina, and T. Todros, "Laparoscopic myomectomy and subsequent pregnancy: results in 54 patients," *Human Reproduction*, vol. 15, no. 9, pp. 1993–1996, 2000.

[7] B. Chigbu, S. Onwere, C. Aluka et al., "Fertility following myomectomy at Aba, Southeastern Nigeria," *Journal of Medical Investigations and Practice*, vol. 9, no. 4, p. 136, 2014.

[8] M. Dahlman, M. Palmer, S. Havstad et al., "Fertility after myomectomy: a retrospective cohort study," *Journal of Minimally Invasive Gynecology*, vol. 19, no. 6, pp. S48–S49, 2012.

[9] J. Frederick, M. Hardie, M. Reid, H. Fletcher, S. Wynter, and C. Frederick, "Operative morbidity and reproductive outcome in secondary myomectomy: a prospective cohort study," *Human Reproduction*, vol. 17, no. 11, pp. 2967–2971, 2002.

[10] G. S. Carls, D. W. Lee, R. J. Ozminkowski, S. Wang, T. B. Gibson, and E. Stewart, "What are the total costs of surgical treatment for uterine fibroids?," *Journal of Women's Health*, vol. 17, no. 7, pp. 1119–1132, 2008.

[11] A. Gaym, "Leiomyoma uteri in Ethiopian women: a clinical study," *Ethiopian Medical Journal*, vol. 42, no. 3, pp. 199–204, 2004.

[12] X. C. Guo and J. H. Segars, "The impact and management of fibroids for fertility: an evidence-based approach," *Obstetrics and Gynecology Clinics*, vol. 39, no. 4, pp. 521–533, 2012.

[13] Y. Zhang and K. Q. Hua, "Patients' age, myoma size, myoma location, and interval between myomectomy and pregnancy may influence the pregnancy rate and live birth rate after myomectomy," *Journal of Laparoendoscopic & Advanced Surgical Techniques*, vol. 24, no. 2, pp. 95–99, 2014.

[14] M. Gavai, E. Berkes, L. Lazar et al., "Factors affecting reproductive outcome following abdominal myomectomy," *Journal of Assisted Reproduction and Genetics*, vol. 24, no. 11, pp. 525–531, 2007.

[15] D. Gehlbach, R. Sousa, S. Carpenter, and J. Rock, "Abdominal myomectomy in the treatment of infertility," *International Journal of Gynecology & Obstetrics*, vol. 40, no. 1, pp. 45–50, 1993.

[16] D. L. Rosenfeld, "Abdominal myomectomy for otherwise unexplained infertility," *Fertility and Sterility*, vol. 46, no. 2, pp. 328–330, 1986.

[17] M. E. F. Dieme, M. M. Niang, O. Gassama et al., "Practice of diagnostic hysteroscopy after myomectomy in the prevention of intrauterine adhesions: experience of Ouakam military hospital (Dakar, Senegal)," *International Journal of Reproduction, Contraception, Obstetrics and Gynecology*, vol. 7, no. 5, p. 1694, 2018.

11

The Role of FSHR SNPs and AMH in Follicular Fluid and Serum in Ovarian Response during COS

Elli Anagnostou, Despina Mavrogianni, Ilectra-Niki Prifti, Evangelia Dimitroulia, Athanasios Protopapas, Peter Drakakis, and Dimitrios Loutradis

1st Department of Obstetrics and Gynecology, Division of Human Reproduction, IVF Unit, Alexandra Hospital, Medical School of National Kapodistrian University of Athens, Athens, Greece

Correspondence should be addressed to Dimitrios Loutradis; loutradi@otenet.gr

Academic Editor: Daniel Vaiman

Background. Several studies have investigated on the polymorphism Ser680Asn of FSHR and its use as a predictive indicator of response to an IVF/ICSI protocol. Furthermore, measurement of AMH in serum and follicular fluid is a useful prognostic indicator for the outcome of an assisted reproduction attempt. The purpose of this study is to examine the FSH receptor Ser680Asn polymorphism in combination with AMH levels in both serum and follicular fluid, on the day of oocyte collection. *Materials and Methods.* A total of 32 women who underwent IVF/ICSI were included. Women were grouped into 2 groups: those who received rFSH ($n = 11$) and those who received hMG ($n = 21$). Serum AMH was measured on day 3 of the cycle, and AMH in the follicular fluid on the day of oocyte retrieval; the same day peripheral blood was collected for the genotyping of Ser680Asn. *Results.* No statistical significant difference was found between serum AMH and follicular fluid AMH regarding the FSH receptor genotype for the Ser680Asn polymorphism. Regarding the sAMH/ffAMH ratio in the 3 genotypes, the value was lower in Asn/Asn women than Ser/Ser and Ser/Asn, but no statistical difference was obtained. Women who carry the Ser allele have a higher number of follicles, retrieved oocytes, and mature oocytes than women who do not contain the Ser allele. Women with AMH < 2.22 ng/ml presented lower AMH follicular fluid levels and lower serum AMH/follicular fluid AMH ratio in a statistically significant manner. Concerning the genotype for the polymorphism Ser680Asn of FSHR in relation to AMH levels, no statistically significant differences were found. *Conclusions.* The identification of polymorphisms, such as Ser680Asn of FSHR, along with the determination of endocrine markers in the follicular fluid, such as AMH, could lead at some point, to the personalized therapy setting per woman.

1. Introduction

Genetic polymorphism is defined as the occurrence of more than one allele in a genetic locus within a population, and in addition, each allele must occur at a rate of at least 1% of the population [1].

Mutations and polymorphisms in the FSH receptor (FSHR) gene could affect the reproductive ability in men and especially in women [2, 3]. Of the eight polymorphisms in the coding region of FSHR, two (Thr307Ala and Ser680-Asn) have been extensively studied in ART protocols, in order to evaluate the stimulation of FSH receptor by gonadotropins [4]. Genetic variants of FSHR are also subject of study in the evolving field of pharmacogenetics, as a tool to select the most appropriate treatment protocol in individuals undergoing *in vitro* fertilization (IVF) [5, 6]. Several studies have investigated on the polymorphism Ser680Asn of FSHR and its use as a predictive indicator of response to an IVF/ICSI protocol. Knowledge of certain polymorphisms, of the FSHR gene or others, could provide information on their role on ovarian stimulation and on the selection of the appropriate protocol which would ensure a sufficient number of mature oocytes for IVF/ICSI [7].

Towards that direction, Perez Mayorga et al. in 2000 demonstrated that the ovarian response to the stimulation with gonadotropins is associated with polymorphisms of the FSHR gene [8]. They observed that women who were homozygous for the Ser allele (Ser/Ser) needed higher doses of exogenously administered FSH, compared with women carrying the Asn allele (Asn/Asn and Ser/Asn). In 2002, Sudo and colleagues reported a statistically significant difference in serum FSH levels between different genotypes [9]. In 2003, de Castro et al. observed higher proportion IVF cycle cancellations in women who were homozygous for Ser (Ser/Ser), a greater distribution of this genotype in poor responders and lower response rate to stimulation to administered recombinant FSH as well [10]. In contrast to the above, the implantation rate and pregnancy rate as stated in the study of Klinkert in 2006 was higher in women with Ser/Ser genotype with respect to the Asn/Asn [11]. The same year, Loutradis and colleagues reported a significant correlation between the dose of gonadotropins in women who participated in an IVF program and levels of FSH [12]. The fact that women with genotype Ser/Ser have elevated levels of FSH and therefore require higher doses of exogenous FSH during an IVF program was also reported by Yao in 2011 [13].

AMH is a dimeric glycoprotein that belongs to the TGF-β family (transforming growth factor-β). In humans, the AMH gene is located at chromosome 19 and consists of five exons [14]. AMH is a product of granulosa cells of the preantral and small antral follicles in women. Follicles of size 5-8 mm follicles make the greatest contribution to serum AMH [15]. Subsequently, as the follicles increase in size, AMH production decreases and pauses [16]. Production of AMH regulates folliculogenesis by inhibiting recruitment of follicles from the resting pool in order to select for the dominant follicle, after which the production of AMH diminishes [17, 18].

Several studies have linked AMH levels with the ovarian reserve, the ovarian response of women in IVF protocols, the outcome of IVF attempt, the age of menopause, and other conditions related to woman's physiology and pathology [19–23].

In a study conducted by Hazout et al. in 2004, a significant correlation was found between serum AMH levels and IVF outcome in women less than 42 years old: higher AMH levels were associated with more mature oocytes, more good quality of embryos, and higher pregnancy rates [24]. It was shown that measurement of AMH in serum and follicular fluid is a useful prognostic indicator for the outcome of an assisted reproduction attempt. Hattori in 2013 examined the AMH levels in serum and follicular fluid as predictive markers in 58 women, excluding women with polycystic ovary syndrome [25]. Higher clinical pregnancy rates occurred in women who had high levels of AMH in the follicular fluid or serum. They concluded that high AMH levels in either serum or follicular fluid appears to be positively associated with the clinical prognosis of pregnancy. In 2013, Lin et al. reported that AMH may serve as a predictive indicator of the number of oocytes and the good quality of embryos, particularly concerning the percentages of blastocyst formation [26]. It has also been observed that there is a positive correlation between AMH serum level and the number of mature oocytes, the number of oocytes fertilized, and the embryos that developed, in women who reached pregnancy and women who did not [27]. In a study by Capkin et al., AMH was measured in serum and follicular fluid on the day of ovulation. There was a statistically significant, positive correlation between the concentration of AMH in the serum and the total number of oocytes collected. Also, it was observed that both AMH concentration in serum and follicular fluid was higher in pregnant women. Finally, the concentration of AMH in serum and follicular fluid had a statistically significant, positive correlation with implantation rates [28].

As for FSH receptor, there are studies in literature investigating the role of AMH and AMH receptor (AMHRII) gene polymorphisms and the response to IVF protocols. These polymorphisms were associated with IVF parameters: basal FSH levels were lower, fertilization rate was statistically higher, the number of follicles was higher, and total dose of gonadotropins was lower among noncarriers of AMHRII polymorphisms [29]. Recently, the combined study of the most frequent polymorphism of FSHR (Ser680Ans) and AMH type II receptor (-482 > G) genes showed that women that carry one polymorphism have on average 5.5 units higher levels of AMH compared to women carrying no polymorphism. In women with no polymorphisms, for each unit of FSH increase, the average concentration of blood AMH is expected to be 72% lower [30].

The purpose of this study is to examine the FSH receptor Ser680Asn polymorphism in combination with AMH levels in both serum and follicular fluid, on the day of oocyte collection.

The key questions to be answered are:

(i) Is there a difference between serum AMH (sAMH) value and FSH receptor genotype (Ser/Ser, Ser/Asn, Asn/Asn)?

(ii) Is there a difference between AMH in the follicular fluid (ffAMH) and the FSH receptor genotype (Ser/-Ser, Ser/Asn, Asn/Asn)?

(iii) Is there a difference between AMH serum and AMH follicular fluid?

(iv) Since the women in the study will receive different treatment protocols for ovarian stimulation, are there differences in serum AMH and follicular fluid AMH levels between the women in the two protocols?

2. Materials and Methods

In this pilot study, a total of 32 women who underwent IVF/ICSI in the 1st Department of Obstetrics/Gynecology of "ALEXANDRA" Maternity Hospital–Division of Reproductive Medicine, Athens Medical School, were included. Inclusion criteria were women 22–42 years of age with no uterine or ovarian anomalies, having normal hormonal profile according to WHO guidelines, a regular menstrual cycle of 21–35 days and both ovaries intact. Each patient underwent a short GnRH-agonist protocol. None of these women had been subjected to ovarian stimulation or any other hormonal treatment for at least three months before entering controlled ovarian stimulation (COS). The protocol was approved by our Ethics Committee, and an informed consent was provided by all participants, according to the Helsinki Declaration.

The following clinical, biochemical, and genetic parameters were recorded: age, years of infertility, number of previous attempts, weight, height, BMI, FSH, LH, AMH serum, AMH follicular fluid, PRL, E2, number of days of stimulation, number of follicles, number of oocytes, maturation rate, number of embryos, fertilization rate, embryo quality, and genotype for the polymorphism Ser680Asn of FSHR.

2.1. COS Protocol. A short GnRH-agonist protocol was used: GnRH-agonist buserelin (Suprefact, Sanofi-Aventis) was started on cycle day 2 at a dose of 0.5 mg and was kept until triggering of final oocyte maturation with hCG. HMG (Menopur, Ferring) (21 women) or rFSH (Gonal F, Merck) (11 women) was administered on day 2 at a dose of 200 IU, and the dose was adjusted according to ovarian response on a daily basis. Serum E2 levels were measured daily starting on day 5 of ovarian stimulation with gonadotropins (day 7 of cycle) until the day of triggering final oocyte maturation with 10,000 IU of hCG (Pregnyl, Merck Sharp & Dohme) given intramuscularly. Follicular monitoring started on day 6 of stimulation (day 8 of cycle), and subsequent ultrasound scans were performed every day until oocyte retrieval. Follicular aspiration and oocyte retrieval took place 36 h after the administration of 10,000 IU hCG by transvaginal ultrasound-guided puncture. Luteal phase support was provided with 200 mg of micronized progesterone administered intravaginally three times daily from the day after egg collection onwards, and serum hCG was measured 14 days later. Ultrasound scans, oocyte retrievals, and embryo-transfers were conducted by two fertility specialists of the centre. Similarly, oocyte grading, fertilization, early embryo development, and embryo grading were conducted by two senior embryologists of the centre.

2.2. Collection of Peripheral Blood and Follicular Fluid. Hormonal assessments were all performed in the same laboratory. Serum FSH, LH, and PRL was performed on day 3 of the cycle by electro chemiluminescence immunoassay (Roche Molecular, Biochemicals, Mannheim, Germany). The estradiol levels (E2) were measured on day 5 of the cycle of controlled ovarian stimulation followed by every day measurement, until the day of hCG administration, by using a specific kit immunoassay with electrochemiluminescence (chemiluminescent microparticle immunoassay—CMIA kit, Abbott Laboratories, Abbott Park, IL, USA). Serum AMH was measured on day 3 of the cycle as well and also in the follicular fluid on the day of oocyte retrieval, using the immunoenzymatic method ELISA (AnshLabs, Webster, United States).

On the day of ovum pick up, peripheral blood was collected from the patients to perform the genotyping, using an EDTA vial. The samples were stored at -20°C. DNA isolation was performed using the kit "pureLink Genomic DNA kit Invitrogen, USA," following the manufacturer's instructions. Real-time polymerase chain reaction (PCR) followed, for the detection of Ser680Asn polymorphism, using the device "LightCycler 480 real-time PCR System"-Roche Applied Science. The primers used were FSH-RS AGTGTG GCTGCTATGAAATGC[S] 196599-619 (56.6°C) and FSH-R A GGCTAAATGACTTAGAGGGACAAGTA[A] 196750-729 (56.9°C). The probe used was SP [A] CCCAGA GTCACCAATGGTXITCCA - PH [S] 196697-718 (62.1°C). The protocol is described elsewhere [31].

2.3. Statistical Analysis. Statistical analysis was performed with the Statistics Package for Social Sciences (SPSS), version 24, while the Sasieni algorithm (1997) and Hardy-Weinberg equilibrium were performed with the online calculator which is available at http://ihg.gsf.de. The statistical methods used for the control of statistical hypothesis were two independent samples t-test, 2 proportion test (normal approximation), and parametric one-way analysis of variance (ANOVA). For qualitative data, the chi-square test was used (Fisher exact test when necessary). The nonparametric tests Mann-Whitney U and Kruskal-Wallis test were used when needed. A p value of less than 0.05 was regarded as statistically significant. All values are presented as mean ± SD, unless otherwise stated.

3. Results

The study included 32 women who were enrolled in an IVF/ICSI program. Two types of gonadotropins were used for ovulation induction: recombinant, human FSH (rFSH, 11 women), and human menopausal gonadotropin (hMG, 21 women). The Ser680Asn polymorphism of the FSH receptor gene and AMH values in both serum and follicular fluid of women were also investigated.

3.1. Ser680Asn Genotyping. The distribution of women according to the genotype for Ser680Asn is as follows: 5/32 (15.6%) women were homozygous for the Ser allele (Ser/Ser), 20/32 (62.5%) women were heterozygous for the polymorphism Ser/Asn, and 7/32 (21.9%) women were homozygous for the Asn allele (Asn/Asn). Although the number of participants in this study was small, the distribution of the three genotypes concurs with the prevalence of previous publications in the Greek population.

3.2. Clinical and Biochemical Characteristics according to the Ser680Asn Polymorphism. The clinical and biochemical characteristics of the 32 women were recorded. Women were grouped into categories, according to the Ser680Asn polymorphism genotype (as shown in Table 1). As shown in Table 1, no statistically significant difference was observed among women with different genotypes in the following characteristics: age, years of infertility, serum AMH, follicular AMH, LH, estradiol on hCG day, and number of follicles and oocytes. Women homozygous for the Ser allele had higher FSH levels (9.14 ± 2.35 mIU/l) compared to the other two genotypes (p value 0.019). Also, the number of mature MII oocytes was lower in Asn/Asn women (4 ± 2), as well as the number of fertilized eggs (4 ± 2) in a statistically significant way (p value 0.035 and 0.026, respectively). Also, fertilization rate was higher in Ser/Asn women (0.75 ± 0.15, p value 0.021).

Table 1: Clinical and biochemical characteristics of women of three groups based on the genotype for the polymorphism Ser680Asn of FSH-R. Values in bold are statistically significant (p value ≤ 0.05). *One-way analysis of variance (Kruskal Wallis).

Parameters	Ser/Ser (N = 5)	Asn/Asn (N = 7)	Ser/Asn (N = 20)	p value*
Age	33 ± 4	34 ± 2	35 ± 4	0.394
Years of infertility	2 ± 1	4 ± 3	4 ± 3	0.076
FSH (mIU/l)	9.14 ± 2.35	7.72 ± 2.24	6.13 ± 1.37	**0.019**
Serum AMH (ng/ml)	2.95 ± 3.85	1.05 ± 0.99	1.28 ± 1.08	0.477
Follicular AMH (ng/ml)	3.94 ± 3.00	3.58 ± 1.75	2.56 ± 1.78	0.186
sAMH/ffAMH (ng/ml)	0.55 ± 0.35	0.37 ± 0.47	0.53 ± 0.29	0.096
LH (mIU/l)	5.39 ± 1.36	4.63 ± 1.91	5.31 ± 2.14	0.562
E2 on day of hCG (pg/ml)	2869.60 ± 2119.40	1437.57 ± 683.54	2249.55 ± 921.54	0.152
Number of follicles	8 ± 2	6 ± 3	9 ± 2	0.094
Number of oocytes	8 ± 2	6 ± 2	8 ± 2	0.09
Number of mature oocytes	6 ± 2	4 ± 2	7 ± 2	**0.035**
Number of fertilized oocytes	5 ± 2	4 ± 2	6 ± 2	**0.026**
Fertilization rate	0.62 ± 0.13	0.64 ± 0.12	0.75 ± 0.15	**0.021**

Table 2: Comparison of clinical profiles of women based on whether or not they carry the Ser allele in their genotype. *Mann-Whitney U.

Parameters	Ser/Ser and Ser/Asn (N = 25)	Asn/Asn (N = 7)	p value*
Number of follicles	8.84 ± 1.91	6.43 ± 2.64	**0.032**
Number of oocytes	8.20 ± 1.94	5.86 ± 2.54	**0.028**
Number of mature oocytes	6.56 ± 1.94	4.29 ± 1.70	**0.01**

Concerning the purpose of the study, no statistical significant difference was found between serum AMH and follicular fluid AMH with FSH receptor genotype for the Ser680Asn polymorphism. Regarding the sAMH/ffAMH ratio in the 3 genotypes, the value was lower in Asn/Asn women (0.37 ± 0.47) than Ser/Ser (0.55 ± 0.35) and Ser/Asn (0.53 ± 0.29), but no statistical significant difference was obtained (p value 0.096).

Grouping patients based on whether or not they have the Ser allele we have two groups: homozygous for normal (Ser/-Ser) and heterozygous (Ser/Asn) compared to homozygous for polymorphism (Asn/Asn). Table 2 presents the results; only values that are statistically significant are shown. Women who carry the Ser allele have a higher number of follicles, retrieved oocytes, and mature oocytes than women who do not contain the Ser allele, and this difference is statistically significant for all three parameters.

3.3. Clinical and Biochemical Characteristics according to AMH. Women were grouped into categories, according to serum AMH levels. According to Fleming's classification [32], women were classified into two groups. The cut-off point was 2.22 ng/ml. Thus, the first group included women with AMH values < 2.22 ng/ml, labeled as poor responders, while the second group included women with AMH values > 2.22 ng/ml.

The two groups were compared for multiple parameters: age, years of infertility, previous attempts, BMI, FSH, follicular fluid AMH, serum AMH/follicular fluid AMH ratio, LH, estradiol on hCG administration day, number of follicles, number of oocytes, maturation rate, number of fertilized oocytes, and fertilization rate (Table 3).

The two groups were found to have statistically significant differences in age, follicular fluid AMH, and serum AMH/follicular fluid AMH ratio. More specifically, women with serum AMH values < 2.22 ng/ml were older (p value 0.015 using t-test and p value 0.019 using Mann-Whitney U), as expected. Also, women with AMH < 2.22 ng/ml presented lower AMH follicular fluid levels (p value 0.000 using t-test and p value 0.001 using Mann-Whitney U) and lower serum AMH/follicular fluid AMH ratio in a statistically significant manner (p value 0.027 using t-test and p value 0.041 using Mann-Whitney U). Concerning the genotype for the polymorphism Ser680Asn of FSHR in relation to AMH levels, no statistically significant differences were found.

Figure 1 presents the distribution of women who participated in the study regarding the type of genotype they carry (Ser/Ser, Ser/Asn, Asn/Asn) and the AMH serum levels. Three AMH classes were defined: class A concerns women with serum AMH values corresponding to menopause (0-0.44 ng/ml), class B concerns women with AMH values corresponding to subfertility (0.44-2.22 ng/ml), and class C concerns women with AMH values corresponding to normal fertility (AMH ≥ 2.22 ng/ml). Due to the limited number of women, no further analysis of the traits of each of the categories concerning the ovarian response was done.

The majority of women was heterozygous for the polymorphism Ser680Asn and had AMH values corresponding to subfertility. The combination that had the lowest

TABLE 3: Clinical and biochemical profiles of women with AMH values < 2.22 ng/ml (poor responders) and women with AMH values > 2.22 ng/ml that underwent IVF. *t-test, **Mann-Whitney U.

Parameters	♀ with AMH < 2.22 ng/ml (N = 24)	♀ with AMH > 2.22 ng/ml (N = 8)	p value
Age	35 ± 3	32 ± 3	**0.015*0.019****
Years of infertility	4 ± 3	3 ± 2	0.417* 0.598**
Previous attempts	1 ± 1	1 ± 1	0.876* 0.180**
BMI	23 ± 3	21 ± 3	0.228* 0.317**
FSH (mIU/l)	7.0 ± 2.1	6.8 ± 1.9	0.863* 0.931**
Follicular AMH (ng/ml)	2.1 ± 1.1	5.5 ± 2.0	**0.000*0.001****
sAMH/ffAMH (ng/ml)	0.4 ± 0.3	0.7 ± 0.4	**0.027*0.041****
LH (mIU/l)	5.2 ± 2.1	5.0 ± 1.5	0.777* 0.879**
E2 on day of hCG (pg/ml)	2006.4 ± 991.9	2656.1 ± 1606.9	0.183* 0.361**
Number of follicles	8 ± 2	9 ± 2	0.661* 0.724**
Number of oocytes	8 ± 2	8 ± 2	0.659* 0.808**
Number of mature oocytes	6 ± 2	6 ± 2	0.924* 0.912**
Maturation rate	0.8 ± 0.1	0.7 ± 0.1	0.256* 0.293**
Number of fertilized oocytes	6 ± 2	5 ± 2	0.716* 0.826**
Fertilization rate	0.7 ± 0.1	0.6 ± 0.2	0.198* 0.228**

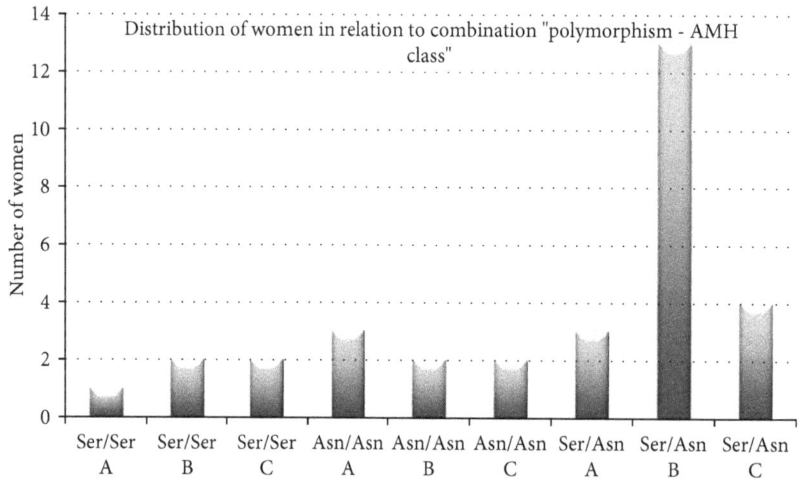

FIGURE 1: Distribution of women in relation to the combination "polymorphism-AMH class" (p value 0.399). Class A corresponds to menopause-related AMH values (0-0.44 ng/ml), class B corresponds to subfertility AMH values (0.44-2.22 ng/ml), and class C symbol corresponds to normal AMH values (2.22 ng/ml).

distribution was the Ser/Ser with AMH values corresponding to menopause.

3.4. Clinical and Biochemical Characteristics according to Gonadotropins Treatment. Women were grouped into categories, according to the gonadotropin regimens which were used for ovulation induction. One group included those who received recombinant human FSH (rFSH) and the other group those who received human postmenopausal gonadotropin (hMG).

The two groups of women were found to have a statistically significant difference in the following parameters: number of follicles, number of retrieved oocytes, number of mature oocytes, number of fertilized oocytes, fertilization rate, and number of good quality embryos (Table 4). More specifically, women who received rFSH treatment presented a better profile concerning all of the above characteristics, in a statistically significant way, in both parametric and nonparametric tests.

Subsequently, they were grouped into three categories: women with AMH levels corresponding to menopause (AMH values: 0-0.44 ng/ml), women with AMH levels corresponding to subfertility (AMH values: 0.44–2.22 ng/ml), and women with AMH levels corresponding to fertility (AMH values: ≥2.22 ng/ml). This grouping resulted in a statistically significant difference and is reported in Table 5.

From the serum AMH values of women, it appears that for rFSH treatment (N = 11), most women had AMH values

TABLE 4: Clinical and biochemical characteristics of women according to the gonadotropin regimens. For all data in the table, p values were calculated with both parametric (t-test—*) and nonparametric tests (Mann-Whitney U—**).

Parameters	Women under rFSH treatment ($N = 11$)	Women under hMG treatment ($N = 21$)	p value
Age	34 ± 4	35 ± 4	0.436* 0.472**
Years of infertility	4 ± 3	4 ± 2	0.708* 0.888**
Previous efforts	1 ± 2	1 ± 1	0.683* 0.908**
BMI	21 ± 3	23 ± 4	0.225* 0.222**
FSH (mIU/l)	6.7 ± 1.3	7.1 ± 2.3	0.508* 0.874**
Serum AMH (ng/ml)	1.3 ± 0.8	1.6 ± 2.2	0.649* 0.321**
Follicular AMH (ng/ml)	2.5 ± 1.5	3.2 ± 2.2	0.321* 0.487**
sAMH/ffAMH (ng/ml)	0.6 ± 0.3	0.4 ± 0.3	0.306* 0.123**
LH (mIU/l)	5.4 ± 2.4	5.1 ± 1.8	0.658* 0.827**
E2 on day of hCG (pg/ml)	2113.4 ± 975.6	2197.9 ± 1297.4	0.851* 0.890**
Number of follicles	10 ± 1	7 ± 2	0.000* 0.002**
Number of oocytes	9 ± 1	7 ± 2	0.003* 0.003**
Number of mature oocytes	7 ± 1	5 ± 2	0.009* 0.014**
Maturation rate	0.8 ± 0.1	0.8 ± 0.1	0.733* 0.842**
Number of fertilized oocytes	7 ± 2	5 ± 2	0.00* 0.002**
Fertilization rate	0.8 ± 0.1	0.7 ± 0.1	0.065* 0.083**
Number of good embryos	6 ± 2	3 ± 3	0.021* 0.053**

TABLE 5: Comparative table of different treatments based on AMH values of the study population. The p value was calculated by the Fisher's exact test.

Serum AMH (ng/ml)	rFSH ($N = 11$)	hMG ($N = 21$)
0-0.44	0 (0%)	7 (33.3%)
0.44-2.22	9 (81.8%)	8 (38.1%)
≥2.22	2 (18.2%)	6 (28.6%)
p value = 0.036		

corresponding to infertility (81.8%) while the rest had AMH values corresponding to fertility (18.2%). On the other hand, the majority of women who received hMG also had AMH values corresponding to infertility (38.1%), while 33.3% were women with AMH values corresponding to menopause and 28.6% were women with AMH values corresponding to fertility.

4. Discussion

The present pilot study was designed to examine the possible combined role of the polymorphism Ser680Asn of FSH receptor and of AMH levels in serum and in follicular fluid, concerning the ovarian response outcome, in women participating in an IVF/ICSI program. It is the first time that the relation of serum AMH and follicular fluid AMH values is evaluated and each of these parameters with the gene polymorphism Ser680Asn of FSHR in women that enrolled in an IVF program. Furthermore, the possible differences in serum AMH and follicular fluid AMH levels between women who received different treatment protocols were investigated.

The identification and determination of the genetic profile of women could be used as a useful tool for predicting the outcome in ART. The future perspective is to individualize the ovarian stimulation and in this direction to personalize the treatment according to each woman's genetic profile. Several studies have focused on the study of gene polymorphism Ser680Asn of FSH receptor, because FSH is a hormone which is necessary for the development and maturation of follicles and acts via its receptor, the granulosa cells of the developing follicle. This particular polymorphism has been associated in many studies with parameters of ovarian stimulation in IVF. The ovarian response to FSH stimulation has been shown to be related to the FSHR genotype [8], and therefore, not only mutations but also polymorphisms in the FSH receptor gene could affect reproductive capacity. Previous studies reported that knowledge of FSHR gene polymorphisms along with other polymorphisms of hormonal receptors could provide information on the effect of ovarian stimulation and the choice of the appropriate protocol [31, 33, 34].

The majority of the study population was heterozygous Ser/Asn (62.5%) for the Ser680Asn polymorphism of the FSHR genc, while the women carrying the Ser/Ser genotype were a minority (15.6%). This frequency is similar to the frequencies described in contemporary literature [8, 31, 33, 35]. Furthermore, the frequencies of these genotypes in the global population according to the meta-analysis of Tang et al. [36] are 40.1% Asn/Asn, 44.6% Asn/Ser, and 16.8% Ser/Ser. In another Greek study, the distribution in the IVF group was

Ser/Ser 24.6%, Ser/Asn 59.8%, and Asn/Asn 24.60% [30]. These data indicate that the frequency distribution Ser/Asn in this study is in accordance with the known distribution in literature and this strengthens this study, even if the number of subjects is low.

Another interesting finding is the FSH levels of the study population. Women with Ser/Ser genotype were found to have statistically significant higher levels of FSH, compared to the other two genotypes. This result is in agreement with other researchers [8, 12, 13]. In the cases that are characterized by higher basal FSH serum concentrations, higher amounts of administered FSH are required [37].

This study also showed that the number of mature oocytes was lower in Asn/Asn women as well as the number of fertilized eggs, in a statistically significant manner. Also, fertilization rate was higher in heterozygotes for polymorphism in women. It is worth noting that the number of follicles and oocytes was lower in Asn/Asn women, with a difference that tended to be statistically significant. Thus, a recommendation to start the ovulation induction protocol with higher doses of gonadotropins seems reasonable in the cases that carry the genotypes Ser/Ser or Asn/Asn.

The results of the present study show that the population of women participating in IVF is favored by the presence of the Ser allele. Specifically, women with the Ser allele had a higher number of follicles, oocytes, and mature MII oocytes than women without the Ser allele, and this difference was statistically significant for all three parameters. This finding is consistent with an earlier study [33], in which a greater number of follicles and oocytes were collected in women who were homozygous for the Ser allele.

Furthermore, we analyzed the distribution of women who participated in the study in relation to the combination " polymorphism-AMH class ", of the 3 genotype and three AMH classes—class A for AMH levels corresponding to menopause, class B for AMH levels corresponding to subfertility, and class C for women with AMH values corresponding to normal fertility. The majority of women was heterozygous for the polymorphism Ser680Asn and had AMH levels corresponding to subfertility. On the other hand, Paschalidou recently studied the -29 (G > A) promoter polymorphism of the FSHR gene, in Greek women undergoing IVF/ICSI. The polymorphic allele for the -29 (G > A) promoter polymorphism correlated with increased number and better quality of oocytes as well. Thus, this observation showed that different polymorphisms of the same gene have different results; thus, we need further studies to identify the appropriate genotype of the phenotypically group of patients that belong to the "subfertility group" or poor responders before IVF attempt, in order to implement special protocols for ovulation induction.

The primary objective of this study was to study the comparison of the serum AMH and of the follicular fluid AMH with the different genotypes of Ser680Asn polymorphism of FSHR. It was observed that AMH levels in both serum and follicular fluid were similar in all three genotypes. Regarding the sAMH/ff AMH ratio in the 3 genotypes, it was observed that the value was lower in Asn/Asn women than in Ser/Ser and Ser/Asn women, but no statistical significant difference was obtained (p value 0.096).

Studies have also reported the use of serum AMH for women initiating IVF, not only as a predictor of pregnancy rate [38] but also as a useful tool to personalize treatment in women undergoing IVF fertilization [39]. The results of the present study are in agreement with current literature research on the association of AMH with the age of women. Our findings showed that women with serum AMH levels < 2.22 ng/ml were older than women with serum AMH levels > 2.22 ng/ml in a statistical significant way, as expected.

Another interesting finding of the present study was the statistically significant, positive relation between serum AMH and AMH in the follicular fluid. More specifically, women with serum AMH values < 2.22 ng/ml (AMH levels corresponding to poor responders) had lower AMH levels in the follicular fluid than women with serum AMH levels > 2.22 ng/ml. In addition, it was observed that women with serum AMH levels corresponding to poor responders had lower sAMH/ff AMH ratio compared with the other group of the women, again in a statistically significant manner. Measurement of AMH in follicular fluid presents great practical difficulties compared to serum measurement, and therefore, there are not many studies on it. This observation is supported by earlier studies [25, 28].

In the present study regarding the genetic profile of FSHR, the heterozygotes group presented the lower level of FSH, the higher number of mature MII oocytes and of fertilized eggs, and fertilization rates as well. Many researchers shed light to other polymorphisms, particularly AMH and AMHRII. These results above are in accordance with our previous study on AMH and AMH type II receptor (AMHRII) single-nucleotide polymorphisms (SNPs) Ile49Ser and -482A > G where basal FSH levels were lower, fertilization rate was statistically higher, the number of follicles was higher, and the total dose of gonadotropins was among noncarriers of AMHRII polymorphism [29]. Taking all these under consideration, one could assume that these genetic observations in different SNPs support the notion that the combination of certain genes as AMH and AMHRII polymorphisms, or ESR1,2 polymorphisms, along with the FSHR SNPs in association with parameters of controlled ovarian stimulation may provide means for the prediction of ovarian response in specific subgroups of women entering an IVF/ICSI program. The effort could be even more tempting if the target is the identification of women of poor prognosis.

Regarding the type of gonadotropins that were used for ovulation induction, recombinant or urine, we observed that women that were treated with rFSH predominated in the number of follicles, the number of oocytes, the number of mature MII oocytes, the number of fertilized oocytes, the fertilization rate, the number of good quality embryo, and the thickness of the endometrium. Several systematic studies in the current literature have investigated comparing rFSH and hMG, in *in vitro* fertilization protocols, with the obtained results remaining controversial [40–42]. In the present study, it appears that women treated with rFSH had AMH values corresponding to "infertility" (81.8%) while the rest had

AMH values corresponding to "fertility" (18.2%). It is interesting that even if the 81.8% of rFSH group had low AMH value, they showed very good response to ovulation induction regarding the number of follicles, the number of oocytes, and fertilization rate. Nevertheless, we must also underline that none of the women in the rFSH group had very low AMH. This alone is a bias for our conclusions, because this may be the reason why the women that received rFSH presented better outcome (more oocytes, etc.), while women that received hMG had worst AMH values and thus worst outcome concerning the ovarian stimulation protocol.

Day 3 serum FSH, indeed, is considered to be a predictive marker for ovarian function. Also, higher serum AMH levels are associated with great number of retrieved oocytes, and lower serum levels of AMH can predict poor ovarian response. The question that rises is if AMH and/or FSH are reliable for the prediction of outcome of the ovulation induction protocol? Recently, the study of polymorphisms on the receptors of those two hormones in combination, FSHR (Ser680Ans) and AMHR II (-482 > G), showed that women with one polymorphic allele have on average 5.5 units higher levels of AMH compared to women carrying no polymorphic allele. In women with no polymorphisms, for each unit of FSH increase, the average concentration of blood AMH is expected to be 72% lower [30]. However, if we get ahead of this observation, then FSH and AMH values and their gene receptor polymorphisms could be both used as biomarkers for projection of ovarian stimulation outcome.

5. Conclusions

The design of this study highlights the possible role of certain markers in the follicular fluid and offers an interesting point of view regarding the value of AMH for the evaluation of the ovarian outcome. The main problem is the small number of the sample; it is obvious that similar questions for the role of SNPs along with markers such as AMH need to be confirmed by other groups of researchers and in larger samples in order to gain more statistical power.

The ideal goal in the future would be to use the appropriate genetic markers to better predict the ovarian response to ovulation induction protocol and offer better results to our patients. The identification of polymorphisms, such as Ser680Asn of FSHR in this study, along with the determination of endocrine markers in the follicular fluid, such as AMH, could lead at some point, to the personalized therapy setting per woman, based on DNA sequencing. Particularly useful is the science of biostatistics, which uses algorithms in information programs, and enables simultaneous and rapid analysis of multiple gene loci and their association with the factors involved in follicular development, implantation, and pregnancy (genome-wide association studies—WGAS).

References

[1] P. Hedrick, *Genetics of Populations*, Jones & Bartlett Learning, 2011.

[2] G. S. Conway, "Clinical manifestations of genetic defects affecting gonadotrophins and their receptors," *Clinical Endocrinology*, vol. 45, no. 6, pp. 657–663, 1996.

[3] J. Gromoll and M. Simoni, "Genetic complexity of FSH receptor function," *Trends in Endocrinology and Metabolism*, vol. 16, no. 8, pp. 368–373, 2005.

[4] S. S. Desai, S. K. Achrekar, S. R. Paranjape, S. K. Desai, V. S. Mangoli, and S. D. Mahale, "Association of allelic combinations of _FSHR_ gene polymorphisms with ovarian response," *Reproductive Biomedicine Online*, vol. 27, no. 4, pp. 400–406, 2013.

[5] D. Loutradis, A. Vlismas, P. Drakakis, and A. Antsaklis, "Pharmacogenetics in ovarian stimulation–current concepts," *Annals of the New York Academy of Sciences*, vol. 1127, no. 1, pp. 10–19, 2008.

[6] M. Laan, M. Grigorova, and I. T. Huhtaniemi, "Pharmacogenetics of follicle-stimulating hormone action," *Current Opinion in Endocrinology, Diabetes, and Obesity*, vol. 19, no. 3, pp. 220–227, 2012.

[7] F. de Castro, F. J. Morón, L. Montoro et al., "Human controlled ovarian hyperstimulation outcome is a polygenic trait," *Pharmacogenetics*, vol. 14, no. 5, pp. 285–293, 2004.

[8] M. Perez Mayorga, J. Gromoll, H. M. Behre, C. Gassner, E. Nieschlag, and M. Simoni, "Ovarian response to follicle-stimulating hormone (FSH) stimulation depends on the FSH receptor genotype," *The Journal of Clinical Endocrinology and Metabolism*, vol. 85, no. 9, pp. 3365–3369, 2000.

[9] S. Sudo, M. Kudo, S. Wada, O. Sato, A. J. Hsueh, and S. Fujimoto, "Genetic and functional analyses of polymorphisms in the human FSH receptor gene," *Molecular Human Reproduction*, vol. 8, no. 10, pp. 893–899, 2002.

[10] F. de Castro, R. Ruiz, L. Montoro et al., "Role of follicle-stimulating hormone receptor Ser680Asn polymorphism in the efficacy of follicle-stimulating hormone," *Fertility and Sterility*, vol. 80, no. 3, pp. 571–576, 2003.

[11] E. R. Klinkert, E. R. te Velde, S. Weima et al., "FSH receptor genotype is associated with pregnancy but not with ovarian response in IVF," *Reproductive Biomedicine Online*, vol. 13, no. 5, pp. 687–695, 2006.

[12] D. Loutradis, E. Patsoula, V. Minas et al., "FSH receptor gene polymorphisms have a role for different ovarian response to stimulation in patients entering IVF/ICSI-ET programs," *Journal of Assisted Reproduction and Genetics*, vol. 23, no. 4, pp. 177–184, 2006.

[13] Y. Yao, C. H. Ma, H. L. Tang, and Y. F. Hu, "Influence of follicle-stimulating hormone receptor (_FSHR_) Ser680Asn polymorphism on ovarian function and in-vitro fertilization outcome: a meta- analysis," *Molecular Genetics and Metabolism*, vol. 103, no. 4, pp. 388–393, 2011.

[14] R. Hampl, M. Šnajderová, and T. Mardešić, "Antimüllerian hormone (AMH) not only a marker for prediction of ovarian reserve," *Physiological Research*, vol. 60, no. 2, pp. 217–223, 2011.

[15] J. V. Jeppesen, R. A. Anderson, T. W. Kelsey et al., "Which follicles make the most anti-Mullerian hormone in humans? Evidence for an abrupt decline in AMH production at the time of follicle selection," *Molecular Human Reproduction*, vol. 19, no. 8, pp. 519–527, 2013.

[16] C. Weenen, J. S. Laven, A. von Bergh et al., "Anti-Müllerian hormone expression pattern in the human ovary: potential implications for initial and cyclic follicle recruitment," *Molecular Human Reproduction*, vol. 10, no. 2, pp. 77–83, 2004.

[17] J. A. Visser, F. H. de Jong, J. S. Laven, and A. P. N. Themmen, "Anti-Müllerian hormone: a new marker for ovarian function," *Reproduction*, vol. 131, no. 1, pp. 1-9, 2006.

[18] D. Dewailly, C. Y. Andersen, A. Balen et al., "The physiology and clinical utility of anti-Mullerian hormone in women," *Human Reproduction Update*, vol. 20, no. 3, pp. 370–385, 2014.

[19] S. L. Broer, M. J. Eijkemans, G. J. Scheffer et al., "Anti-mullerian hormone predicts menopause: a long-term follow-up study in normoovulatory women," *JCEM*, vol. 96, no. 8, pp. 2532–2539, 2011.

[20] S. L. Broer, F. J. Broekmans, J. S. Laven, and B. C. J. M. Fauser, "Anti-Müllerian hormone: ovarian reserve testing and its potential clinical implications," *Human Reproduction Update*, vol. 20, no. 5, pp. 688–701, 2014.

[21] S. Brugo Olmedo, S. de Vincentiis, E. de Martino et al., "Prediction of reproductive outcomes according to different serum anti-Müllerian hormone levels in females undergoing intracystoplasmic sperm injection," *PLoS One*, vol. 8, no. 9, article e75685, 2013.

[22] L. Casadei, A. Madrigale, F. Puca et al., "The role of serum anti-Müllerian hormone (AMH) in the hormonal diagnosis of polycystic ovary syndrome," *Gynecological Endocrinology*, vol. 29, no. 6, pp. 545–550, 2013.

[23] M. A. Ganidou, E. M. Kolibianakis, C. A. Venetis et al., "Is assessment of anti-Müllerian hormone and/or antral follicle count useful in the prediction of ovarian response in expected normal responders treated with a fixed dose of recombinant FSH and GnRH antagonists? A prospective observational study," *Gynecological Endocrinology*, vol. 30, no. 11, pp. 817–821, 2014.

[24] A. Hazout, P. Bouchard, D. B. Seifer, P. Aussage, A. M. Junca, and P. Cohen-Bacrie, "Serum antimullerian hormone/mullerian-inhibiting substance appears to be a more discriminatory marker of assisted reproductive technology outcome than follicle-stimulating hormone, inhibin B, or estradiol," *Fertility and Sterility*, vol. 82, no. 5, pp. 1323–1329, 2004.

[25] Y. Hattori, T. Sato, H. Okada, C. Saito, and M. Sugiura-Ogasawara, "Comparison of follicular fluid and serum anti-Mullerian hormone levels as predictors of the outcome of assisted reproductive treatment," *European Journal of Obstetrics, Gynecology, and Reproductive Biology*, vol. 169, no. 2, pp. 252–256, 2013.

[26] W. Q. Lin, L. N. Yao, D. X. Zhang, W. Zhang, X. J. Yang, and R. Yu, "The predictive value of anti-Mullerian hormone on embryo quality, blastocyst development, and pregnancy rate following in vitro fertilization-embryo transfer (IVF-ET)," *Journal of Assisted Reproduction and Genetics*, vol. 30, no. 5, pp. 649–655, 2013.

[27] M. Ferrario, R. Secomandi, M. Cappato et al., "Ovarian and adrenal androgens may be useful markers to predict oocyte competence and embryo development in older women," *Gynecological Endocrinology*, vol. 31, no. 2, pp. 125–130, 2014.

[28] S. I. Capkin, S. Ozyer, R. Karayalcin, O. Moraloglu, S. Ozcan, and M. Ugur, "Serum and follicular fluid anti-Mullerian hormone concentrations at the time of follicle puncture and reproductive outcome," *Journal of the Turkish German Gynecological Association*, vol. 13, no. 1, pp. 21–26, 2011.

[29] I. Karagiorga, G. A. Partsinevelos, D. Mavrogianni et al., "Single nucleotide polymorphisms in the anti-Müllerian hormone (AMH Ile49Ser) and anti-Müllerian hormone type II receptor (AMHRII -482 A>G) as genetic markers in assisted reproduction technology," *Journal of Assisted Reproduction and Genetics*, vol. 32, no. 3, pp. 357–367, 2015.

[30] I. G. Papanikolaou, P. Giannelou, E. Anagnostou, D. Mavrogianni, P. Drakakis, and D. Loutradis, "Combined study on the single nucleotide polymorphisms in the follicle-stimulating hormone receptor (Ser680Asn) and anti-Müllerian hormone receptor type II (-482A>G) as genetic markers in assisted reproduction," *Hormone Molecular Biology and Clinical Investigation*, vol. 38, no. 1, 2019.

[31] C. Paschalidou, E. Anagnostou, D. Mavrogianni et al., "The effects of follicle-stimulating hormone receptor (FSHR) -29 and Ser680Asn polymorphisms in IVF/ICSI," *Hormone Molecular Biology and Clinical Investigation*, vol. 41, 2020.

[32] R. Fleming, F. Broekmans, C. Calhaz-Jorge et al., "Can anti-Mullerian hormone concentrations be used to determine gonadotrophin dose and treatment protocol for ovarian stimulation?," *Reproductive Biomedicine Online*, vol. 26, no. 5, pp. 431–439, 2013.

[33] E. Anagnostou, D. Mavrogianni, C. Theofanakis et al., "ESR1, ESR2 and FSH receptor gene polymorphisms in combination: a useful genetic tool for the prediction of poor responders," *Current Pharmaceutical Biotechnology*, vol. 13, no. 3, pp. 426–434, 2012.

[34] L. Lazaros, E. Hatzi, N. Xita et al., "Influence of FSHR diplotypes on ovarian response to standard gonadotropin stimulation for IVF/ICSI," *The Journal of Reproductive Medicine*, vol. 58, no. 9-10, pp. 395–401, 2013.

[35] C. Daelemans, G. Smits, V. de Maertelaer et al., "Prediction of severity of symptoms in iatrogenic ovarian hyperstimulation syndrome by follicle-stimulating hormone receptor Ser680Asn polymorphism," *The Journal of Clinical Endocrinology and Metabolism*, vol. 89, no. 12, pp. 6310–6315, 2004.

[36] H. Tang, Y. Yan, T. Wang et al., "Effect of follicle-stimulating hormone receptor Asn680Ser polymorphism on the outcomes of controlled ovarian hyperstimulation: an updated meta-analysis of 16 cohort studies," *Journal of Assisted Reproduction and Genetics*, vol. 32, no. 12, pp. 1801–1810, 2015.

[37] M. Simoni, C. B. Tempfer, B. Destenaves, and B. C. Fauser, "Functional genetic polymorphisms and female reproductive disorders: Part I: Polycystic ovary syndrome and ovarian response," *Human Reproduction Update*, vol. 14, no. 5, pp. 459–484, 2008.

[38] H. M. Kamel, A. H. Amin, and A. R. Al-Adawy, "Basal serum anti-Mullerian hormone (AMH) is a promising test in prediction of occurrence of pregnancy rate in infertile women undergoing ICSI cycles," *Clinical Laboratory*, vol. 60, no. 10, pp. 1717–1723, 2014.

[39] T. S. Patrelli, S. Gizzo, N. Sianesi et al., "Anti-Müllerian hormone serum values and ovarian reserve: can it predict a decrease in fertility after ovarian stimulation by ART cycles?," *PLoS One*, vol. 7, no. 9, article e44571, 2012.

[40] M. van Wely, I. Kwan, A. L. Burt et al., "Recombinant versus urinary gonadotrophin for ovarian stimulation in assisted reproductive technology cycles," *Cochrane Database of Systematic Reviews*, vol. 2, article CD005354, 2011.

[41] Z. Petanovski, G. Dimitrov, B. Aydin et al., "Recombinant FSH versus HP-HMG for controled ovarian stimulation in intracitoplasmic sperm injection cycles," *Medicinski Arhiv*, vol. 65, no. 3, pp. 153–156, 2011.

[42] C. Theofanakis, V. Athanasiou, E. Liokari et al., "The impact of HCG in IVF treatment: does it depend on age or on protocol?," *Journal of Gynecology Obstetrics and Human Reproduction*, vol. 48, no. 5, pp. 341–345, 2019.

12

Adherence to Iron-Folic Acid Supplementation and Associated Factors among Pregnant Women in Kasulu Communities in North-Western Tanzania

Winfrida B. Lyoba,[1,2] Joyce D. Mwakatoga,[3] Charles Festo,[1] Jackline Mrema,[1] and Ester Elisaria[1]

[1]*Department of Impact Evaluation, Health System and Policy Analysis, Ifakara Health Institute, Dar es Salaam, Tanzania*
[2]*Department of Global Health and Bio-Medical Sciences, College of Life Science and Bioengineering, The Nelson Mandela Institution of Science and Technology, Arusha, Tanzania*
[3]*Department of Agricultural Extension and Community Development, College of Agriculture, Sokoine University of Agriculture, Morogoro, Tanzania*

Correspondence should be addressed to Winfrida B. Lyoba; lyobaw@nm-aist.ac.tz

Academic Editor: Samir Hamamah

Introduction. Pregnant women are at a high risk of anaemia, with iron-folate deficiency being the most common cause of anaemia among pregnant women. Despite the well-known importance of iron and folic acid supplementation (IFAS) during pregnancy, adherence to these supplements is relatively low and associated factors were not well identified in the study area. This study is aimed at investigating adherence to IFAS and associated factors among pregnant women in Kasulu district, north-western Tanzania. *Methods.* A health facility cross-sectional survey with a mixed-method approach was conducted in Kasulu district from March to April 2019. A structured questionnaire was given to 320 women with children aged 0-6 months to assess factors associated with adherence to IFAS among pregnant women. Data were entered into SPSS version 22.0 for analysis. Binary logistic regression was further employed to determine the factors associated with adherence to IFAS. Focus group discussions were done with 19 pregnant women and 15 mothers of children aged 0-6 months to obtain more clarifications on the factors associated with adherence to IFAS. Furthermore, in-depth interviews were done with six health care providers to explore their perceptions of IFAS. *Results.* Out of the 320 respondents of the survey, 20.3% ($n = 65$) adhered to IFAS. Factors associated with adherence to IFAS among pregnant women included time to start ANC (AOR = 3.72, 95% CI: 1.42, 9.79), knowledge of anaemia (AOR = 3.84, 95% CI: 1.335, 10.66), counseling on the importance of the iron-folic acid (AOR = 3.86, 95% CI: 1.42, 10.50), IFAS given during clinical visit (AOR = 15.72, 95% CI: 5.34, 46.31), number of meals consumed (AOR = 3.44, 95% CI: 1.28, 9.21), number of children (AOR = 3.462, 95% CI: 1.035, 11.58), and distance to health facility (AOR = 0.34, 95% CI: 0.131, 0.886). Qualitative findings revealed that delayed first ANC visit, lack of remainder for pregnant women to take IFAS, low awareness about the negative effects of anaemia, low of knowledge of IFAS and management of side effects, negative beliefs about the use of IFAS, and follow-up mechanism were major reasons for poor adherence. *Conclusion.* Adherence to iron-folic acid supplementation during pregnancy was low. Strengthening systems for creating reminding mechanism, raising community awareness through educational programs to pregnant women and health providers could improve adherence to IFAS.

1. Introduction

Anaemia affects more than two billion people, 30-50% of whom are from developing countries including Tanzania [1]. Nearly 50% of all anaemia can be attributed to iron deficiency [1, 2]. Folic acid is also a vital micronutrient required for the metabolism, foetal growth, and the development of the neural tube [3]. Globally, the estimated prevalence of anaemia among nonpregnant and pregnant women was 29% and 38%, respectively, whereas, in Africa, the estimated proportions were 37.8% and 46.3%, respectively [2]. In Tanzania, the burden of iron deficiency accounts for approximately 57% among pregnant mothers and 46% among breastfeeding mothers [4]. Similarly, the prevalence of anaemia among women of reproductive age between 15 and 49 years is 45% in Tanzania and Kigoma region alone disproportionately carrying over half (55.1%) of the burden [4].

Pregnant women are more vulnerable to anaemia because of various factors. These include biological changes (menstrual period), undernutrition attributed to poverty, food insecurity, gender inequalities, inadequate knowledge of proper dietary practices, and increased iron and folic acid deficiency [5]. Furthermore, pregnant women experience increased micronutrient demand especially iron for the growth of foetus and metabolism which cannot be easily met by diet alone because of the poor intake and low absorption of iron [3].

Women who failed to consume the tablets according to the IFAS recommendation would experience iron and folic acid (IFA) deficiency anaemia and associated negative effects on mothers and newborns. Folic acid deficiency in pregnant women is associated with preeclampsia and, preterm delivery. It is also related to neural tube defects, foetal malformation, type 2 diabetes, and obesity in the newborn [6–8]. Similarly, iron deficiency anaemia is connected with maternal risks including haemorrhage, premature delivery, rupture membrane, decreased work capacity, and maternal deaths. Correspondingly, small for gestational age, low birth weight, poor cognitive development, stillbirth, and cardiovascular disease were risks associated with iron anaemia in the newborn [2, 9, 10]. Anaemia leads to approximately 50,000 deaths during childbirth each year globally [9] and iron deficiency alone accounts for 22% of all anaemia deaths [7]. In sub-Saharan Africa, anaemia contributed to approximately 28.6% of maternal deaths [11] and 10% in Tanzania [12].

The World Health Organization (WHO) recommends uptake of iron and folic acid supplement during pregnancy for at least six months [13]. Tanzania adopted the WHO recommendation and requires all pregnant women to consume 30-60 mg of a dose of iron and 400 μg of folic acid daily starting early at first antenatal visit [2, 4, 13]. Despite the national guideline emphasis, adherence to iron-folic acid supplements during pregnancy is still low [4].

The proportion of pregnant women who reported to uptake iron and folic acid supplementation in Tanzania for at least 90 days was less than a quarter (21%) with only 7% in Kigoma region [4]. IFAS is considered the best strategy to control anaemia during pregnancy, but low adherence to IFAS compromises the effectiveness of this strategy [4]. Based on these facts, describing adherence to IFAS and associated factors among pregnant women would be the potential for evidence-based interventions.

Moreover, various studies have been conducted in Tanzania about IFAS; however, the majority of these focused on the effects of IFAS in newborn and pregnant women and only limited studies assessed the adherence to IFAS and associated factors among pregnant women. With these inadequate studies, the available data may also be outdated. Currently, studies conducted on IFAS in Kasulu district are limited. Therefore, this study is aimed at assessing adherence to IFAS and associated factors in the Kasulu district in north-western Tanzania.

2. Methods and Materials

2.1. Study Design and Study Area. A health facility-based cross-sectional study using a mixed-method approach was conducted in Kasulu district in Kigoma region, 4°44′0° S and 30°44′0° E Tanzania from March to April 2019 [14]. The district has two administrative areas with a total population of 634,038 people [15]. Kasulu district is predominately occupied by the "Waha" ethnic group. The main activities are subsistence and small-scale farming and medium-scale business, particularly in Kasulu town. The other tribe found in the district is Sukuma, who engaged in pastoralism activities [14]. The average of pregnant women registered in Kasulu district per year was 38,951, and nearly three quarters were from Kasulu rural. A total of 34,365 of women with children aged 0-6 months were also recorded, and over seventy percent were from Kasulu rural.

2.2. Study Population. The study population consisted of health care providers, pregnant women, and mothers with children aged 0-6 months, who attended antenatal clinic (ANC) and postnatal services during the study. Women with children aged 0-6 months, attended ANC visits during their last pregnancy, and supplied with IFAS were included in the quantitative study. The qualitative study involved pregnant women, women with children aged 0-6 months, and health care providers working at the reproductive and child health department. Health care providers and all mothers came from two health facilities in Kasulu district; these were Kasulu Hospital (KH) and Kiganamo Health Center (KHC). All women with children aged 0-6 months who did not attend ANC visit during pregnancy, all women having less than three ANC visits, and all women who were not supplied with IFAS, unable to speak/hear, or with mental disorders were excluded from the study. Detailed information in Figure 1.

2.3. Sample Size and Sampling Procedures. A total of 320 mothers of children aged 0-6 months were included in the study. The sample size was determined based on a single population proportion formula $(Z^2P(1-P)/(e)^2)$ with a 95% CI, 5% margin error $(Z\alpha/2 = 1.96)$ by considering the national adherence to IFAS $(P = 21\%)$ [4] at 80% desired power $(B\alpha)$ and 10% of the estimated nonresponse rate. Nonresponse was considered to maximize the sample size of 320 study respondents.

Mothers of children aged 0-6 months were systematically sampled from a list of clients attending postnatal services in the two facilities. These included Kasulu Hospital and Kiganamo Health Center which are well known to accommodate and provide maternal services to a large number of pregnant women compared to other health facilities in Kasulu town. This study was done between March and April 2019.

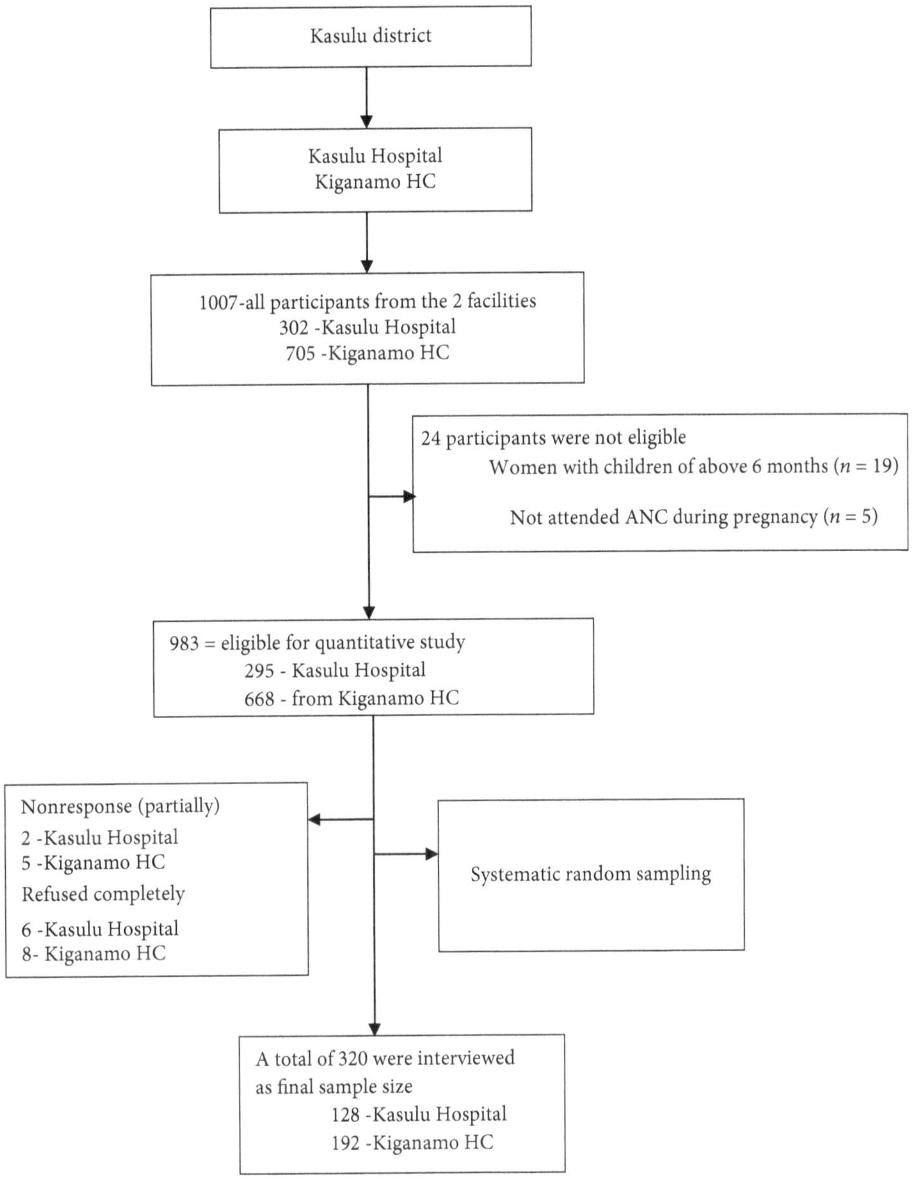

Figure 1: Participants' flow diagram.

In addition, 40 respondents were purposively selected and involved in a qualitative study. These included six health care providers who participated in in-depth interviews (IDIs), 19 pregnant women, and 15 mothers with children aged 0-6 months who participated in focus group discussions (FGDs). A total of four FGDs were conducted of which two comprised of pregnant women and two comprised of mothers of children aged 0-6 months. Each FDG included 7-11 respondents.

2.4. Data Collection Procedures and Quality Control. A structured questionnaire established based on information from Tanzania Demographic Health Survey (TDHS) and published articles was administered to women who had children aged 0-6 months [4, 16–18]. The structured questionnaire captured sociodemographic information, maternal factors, health facility factors, household factors, medication factors, access to health care, perception of the quality of services, knowledge of anaemia, knowledge of IFAS, and adherence to IFAS. All tools were developed in English and translated into Swahili (a local language) for simplicity and understanding and then back-translated to English by language researchers conversant in both languages to facilitate consistency. Data collectors and supervisors were trained on the objectives, how to keep confidential information, and filling of information. Tools were pretested, and all necessary changes were made before the start of actual data collection. An interview guide was used for the focused group discussion and in-depth interviews.

2.5. Operational Definition

2.5.1. Adherence to IFAS. Adherence to IFAS was self-reported and assessed by considering the total numbers of IFAS tablets consumed during their last pregnancy. Pregnant women were recommended to consume one tablet of iron and folic acid tablets containing 30-60 mg of iron and

400 μg of folic acid daily for at least 90 days [2, 4, 13]. Six questions were added together to assess adherence to IFAS. These include information about the number of ANC visits, the number of sachets given in each visit, and the total number of tablets given for the whole period of pregnancy. The number of tablets consumed and remaining before childbirth was also recorded. All women who took tablets for at least 90 days were considered to adhere to the IFAS program and vice versa.

2.5.2. Knowledge of Anaemia. The knowledge of anaemia was assessed by adding up the four multiple-choice items including causes, symptoms, consequences, and prevention methods of anaemia. The correct answer was labeled, and the wrong answer was not labeled. Answers were categorized into two groups; those who scored medium and above were considered to have high knowledge and low knowledge when scored below medium.

2.5.3. Knowledge of Iron-Folic Acid Supplementation. To understand the knowledge of IFAS among respondents, six multiple-choice questions were added together including physical appearance (color), time to start using IFAS, the recommended number of tablets, benefits of IFAS, and negative effects to mothers and children when the adequate tablets were not consumed. The correct answer was labeled, and the wrong answer was not labeled. Answers were classified into two groups and labeled high knowledge if scored medium and above and low knowledge of IFAS if scored below medium.

2.5.4. Perception of the Quality of Services. To measure perception, five multiple-choice questions were added up including the number of tablets provided, general physical checkup, service satisfaction, being given IFAS for free, and customer care. The answer was ordered into two groups and labeled positive perception when scoring medium and above and negative perception when scoring below medium.

2.6. Data Processing and Analysis. Quantitative data were checked, coded, and entered into SPSS software version 22 with a statistical significance decided at P value < 0.05. Descriptive analysis, including frequencies, percentages, and chi-square testing, was employed when determining the association among variables and adequacy of cells. A binary logistic regression model was fitted after multicollinearity diagnosis to establish factors to IFAS adherence. Adjusted odds ratio (AOR) with 95% CI, P value < 0.05 was considered statistically significant.

The recall bias was managed through interviewing the mothers who gave birth within a short time, six months prior to the study (women with children aged 0-6 months). Also, a sachet of iron and folic acid supplementation was demonstrated to mothers during the interview to aid their memories.

All audio records from qualitative interviews were transcribed and translated to English before analysis. The authors transcribed each discussion verbatim and carefully checked each transcript for accuracy by simultaneously listening to the audio recording and reading transcript. Notes taken during the discussions or interviews were incorporated in the final transcripts. Data were coded and analyzed using NVIvo software version 10. Thematic analysis was employed to explore the themes raised during focus group discussions and in-depth interviews. Finally, the themes that stemmed from both FGD and IDI were triangulated with quantitative findings.

2.7. Ethical Consideration. Ethical clearance and approval of the study were obtained from Ifakara Health Institute Review Board on 9th February 2019 (IHI/IRB/No: 9-2019). Introduction letter from the Department of Research and Training of Ifakara Health Institute was also provided to investigators. The study team made a courtesy visit to the district administration prior to data collection. Furthermore, the purpose of the study was explained to all respondents and written informed consent forms were provided and signed before the interview. The verbal consent was also enquired before the group discussion. The informed consent was read to respondents loudly in front of the witness. Respondents who were unable to read and write were asked to sign using a thumb fingerprint before the study. The confidentiality of their information was assured among respondents.

3. Results

3.1. Social and Demographic Characteristics of Women with Children Aged 0-6 Months. The summary of the sociodemographic information of the respondents is provided in Table 1. Of the 320 respondents of the survey, 128 were from Kiganamo Health Center and 192 from Kasulu Hospital. A majority of the respondents were aged 15-24 years 140 (43%). More than half of the respondents (53.75%) completed primary education, and nearly three quarters ($n = 232$, 72.5%) were not employed in formal sectors (Table 1).

3.2. Knowledge about Anaemia. Out of 320 respondents, two hundred twenty-two (69.4%) had high knowledge of anaemia. The findings from qualitative study concerning the causes of anaemia were thought to be sitting under the sun, infectious diseases (malaria, UTI, HIV, and worms), poor diet, and inadequate consumption of vegetables and fruits. The symptoms of anaemia include dizziness, fatigue, feeling sick, and edema. The majority of respondents found that the consequences of anaemia among pregnant women were death attributed to bleeding during childbirth and miscarriage. On the other hand, health care providers had different understanding regarding the meaning of anaemia in pregnant women. Anaemia in pregnant was implied when Hb was below 7.5 mg/l, and others said pregnant women were considered to have anaemia when Hb was below 12 mg/l.

3.3. Knowledge of Iron-Folic Acid Supplementation (IFAS). Awareness of IFAS among women with children aged 0-6 months was demonstrated by attending antenatal clinics. Among all respondents, less than half ($n = 110$, 34.4%) had high knowledge of IFAS and were primarily received during the ANC visit. A total of two hundred fifty-nine (80.9%) women had an understanding that IFAS increases blood level during pregnancy. Similarly, seventeen women (5.3%) had

Table 1: The sociodemographic characteristics of respondents in Kasulu district, north-western Tanzania, March-April 2019 ($N = 320$).

Variables	Categories	Frequency (n)	Percent (%)
Mothers age (years)	15-24 years	140	43.8
	25-34 years	121	37.8
	35-49 years	59	18.4
Mothers education	No formal education	69	21.5
	Completed primary	172	53.8
	Completed secondary +	79	24.7
Mothers occupation	Not employed	232	72.5
	Employed	88	27.5
Marital status	Single	35	10.9
	Married	285	89.1
Family size	1-3	89	27.8
	4-6	136	42.5
	6+	95	29.7

+ = Above.

knowledge of IFAS that it works best to improve the health of the newborn. Qualitative findings revealed that a belief on IFAS to increase blood level influenced the women's adherence to IFAS. It was also reported that deaths and abnormalities like neural tube defects among newborns were reduced when IFAS is consumed properly during pregnancy. On the other hand, pregnant women built trust in the performance of health care providers. In the same manner, both women and health care providers had low awareness about the timing of starting IFAS. Further, the time spent to educate women about the importance of IFAS was not enough (30 minutes) as quoted below:

"We could not provide a detailed explanation to pregnant women; we often tell them, IFAS prevents you from giving birth to a child with a big head, but when asked how it works, it becomes difficult to explain because we have no further information". .....She emphasized, "We need to update our knowledge" (a health care provider at KH).

3.4. Factors Related to Adherence to Iron-Folic Acid Supplementation among Pregnant Women. Over ninety percent of respondents ($n = 296$) were given IFAS from two clinics, and the adherence to IFAS was 20.3% ($n = 65$). The reasons related to poor adherence were delayed initiation of ANC, distance to the health facilities, availability of IFAS, perceived quality of health facility services, being healthy, women's experiences with multiple births, misconception about pregnancy and IFAS, lack of knowledge on the benefits of IFAS, negligence, forgetfulness, and side effects, including nausea, dizziness, and vomiting. See the quote below:

"If not sick, why should we take it". "....we were also told by women in our communities that, whoever takes IFAS, experiences more bleeding during delivery and gave birth to blaze skinny babies" (FGD: women with a child aged 0-6 months at KHC).

3.4.1. Timing of ANC Services. Most of the women, approximately two hundred and seventeen (67.8%), started the first antenatal clinic (ANC) visit during the second or third trimester (Table 2). Delayed ANC attendance was associated with women's perception. Attending to ANC early was attributed with the negative perception that woman was weak, fear of being pregnant, and pregnancy was designated as secret. It was also associated with notion around HIV testing to both partners as part of prevention of mother-to-child transmission (PMTCT) program accompanied by partners to attend ANC as quoted below:

"We want to be sure of what is inside the womb by sensing fetal movement first before going to the clinic for the first visit because if you go early many will laugh at you and say it's like you are making an advertisement that you have pregnant, it is a show up" (FGD: women with children aged 0-6 months at KH).

During the discussion, a prime woman with the age of 28 years emphasized that the PMTCT program and related attributes were associated with delayed ANC visits.

"The first time I came to the clinic, I found a case of pregnant women who came with a motorcycle driver acting to be her husband. After testing for HIV, a driver was infected. During the counseling session, a pregnant woman confirmed that a man was not her husband. Therefore, this strategy puts pressure on women leading them to tell lie and delay to attend ANC services" (FGD: pregnant women at KH).

3.4.2. Distance to the Health Facility. Distance was estimated by using the time spent from residents to the health facility. Over half of the women spent 30 minutes or less to reach the health facility ($n = 172$, 53.8%), and one hundred forty-eight respondents spent 60 minutes and above (46.2%) as presented in Table 2. On the other hand, the cost of transportation is attributed between 1000 and 3000 Tshs per each ANC visit. The challenge of distance to attend ANC during pregnancy was also revealed from qualitative findings as quoted below:

"Please help us to have a clinic close to residential areas, it is difficult for a pregnant woman to walk more than one hour to access ANC services" (FGD: pregnant women at KHC).

Table 2: Characteristics related to supplementation among respondents in Kasulu district, north-western Tanzania, March-April 2019 ($N = 320$).

Variables	Categories	Frequency (n)	Percent (%)
Distance to the health facility (minutes)	0-30 minutes	172	53.8
	60+ minutes	148	46.2
Number of children	1-3 children	221	69.1
	4+ children	99	30.9
Time at first ANC visit	0-3 months	103	32.2
	4-6 months	197	61.6
	7-9 months	20	6.2
Access to IFAS	ANC	296	92.5
	Not ANC	24	7.5
IFAS given each visit	Yes	128	40
	No	192	60
Reminded by a husband to take IFAS	Reminded	28	8.8
	Not reminded	292	91.3
Side effects	Side effects	108	33.8
	No side effects	212	66.2
Knowledge of anaemia	High knowledge	222	69.4
	Low knowledge	98	30.6
Knowledge of IFAs	High knowledge	110	34.4
	Low knowledge	210	65.6
Time spent to educated IFAS	Enough	92	28.8
	Not enough	228	71.2
Perception of health services	Positive	230	71.9
	Negative	90	28.1
Adherence level	Adherence	65	20.3
	No adherence	255	79.7

3.4.3. Support from a Partner. Nine percent ($n = 28$) of women reported being reminded by their husband about taking IFAS during pregnancy (Table 2). A similar finding was reported in the qualitative data as quoted below:

"How do they remind us when they do not understand its benefits..., they even not bother..., they don't care..., they are less concerned" (FGD: pregnant women at KH).

3.4.4. Perception of the Health Services. Nearly three-quarters of the women ($n = 230$, 71.9%) had a positive perception of health services provided at health facilities (Table 2). A majority of the respondents perceived the quality of services provided at both health facilities to be good. Challenges reported were much time spent at the ANC that was attributed to the large number of women presented at each visit and an inadequate amount of tablets provided at each visit that sometimes was not enough to meet the next visit. It was also reported that being instructed to come with partners at ANC during the first visit was another challenge thought by respondents. These were different to health care providers; challenges of the IFAS program and services were attributed with a few staffs and poor working environment as quoted below:

"IFAS does not belong to anybody, because other services like malaria, family planning, and HIV have special people working closely with the ANC and community to ensure the community understands better. No effort has been put in place to advocate on the importance of IFAS in and out of clinics" (a health care provider at KH).

3.4.5. Availability of IFAS. IFAS was provided at ANC for free; however, forty percent ($n = 128$) of the respondents attended ANC visits only were given IFAS on each visit. Women who were provided 90 IFAS tablets or more was low compared to the women who were given IFAS during their ANC visit ($n = 296$, 92.5%) with frequently IFAS stock out in health facilities.

3.5. Factors Associated with Adherence to Iron-Folic Acid Supplementation (IFAS) among Pregnant Women Attended ANC Services. In this study, IFAS given in each visit, knowledge of IFAS, knowledge of anaemia, gestation period at first ANC visit, the number of meals, and number of children

TABLE 3: Factors associated with adherence of IFAS among respondents in Kasulu district, north-western Tanzania, March-April 2019 ($N = 320$).

Variables	Adherence level		COR (CI at 95%)	AOR (CI at 95%)
	Adhered *N* (%)	Not adhered *N* (%)		
Distance to the health facility (minutes)				
60+ minutes	27 (16.77)	134 (83.23)	1.271 (0.732, 2.205)	0.338 (0.131, 0.886)*
0-30 minutes	38 (23.90)	121 (76.1)		1
Number of ANC visits				
4+	49 (24.62)	150 (75.38)	0.466 (0.256, 0.865)	0.6106 (0.220, 1.692)
Less than 4	16 (13.22)	105 (86.78)		1
Knowledge of IFAS				
High knowledge	35 (31.82)	75 (68.18)	2.80 (1.604, 4.890)	3.864 (1.422, 10.500)*
Low knowledge	30 (14.29)	180 (85.71)		1
Knowledge of Anaemia				
High knowledge	56 (38.62)	89 (61.38)	3.336 (1.577, 7.059)	3.840 (1.335, 10.685)*
Low knowledge	09 (5.14)	166 (94.86)		1
IFAS given each visit				
Given each visits	52 (40.62)	76 (59.38)	9.421 (4.848, 18.307)	15.718 (5.335, 46.311)*
Not given each visits	13 (6.77)	179 (93.23)		1
Number of meals				
Twice and below	49 (28.32)	124 (71.68)	3.385 (1.721, 5.894)	3.439 (1.284, 9.212)*
Three times or more	16 (10.88)	131 (89.12)		1
Time at first visit				
1st trimester	33 (32.04)	70 (67.96)	2.725 (1.559, 4.765)	3.724 (1.417, 9.791)*
2nd+ trimester	32 (14.75)	185 (85.25)		1
Side effect				
Side effects	12 (11.11)	96 (88.89)	0.375 (0.191, 0.757)	0.132 (0.043, 0.406)
No side effects	53 (25)	159 (75)		1
Reminded by husband				
Yes	55 (18.84)	237 (81.16)	2.394 (1.047, 5.473)	1.157 (0.454, 2.946)
No	10 (35.71)	18 (64.29)		1
Number of children				
Less than 4 children	57 (25.79)	164 (74.21)	3.185 (1.807, 8.651)	3.462 (1.035,11.582)*
4+ children	8 (8.08)	91 (91.92)		1

AOR = adjusted odds ratio; CI = confidence interval; COR = crude odds ratio; *statistically significant; 1 = reference. Note Hosmer and Lemeshow Test = 0.925; therefore, the model is fitted to predict the factors associated with adherence.

were the factors associated with adherence of IFAS among pregnant women. The details on the associated factors of IFAS are shown in Table 3.

4. Discussion

In this study, the adherence to IFAS was low among pregnant women and factors associated with adherence to IFAS were included: the knowledge of anaemia, knowledge of IFAS, time a woman attended at ANC visit, number of IFAS tablets provided, number of meals, number of children, and distance to the health facility. Details are found in Table 2.

The result of adherence to IFAS in this study was consistent with national adherence (21%) [4]. Similarly, studies conducted in Kiambu, Kenya (32.7%), and Amhara, Western Ethiopia (20.4%), also found the low adherence to IFAS among pregnant women [19, 20]. Also, adherence to IFAS was modestly higher compared to the studies conducted in Eastern Kenya (18.3%), Uganda (12%), Norway (16%), and Northern Tanzania (16.1%) [21–24] and lower compared to studies conducted in Senegal (51%), Kathmandu-Nepal (73.2%), Tamil Nadu-India (60.6%), and Mizan-Aman-Ethiopia (70.6%) [25–28]. Some of the probable reasons of inconsistency might be a different study subject, sociodemographic characteristics, locality, follow-up and reminding mechanism, knowledge of IFAS, and qualities of health services offered in the health facilities including counseling on its benefits, the average number of IFAS recommended during pregnancy, and belief on the use of IFAS.

The findings of this study indicated that women who had high knowledge of IFAS were 3.9 times more likely to adhere to the IFAS program compared to the women who had low knowledge. The study was reliable with the studies conducted in Northern Wollo, Ethiopia, and Misha district, Ethiopia [29, 30]. The time spent to counsel pregnant mothers about the benefits of IFAS, consequences of not using IFAS, proper prescription, and awareness of side effect management were the reasons for adherence to the IFAS program.

Women with high knowledge of anaemia were 3.8 times more likely to adhere to the program compared to women with low knowledge of anaemia. This was consistent with studies conducted in Aykel, Ethiopia, and Nepal [26, 31]. The probable reasons for adherence might be the proper counseling about the prevention measures, consequences of anaemia at ANC, and availability of media used to create awareness in communities.

Similarly, women provided with IFAS tablets in each visit were 15.7 times more likely to adhere to the program compared to women who were not provided with IFAS each visit. These findings corroborated with studies conducted in Mizan-Aman, Ethiopia, and Pakistan [28, 32]. Studies conducted in Uganda, Pakistan, and South Africa found that less supply of IFAS had low adherence to IFAS [24, 32, 33]. Other studies conducted in Ismailia government and Assela town-Ethiopia reported that crowding of tablets was associated with the low adherence to supplementation [34, 35]. The reasons might be associated with the availability of tablets at ANC, the number of ANC visits, knowledge of health care providers about time to start IFAS, and awareness of the average number of IFAS required for adherence.

Other studies have indicated that women with high wealth quintile and eating three and above meals per day were likely to adhere to IFAS compare to women from low wealth quintile [36, 37]. However, in the present study, women from the families eating twice or less were found to be 3.4 times more likely to adhere to IFAS as compared to women from the families who ate three times and more. This was contrary to a study conducted in India, which showed that women from households with high wealth quintile were less likely to adhere to IFAS due to good health and able to access them when needed [27]. The reasons might be education level, occupation of women and their partners or household income, location, and verse versa.

The time to start ANC visits was associated with adherence to the IFAS program. The present study revealed that women who attended ANC visit in the first trimester were likely to adhere to the IFAS program 3.7 times more compared to those who started ANC visit in the second trimester and third trimester. This was consistent with studies conducted in North Wollo Zone-Ethiopia, Ibadan-Nigeria, Bangladesh, and Tamil Nadu-India, which reported that early registration in the first and second trimester has a positive effect to adherence to IFAS program than in the third trimester [16, 27, 29, 38]. The possible reasons for adherence might be the knowledge on the time to start ANC, beliefs, perception, distance to the health facility, and delayed ANC visit attributed to HIV testing to both women and their partners. This might affect directly the duration and number of tablets consumed to adhere to the IFAS program.

In this study, women with 1-3 children were 3.5 times more likely to adhere to the program compared to women with 4 and above children. This was consistent with studies conducted in India and Tanzania, which showed that women with two children and below were likely to adhere to the program compared to women with more children [21, 39]. According to a study conducted in Assela town, Ethiopia, it was reported that having fewer children had less likely to adhere compared with women with more children [35]. The probable reasons for adherence to IFAS could be the maternal-related experience. Studies conducted in Debre Tabor-Ethiopia and Ismailia government reported that gravidity had an association with adherence to IFAS [17, 34].

The distance from residential to the health facilities was associated with adherence to the IFAS program. Women living 60 minutes or more from the health facilities were less likely to adhere to the IFAS program 0.34 times compared to the women living near the health facilities. In other studies, women who were living close to health facilities or private pharmacies had more chance to adhere to the IFAS program more times compared to women who were living far from health facilities [25, 36, 40]. The reasons might be the lack of close health facilities and less economic index; less availability of pharmacies used to sell IFAS and negligence among mothers were the reasons for low adherence to the IFAS program.

The other reasons for low adherence to IFAS were revealed from the qualitative analysis including women's experiences, lack of knowledge about the benefits of IFAS, negligence, forgetfulness, and the side effects including nausea, dizziness, and vomiting. The other reason was misinformation about pregnancy and misperception around the IFAS, including giving birth to a child with burned skin. It was also reported that the majority did not consume IFAS if they were feeling healthy and become less motivated. This study corroborates with the study conducted in Ethiopia [41, 42]; however, the other studies reported that fear of being sick or being sick was associated with adherence to the IFAS program [21, 26, 28, 43]. On the other hand, misinformation included fear to give birth to big baby, spot-on teeth of children and face of mothers, difficult delivery, not beneficial to babies, mothers experience with no history of having children with neural tube defects, and more bleeding during delivery was associated with low adherence to IFAS [10, 20, 33, 35, 44]. Regarding forgetfulness, the study was consistent with various studies conducted in various regions including Kenya, Vietnam, Pakistan, Ethiopia, and Iran [23, 32, 43, 45, 46].

4.1. Limitation of Study. The study had its limitations and needs to be considered during the interpretation of the results. First, adherence to IFAS was determined by self-report which might affect the actual adherence due to the possibility of over- or underreporting of ingested tablets. Second, pill counts and measuring of haemoglobin concentration and biomarkers may predict better the adherence to IFAS; however, it was not done in this study.

5. Conclusion

Adherence to iron and folic acid among pregnant women was low. Factors associated with adherence to IFAS included time to start ANC, knowledge of anaemia among women, counseling on the importance of the iron-folic acid, number of IFAS provided each visit, and number of children. However, the side effects and distance to the health facility had less effect on adherence to IFAS. Therefore, the prevention of iron-folic acid deficiency through strengthening the system to create community awareness; health promotion and counseling; education programs among health care providers, males, and pregnant women; and reminding mechanisms is paramount to improve adherence to IFAS.

Abbreviations

ANC: Antenatal care
DHS: Demographic and Health Survey
DST: Daylight saving time
FGD: Focused group discussion
GMT: Greenwich Mean Time
HIV: Human infection virus
HSSP: Health Sector Strategic Plan
IDI: In-depth interview
IERB: Institutional Ethical Review Board
IFAS: Iron and folic acid supplementation
KH: Kasulu Hospital
KHC: Kiganamo Health Center
MSD: Medical Store Department
NBS: National Bureau of Statistics
PMTCT: Prevention of mother-to-child transmission of HIV
OR: Odds ratio
TDHS: Tanzania Demographic and Health Survey
URT: United Republic of Tanzania
UTI: Urinary tract infection
VIF: Variable interaction factor
WFP: World Food Program
WHO: World Health Organization.

Disclosure

A university and funder were not involved in manuscript writing, editing, approval, or decision to where the article would be published.

Authors' Contributions

Winfrida Benedicto Lyoba designed and conducted the research and drafted the manuscript. Winfrida Benedicto Lyoba in collaboration with Joyce Donald Mwakatoga has contributed to the analysis and interpretation of data. Ester Elisaria has contributed to the study design and critically reviewed the manuscript and edited the paper. Charles Festo and Jackline Mrema were actively involved in the review of the manuscript, and all authors agreed to be accountable for all aspects of the work in ensuring that the accuracy or integrity of any part of the manuscript was correctly examined and determined.

Acknowledgments

Our special thanks goes to the African Development Bank for financial support; The Nelson Mandela Institution of Science and Technology; Ifakara Health Institute; Kasulu District Executive Directors; Health Facility Administration; Dr. Manuel Battegay and Dr. Martin Rohacek for the advice on designing, drafting of the paper, and reviewing; all women and health care providers who participated in this research.

References

[1] G. A. Stevens, M. M. Finucane, L. M. de-Regil et al., "Global, regional, and national trends in haemoglobin concentration and prevalence of total and severe anaemia in children and pregnant and non- pregnant women for 1995–2011: a systematic analysis of population- representative data," *The Lancet Global Health*, vol. 1, no. 1, pp. e16–e25, 2013.

[2] WHO, *The global prevalence of anaemia in 2011*, World Health Organization Geneva, 2015.

[3] M. Naithani, V. Saxena, A. A. Mirza, R. Kumari, K. Sharma, and J. Bharadwaj, "Assessment of folic acid supplementation in pregnant women by estimation of serum levels of tetrahydrofolic acid, dihydrofolate reductase, and homocysteine," *Scientifica (Cairo)*, vol. 2016, article 1520685, 5 pages, 2016.

[4] TDHS, *Tanzania*2015-16 Demogr. Heal. Surv. Malar. Indic. Surv.

[5] M. Y. Yakoob, Y. P. Khan, and Z. A. Bhutta, "Maternal mineral and vitamin supplementation in pregnancy," *Expert Review of Obstetrics & Gynecology*, vol. 5, no. 2, pp. 241–256, 2010.

[6] A. J. Copp and N. D. E. Greene, "Genetics and development of neural tube defects," *The Journal of Pathology*, vol. 220, no. 2, pp. n/a–230, 2009.

[7] V. Sengpiel, J. Bacelis, R. Myhre et al., "Folic acid supplementation, dietary folate intake during pregnancy and risk for spontaneous preterm delivery: a prospective observational cohort study," *BMC Pregnancy Childbirth*, vol. 14, no. 1, p. 375, 2014.

[8] D. N. Tosh, Q. Fu, C. W. Callaway et al., "Epigenetics of programmed obesity: alteration in IUGR rat hepatic IGF1 mRNA expression and histone structure in rapid vs. delayed postnatal catch-up growth," *American Journal of Physiology-Gastrointestinal and Liver Physiology*, vol. 299, no. 5, pp. G1023–G1029, 2010.

[9] T. Alemu and M. Umeta, "Reproductive and Obstetric Factors Are Key Predictors of Maternal Anemia during Pregnancy in Ethiopia: Evidence from Demographic and Health Survey (2011)," *Anemia*, vol. 2015, Article ID 649815, 8 pages, 2015.

[10] R. Galloway and J. McGuire, "Determinants of compliance with iron supplementation: supplies, side effects, or psychology?," *Social Science & Medicine*, vol. 39, no. 3, pp. 381–390, 1994.

[11] L. Say, D. Chou, A. Gemmill et al., "Global causes of maternal death: a WHO systematic analysis," *The Lancet Global Health*, vol. 2, no. 6, pp. e323–e333, 2014.

[12] B. C. Hanson, G. Mbaruku, and F. Manzi, "High risk of maternal death in southern Tanzania," *Ifakara Health Institute*, no. 18, pp. 1–4, 2014.

[13] WHO, "Guideline : Daily Iron and Folic Acid Supplementation in Pregnant Women," *World Heal. Organ*, vol. 46, pp. 323–329, 2012.

[14] Kasulu District Report, *Information of demographics, economy and wards*, 2012, https://en.wikipedia.org/wiki/Kasulu_District.

[15] The National Bureau of Statistics, "2012 population and housing census. Population distribution by administrative areas," *Dar-es-Salaam: National Bureau of Statistics*, 2013.

[16] P. H. Nguyen, H. Nguyen, I. Gonzalez-Casanova et al., "Factors influencing maternal nutrition practices in a large scale maternal, newborn and child health program in Bangladesh," *PLoS One*, vol. 12, no. 7, pp. 1–17, 2017.

[17] A. D. Gebremariam, S. A. Tiruneh, B. A. Abate, M. T. Engidaw, and D. T. Asnakew, "Adherence to iron with folic acid supplementation and its associated factors among pregnant women attending antenatal care follow up at Debre Tabor General Hospital, Ethiopia, 2017," *PLoS One*, vol. 14, no. 1, p. e0210086, 2019.

[18] J. Kimiywe, B. Ahoya, J. Kavle, and A. Nyaku, "Barriers to maternal iron-folic acid supplementation and compliance in Kisumu and Migori, Kenya," USAID Maternal and Child Survival Program, Nairobi, Kenya, 2017.

[19] M. W. Kamau, W. Mirie, and S. Kimani, "Compliance with Iron and folic acid supplementation (IFAS) and associated factors among pregnant women: results from a cross-sectional study in Kiambu County, Kenya," *BMC Public Health*, vol. 18, no. 1, p. 580, 2018.

[20] B. Taye, G. Abeje, and A. Mekonen, "Factors associated with compliance of prenatal iron folate supplementation among women in Mecha district, western Amhara: a cross-sectional study," *Pan Afr. Med. J.*, vol. 20, no. 1, 2015.

[21] O. Ogundipe, C. Hoyo, T. Østbye et al., "Factors associated with prenatal folic acid and iron supplementation among 21,889 pregnant women in northern Tanzania: a cross-sectional hospital-based study," *BMC Public Health*, vol. 12, no. 1, p. 481, 2012.

[22] J. H. S. Mortensen, N. Øyen, R. M. Nilsen, T. Fomina, S. Tretli, and T. Bjørge, "Paternal characteristics associated with maternal periconceptional use of folic acid supplementation," *BMC Pregnancy and Childbirth*, vol. 18, no. 1, pp. 188–188, 2018.

[23] M. Juma, S. O. Oiye, and S. O. Konyole, "Predictors of optimum antenatal iron-folate supplementation in a low resource rural set-up in eastern Kenya," *Journal of Public Health and Epidemiology*, vol. 7, no. 11, pp. 337–345, 2015.

[24] T. S. Kiwanuka, S. Ononge, P. Kiondo, and F. Namusoke, "Adherence to iron supplements among women receiving antenatal care at Mulago National Referral Hospital, Uganda-cross-sectional study," *BMC Research Notes*, vol. 10, no. 1, pp. 510–516, 2017.

[25] K. Niang, A. Faye, J. A. Diégane Tine et al., "Determinants of iron consumption among pregnant women in southern Senegal," *Open Journal of Obstetrics and Gynecology*, vol. 7, no. 1, pp. 41–50, 2017.

[26] R. Ss, T. Ratanasiri, T. Arkaravichien, P. Thapa, and R. Koju, "Compliance and its determinants regarding iron and folic acid supplementation during pregnancy in Kathmandu, Nepal," *Kathmandu University Medical Journal*, vol. 14, no. 56, pp. 311–317, 2016.

[27] K. Selvaraj, P. Arumugasamy, and S. Sarkar, "Compliance and patterns of iron-folic acid intake among adolescent girls and antenatal women in rural Tamil Nadu," *CHRISMED Journal of Health and Research*, vol. 4, no. 2, pp. 87–93, 2017.

[28] S. Shewasinad and S. Negash, "Adherence and associated factors of prenatal iron folic acid supplementation among pregnant women who attend ante natal care in health facility at Mizan-Aman Town, Bench Maji Zone, Ethiopia, 2015," *Journal of Pregnancy and Child Health*, vol. 4, no. 3, 2017.

[29] A. Demis, B. Geda, T. Alemayehu, and H. Abebe, "Iron and folic acid supplementation adherence among pregnant women attending antenatal care in North Wollo Zone northern Ethiopia: institution based cross-sectional study," *BMC Res. Notes*, vol. 12, no. 1, p. 107, 2019.

[30] A. A. Sadore, L. A. Gebretsadik, and M. A. Hussen, "Compliance with Iron-Folate Supplement and Associated Factors among Antenatal Care Attendant Mothers in Misha District, South Ethiopia: Community Based Cross-Sectional Study," *Journal of Environmental and Public Health*, vol. 2015, Article ID 781973, 7 pages, 2015.

[31] H. Assefa, S. M. Abebe, and M. Sisay, "Magnitude and factors associated with adherence to iron and folic acid supplementation among pregnant women in Aykel town, northwest Ethiopia," *BMC Pregnancy and Childbirth*, vol. 19, no. 1, pp. 296–298, 2019.

[32] Y. B. Nisar, A. Alam, B. Aurangzeb, and M. J. Dibley, "Perceptions of antenatal iron-folic acid supplements in urban and rural Pakistan : a qualitative study," *BMC Pregnancy and Childbirth*, vol. 14, no. 1, pp. 1–12, 2014.

[33] X. Mbhenyane and M. Cherane, "Compliance with the consumption of iron and folate supplements by pregnant women in Mafikeng local municipality, north west province, South Africa," *African Health Sciences*, vol. 17, no. 3, pp. 657–670, 2017.

[34] Z. M. Ibrahim, S. A. B. D. El-hamid, H. Mikhail, and M. S. Khattab, "Assessment of adherence to iron and folic acid supplementation and prevalence of anemia in pregnant women," *The Medical Journal of Cairo University*, vol. 79, no. 2, 2011.

[35] W. Niguse and R. Murugan, "Determinants of adherence to iron-folic acid supplementation among pregnant women attending antenatal clinic in Asella town, Ethiopia," *International Journal of Therapeutic Applications*, vol. 35, pp. 60–67, 2018.

[36] N. G. Onyeneho, N. I'Aronu, N. Chukwu, U. P. Agbawodikeizu, M. Chalupowski, and S. V. Subramanian, "Factors associated with compliance to recommended micronutrients uptake for prevention of anemia during pregnancy in urban, peri-urban, and rural communities in southeast Nigeria," *Journal of Health, Population and Nutrition*, vol. 35, no. 1, p. 35, 2016.

[37] R. Ejaz, A. Khan, and M. A. Raza, "Maternal health care : the case of iron supplementation in India," *Pakistan Journal of Commerce and Social Sciences*, vol. 7, no. 2, pp. 263–275, 2013.

[38] T. A. Lawal and A. O. Adeleye, "Determinants of folic acid intake during preconception and in early pregnancy by mothers in Ibadan, Nigeria," *Pan African Medical Journal*, vol. 19, 2014.

[39] A. Chourasia, C. M. Pandey, and A. Awasthi, "Factors influencing the consumption of iron and folic acid supplementations in high focus states of India," *Clinical Epidemiology and Global Health*, vol. 5, no. 4, pp. 180–184, 2017.

[40] S. L. Young, S. S. Khalfan, T. H. Farag et al., "Association of pica with anemia and gastrointestinal distress among pregnant women in Zanzibar, Tanzania," *The American Journal of Tropical Medicine and Hygiene*, vol. 83, no. 1, pp. 144–151, 2010.

[41] A. Gebre, "Assessment of factors associated with adherence to iron-folic acid supplementation among urban and rural pregnant women in north western zone of Tigray, Ethiopia: comparative study," *International Journal of Nutrition and Food Sciences*, vol. 4, no. 2, p. 161, 2015.

[42] B. Gebreamlak, A. F. Dadi, and A. Atnafu, "High adherence to iron/folic acid supplementation during pregnancy time among antenatal and postnatal care attendant mothers in governmental health centers in Akaki Kality Sub City, Addis Ababa, Ethiopia: hierarchical negative binomial poisson regression," *PLOS ONE*, vol. 12, no. 1, p. e0169415, 2017.

[43] N. Boti, T. Bekele, W. Godana et al., "Adherence to iron-folate supplementation and associated factors among pastoralist's pregnant women in Burji Districts, Segen Area People's Zone, southern Ethiopia: community-based cross-sectional study," *International Journal of Reproductive Medicine*, vol. 2018, Article ID 2365362, 8 pages, 2018.

[44] D. Rofail, A. Colligs, L. Abetz, M. Lindemann, and L. Maguire, "Factors contributing to the success of folic acid public health campaigns," *Journal of Public Health*, vol. 34, no. 1, pp. 90–99, 2012.

[45] M. Nechitilo, P. Nguyen, A. Webb-Girard et al., "A qualitative study of factors influencing initiation and adherence to micronutrient supplementation among women of reproductive age in Vietnam," *Food and Nutrition Bulletin*, vol. 37, no. 4, pp. 461–474, 2016.

[46] S. Siabani, S. Siabani, H. Siabani, M. Moeini Arya, F. Rezaei, and M. Babakhani, "Determinants of compliance with iron and folate supplementation among pregnant women in west Iran: a population-based cross-sectional study," *Journal of Family & Reproductive Health*, vol. 12, no. 4, pp. 197–203, 2018.

13

Mother's Satisfaction towards Childbirth Care at Public Health Centers in Bench-Maji Zone, Ethiopia: A Facility-Based Cross-Sectional Study

Shewangizaw Hailemariam,[1] **Amare Genetu**,[1] **and Ermiyas Sahile**[2]

[1]*Department of Midwifery, College of Health Science, Mizan-Tepi University, Mizan-Teferi, Ethiopia*
[2]*Department of Midwifery, College of Health Science, Kotebe Metropolitan University, Addis Ababa, Ethiopia*

Correspondence should be addressed to Shewangizaw Hailemariam; shewa1278@gmail.com

Academic Editor: Hind A. Beydoun

Background. Assessing the level of maternal satisfaction towards maternal health care services has a paramount importance in improving the service quality and enhancing service utilization. Hence, the aim of this study was to assess maternal satisfaction towards childbirth care and its determinants at public health facilities in Bench-Maji Zone, Ethiopia. *Methods.* A facility-based cross-sectional study was conducted from May 20, 2018, to July 11, 2018 in Bench-Maji Zone, Ethiopia. A total of 845 mothers were selected by employing a systematic random sampling technique. Data were collected using a pretested and structured questionnaire. Satisfaction was measured by the five-point Likert scale from very dissatisfied (1) to very satisfied (5). Data were entered in to Epi data version 3.1 and analyzed using SPSS version 20. A P value < 0.05 was considered to declare statistical significance. *Result.* About 506 (63.25%) of the mothers were satisfied by the overall care provided during childbirth. Factors associated with mothers' satisfaction with childbirth care includes attending no formal education [AOR = 3.69; 95% CI (1.99, 7.91)], rural residency [AOR = 2.63; 95% CI (1.43, 5.80)], perceived measure taken to assure privacy [AOR = 3.56; 95% CI (1.25, 7.41)], and attending antenatal care [AOR = 6.23; 95% CI (3.42, 12.87)]. *Conclusion.* The overall satisfaction of mothers with childbirth care in public health centers of Bench-Maji Zone is low when compared with other studies. Hence, understanding mothers' expectations, assuring privacy, and enhancing antenatal care attendance might improve maternal satisfaction with childbirth care.

1. Background

Mothers' satisfaction with childbirth care is a multidimensional construct comprising satisfaction with technical aspects, environmental aspects, and communication and interpersonal aspects [1]. The assessment of mothers' satisfaction adds an important "consumer" perspective to evaluations. Feedback from mothers can influence the whole quality improvement agenda within the institution or organization [2]. Mothers who perceive the quality of care as good, are more likely to visit it again, thereby increasing demand for the service [3, 4]. Maternal health service utilization and neonatal outcome can be considerably enhanced by improving the quality of facility childbirth care.

Globally, low-middle-income countries continue to account for almost all of the pregnancy-related mortalities that are largely preventable through adequate utilization of essential maternal health care services such as skilled birth assistance (SBA) and antenatal care (ANC) [5]. Studies suggest that utilization of SBA and ANC is highly influenced by mothers' satisfaction [6]. Hence, the World Health Organization (WHO) recommend mothers' service satisfaction be assessed to improve the quality and effectiveness of health care [7].

It is a well-established fact that maternal satisfaction on the provided service could enhance subsequent utilization and compliance with medical treatments [8–10]. However, there is a limited study regarding the extent of mothers' satisfaction with delivery service in Ethiopia. Hence, this study will provide evidence regarding mothers' satisfaction with childbirth care and its determinants.

2. Methods

2.1. Study Area and Design. Facility-based cross-sectional study was conducted from May 20 to July 11, 2018, in Bench-Maji Zone which is located 561 km away from Addis Ababa, the capital city of Ethiopia, in Southwest direction with an estimated population of 829,493 out of which 418,213 are women; 129,500 are children under five; and 26,462 are under 1 year. The zone has 39 functional public health centers. Additionally, there are 182 functional health posts and 9 under construction, one university, and one health science college. The zone has 182 midwives, 329 nurses, and 476 health extension workers [11].

2.2. Source and Study Population. Source population were all mothers who gave birth in public health centers of Bench-Maji Zone, and the study population were all mothers who gave birth in selected public health centers of Bench-Maji Zone from May 20, 2018, to July 11, 2018.

2.3. Sample Size and Sampling Procedure. During the calculation of the sample size, the proportion of mothers satisfied with delivery service in Bench–Maji Zone was assumed to be 50%. Based on the assumption that the actual sample size for the study was determined using a single-population proportion formula with a marginal error of 5% and 95% confidence level, the sample size became 384. Considering design effect, the sample size was multiplied by 2 and a 10% nonresponse rate was added and the final sample size became 845.

A two-stage sampling technique was employed to select study participants. At the first stage, twelve public health centers (30% of the public health centers) were selected from a total of 40 public health centers found in Bench-Maji Zone. Second, the total sample size was proportionally allocated to each of the selected public health centers based on the average number of delivery in the most recent quarterly report of each health centers. Finally, after calculating "*K*" for each public health centers, the study participants were selected by using a systematic random sampling technique.

2.4. Data Collection Tool and Procedure. Exit interview was made by using a structured tool having four sections: the first section contains sociodemographic characteristics of the mother, the second section contains obstetric characteristics of the mother, the third was about mother's perception of health care service, and the forth section contains satisfaction-related questions. Client satisfaction measuring instrument was adapted from Ethiopian Ministry of Health and contextualized to labor and delivery setting. The satisfaction items were grouped into three categories: technical aspects, environmental aspects, and communication and interpersonal aspects. Each components of satisfaction were measured by 6 items. Overall mothers' satisfaction was measured by 18 items each having a five-point Likert scale from very dissatisfied (1) to very satisfied (5). The overall satisfaction scale had an internal consistency or reliability score of 0.83. Data were collected by twelve midwives after having 3 days of training about the data collection process and the purpose of the study. During data collection, the data was checked for completeness and consistency of information. The overall data collection process was supervised by three public health officers. The local language Amharic was used to collect the data.

2.5. Operational Definition. Client overall satisfaction and component-wise client satisfaction were dichotomized into satisfied and dissatisfied depending on the threshold which was computed using the demarcation threshold formula: ((total highest score − total lowest score)/2) + total lowest score [10].

2.6. Data Processing and Analysis. Data were checked for completeness, edited, cleaned, coded, and entered in to EpiData version 3.1 and then was exported to SPSS version 20 for analysis. In the descriptive statistics, frequencies, proportion, and mean was calculated and the results of the analysis were presented in text and tables. Binary logistic regression was carried out to assess the association of different independent variables with the dependent variable. Independent variables having $P < 0.25$ on the binary logistic regression analysis were considered candidates for the final multivariate logistic regression analysis. Multivariate logistic regression analysis was carried out to identify factors having statistically significant associations with mothers' overall satisfaction with childbirth care.

2.7. Data Quality Assurance. The questionnaire prepared in English was translated into Amharic and then back translated into English to ensure consistency. The questionnaire was pretested on 5% of the actual sample size in Maji district. There was supervision on a daily basis and checking on 10% of the collected questionnaire. Finally, error reports were checked after entry to EpiData using each case code.

2.8. Ethical Consideration. Ethical clearance was obtained from Mizan-Tepi University. Permission was also obtained from Bench-Maji zone Health department and health centers as well. Efforts were made to keep confidentiality of the data; all participants were reassured that no personal identifier will be used. Verbal informed consent was sought from all study participants.

3. Result

3.1. Sociodemographic Characteristics of the Respondents'. A total of 94.7%, $n = 800$, mothers willingly responded to the interviewer-administered structured questionnaire. The mean age of the respondents' was 24.7 (±3.26) years. The minimum and the maximum age of the respondents' were 18 and 39, respectively. Of the total respondents, 404 (50.5%) had no formal education and 344 (43%) were housewives. The majority 729 (91.1%) of respondents were married, over 330 (41.25%) of respondents were Protestant Christians, and 305 (38%) of the respondents were Orthodox Christians. Twenty-six percent of the respondents reside in urban areas (Table 1).

3.2. Obstetrics and Other Maternal Factors. Regarding obstetrics characteristics, 723 (90.4%) had antenatal care follow-up,

Table 1: The sociodemographic characteristics of mothers who gave birth in selected public health centers of Bench-Maji Zone, Ethiopia. May 2018. $n = 800$.

Variable	Response	Frequency	Percentage	P value
Age	<20	50	6.25	
	20-24	269	33.62	0.345
	25-29	328	41.0	0.269
	30-34	104	13	0.540
	>35	49	6.12	0.641
Residence	Urban	212	26.5	
	Rural	588	73.5	0.001
Marital status	Single	71	8.9	
	Married	729	91.1	0.461
Ethnicity	Bench	307	38.37	
	Keffa	202	25.25	0.913
	Amhara	239	29.9	0.822
	Oromo	40	5	0.322
	Tigra	7	0.87	0.252
	Gurage	5	0.62	0.716
Educational status	No formal education	404	50.5	0.001
	Primary school	267	33.37	0.004
	Secondary school	99	12.37	0.002
	Diploma and above	30	3.75	
Religion	Orthodox	305	38	
	Muslim	158	19.75	0.632
	Protestant	330	41.25	0.461
	Catholic	5	0.62	0.357
	Traditional beliefs	2	0.25	—
Occupational status	Government worker	27	3.4	
	Non-government worker	190	23.8	0.376
	Merchant	60	7.5	0.420
	Housewife	344	43	0.652
	Daily laborer	123	15.4	0.516
	Student	56	7	0.441

324 (40.5%) were parity I, 44 (5.5%) claimed to had abortion, and 73 (9.1%) were unwanted pregnancy, and 320 (40%) mothers had previous facility-based childbirth experience. Five hundred sixty-seven (70.9%) of the mothers were prepared for labor and delivery, 704 (88%) of the deliveries were attended by female service provider, 136 (17%) of the deliveries end up in immediate maternal complication, and 35 (4.4%) of the deliveries became still birth as shown in (Table 2).

3.3. Maternal Perception of Health Care Service. With respects to maternal perception of facility service availability, 734 (91.8%) of the mothers mentioned the presence of waiting area, and 678 (84.8%) mentioned the presence of toilet in the facility. Five hundred thrifty-four (66.8%) of the mothers claimed the presence of an attendant throughout delivery, 312 (39%) of the mothers claimed that they have waited more than 15 minute to be seen by the care provider, 659 (82.4%) of the mothers were informed about the wellbeing of their baby following examination, and care providers measure taken to assure privacy were regarded as "good" by 659 (82.4%) of the mothers, summarized in (Table 3).

3.4. Maternal Satisfaction with Delivery Care Services. Regarding the three dimensions of satisfaction (component wise satisfaction), technical aspects had the highest median scores followed by communication and interpersonal aspects and environmental aspects. Pertaining to the overall mothers' satisfaction, 506 (63.25%) of the mothers were satisfied with the overall service provided. Mothers were asked whether they would come again and recommend others to utilize facility-based childbirth care service; more than 88% of the mothers mention that they would come again and 95% of mothers claimed to recommend others to deliver at the public health centers (Table 4).

3.5. Factors Associated with Maternal Satisfaction with Delivery Care. After adjusting for "fetal outcome," "sex of the attendants," "presence of maternal complication," "being prepared for labor and delivery," "client informed about the wellbeing of the baby," and "status of the pregnancy," four variables, namely, educational status, residence, measure taken to assure privacy, and attending ANC were found to be significant in the final multivariate logistic regression analysis as shown in (Table 5). Mothers with no formal education and mothers with secondary school were 3.6 and 1.6 times, respectively, more likely to be satisfied by the overall delivery service provided than mothers with educational status diploma and above (AOR = 3.69; 95% CI (1.99, 7.91) and AOR = 1.60; 95% CI (1.34-2.96), respectively). Mothers from rural residence were AOR = 2.63 (95% CI (1.43, 5.80)) times more likely to be satisfied by the overall delivery service provided than those from urban residence. Mothers who regarded measure taken to assure privacy as "good" were AOR = 3.56 (95% CI (1.25, 7.41)) times more likely to be satisfied by the overall delivery service provided than their counterpart. Mothers who fully attended all the WHO-recommended ANC visits were AOR = 6.23 (95% CI (3.42, 12.87)) more likely to be satisfied by the overall delivery service provided than those who did not.

4. Discussion

The present study assessed the level of mothers' satisfaction with delivery service and the associated factors; the study revealed that 63.25%, 95% CI (60.08%-66.41%), of mothers were satisfied with the overall delivery services provided, and this finding is much lower than studies undertaken in Assela Hospital (80.7%), Wolaita zone (82.9%), Debre Markos town (81.7%), and Omo Nada District, Jimma Zone (77%) [12–15]. Nevertheless, it is higher than studies conducted in Gondar teaching hospital; Northwest Ethiopia

Table 2: The obstetric characteristics of mothers who gave birth in selected public health centers of Bench-Maji Zone, Ethiopia. May 2018. $n = 800$.

Variables	Response	Frequency	Percent	P value
Parity	1	324	40.5	
	2-4	397	49.6	0.398
	≥5	79	9.9	0.382
Ever had abortion	Yes	44	5.5	
	No	756	94.5	0.269
Status of pregnancy	Wanted	727	90.9	
	Unwanted	73	9.1	0.149
Ever delivered in health facility	Yes	320	40	
	No	480	60	0.509
Prepared for labor and delivery	Yes	567	70.9	0.071
	No	233	29.1	
Sex of attendant	Female	704	88	0.205
	Male	96	12	
Maternal complication immediately	Yes	136	17	0.187
	No	664	83	
Fetal outcome	Live birth	765	95.6	
	Still birth	35	4.4	0.097
Privacy	Good	513	64.1	
	Poor	287	35.9	0.001
ANC attended	Yes	723	90.4	
	No	77	9.6	0.001

Table 3: Maternal perception of health care service among mothers who gave birth in selected public health centers of Bench-Maji Zone, Ethiopia. May 2018. $n = 800$.

Variables	Response	Frequency	Percent	P value
Perceived presence of waiting area	Yes	734	91.8	
	No	66	8.2	0.901
Presence of toilet	Yes	678	84.8	
	No	122	15.2	0.551
Care provider measures taken to assure privacy	Good	659	82.4	
	Not good	141	17.6	0.001
Presence of attendant throughout delivery	Yes	534	66.8	
	No	266	33.2	0.641
Mother informed about the baby following examination	Yes	498	62.2	
	No	302	37.8	0.407
Waiting time to be seen by the provider	15 minute	488	61	
	More than 15 minute	312	39	0.312

(31.3%); Nairobi, Kenya (56%); and Sri Lanka (48%) [16–18]. The reason for this discrepancy might be due to socioeconomic characteristic of the study population and the type of facility studied and could also be due to the methodological difference in which we used a threshhold demarcation formula to set the cutoff point for satisfaction.

Table 4: Median satisfaction score of the three dimensions of satisfactions among mothers gave birth in selected public health centers of Bench-Maji Zone, Ethiopia. May 2018.

Dimensions	Median
Technical aspects	
Level of satisfaction with pain management	5
Level of satisfaction with support given during labor & delivery	4
Level of satisfaction with care given to newborn	5
Level of satisfaction with time given by providers	4
Level of satisfaction with continuity of care	5
Level of satisfaction with general care received	5
Communication and interpersonal aspects	
Level of satisfaction with explanation before procedures	4
Level of satisfaction with promptness of response	5
Level of satisfaction with listening concern	4
Level of satisfaction with supportiveness of staff	5
Level of satisfaction with allowing socials to be together	5
Level of satisfaction with respect	4
Environmental aspects	
Level of satisfaction with easily getting maternity ward starting from the gate	4
Level of satisfaction with maternity ward's toilets, hand washing and shower.	3
Level of satisfaction with cleanness of the ward	5
Level of satisfaction with privacy	4
Level of satisfaction with infrastructures like electricity, water	4
Level of satisfaction with easily getting maternity ward starting from the gate	5

When it comes to component-wise satisfaction, technical aspects had the highest median scores followed by communication and interpersonal aspects and environmental aspects. In contrary to this finding, the study conducted in Sri Lanka claimed a lower level of satisfaction with technical aspects compared to any another components [18]. This disparity could be due to study setting difference in which our study was conducted among health centers; higher satisfaction with technical aspect at health centers than hospitals might imply work fatigue as a health care provider at a hospital level attends to many deliveries in a day than one working at health-center level because of high client flow. Environmental aspect had the lowest median score than any other components, and this is consistent with the study undertaken in South Ethiopia and contradicts with the study conducted in India and Bangladesh—in which a relatively high proportion of clients are satisfied with environmental aspect [19, 20]. This could be explained as hospitals are relatively more equipped with facility infrastructures like toilet, water, and electricity compared with health centers.

The current study evidenced a reciprocal relationship between educational status and mother satisfaction; mothers with secondary school and lower educational status were

TABLE 5: Factors significantly associated with overall mothers' satisfaction in multivariate logistic regression, Bench-Maji Zone, Ethiopia. May 2018.

Variables	Level of satisfaction Satisfied Count (%)	Dissatisfied Count (%)	COR (95% CI)	AOR (95% CI)	*P* value
Educational status					
No formal education	317 (78.46%)	87 (21.53%)	11.97 (5.01-29.43)	3.69 (1.99, 7.91)	0.001
Primary school	137 (51.31%)	130 (48.69%)	3.46 (2.91-7.01)	1.27 (1.03, 1.94)	0.034
Secondary school	45 (45.45%)	54 (54.54%)	2.73 (1.59-6.05)	1.60 (1.34-2.96)	0.012
Diploma and above	7 (23.33%)	23 (76.67%)	1	1	
Residence					
Urban	88 (46.22%)	124 (53.78%)	1	1	
Rural	418 (69.39)	170 (30.61%)	3.47 (1.99-10.14)	2.63 (1.43, 5.80)	0.001
Measure taken to assure privacy					
Good	387 (75.43%)	126 (24.57%)	4.33 (2.77-9.01)	3.56 (1.25, 7.41)	0.001
Poor	119 (41.46%)	168 (58.54%)	1	1	
ANC attended					
Yes	435 (65%)	288 (30%)	1	1	
No	71 (46.75%)	6 (53.24%)	7.83 (5.78-19.43)	6.23 (3.42, 12.87)	0.001
Fetal outcome					
Live birth	476 (62.22)	289 (37.78)	1	1	
Still birth	30 (85.71%)	5 (14.29)	3.64 (1.07-6.03)	1.27 (0.87, 29.11)	0.631
Sex of the attendants					
Female	462 (65.62%)	242 (34.37%)	1	1	
Male	44 (45.83%)	52 (54.16%)	0.44 (0.16-0.71)	0.19 (0.01-1.06)	0.701
Presence of maternal complication					
Yes	75 (55.14%)	61 (44.85%)	0.65 (0.29, 0.9)	0.25 (0.11, 1.09)	0.167
No	437 (65.22%)	233 (34.78%)	1	1	
Being prepared for labor and delivery					
Yes	386 (68.08)	181 (31.92%)	1	1	
No	120 (51.5%)	113 (48.49%)	0.49 (0.06, 1.04)	1.09 (0.24, 29.07)	0.408
Client informed about the wellbeing of the baby					
Yes	314 (63.05%)	184 (36.95%)	0.98 (0.11, 1.52)	0.41 (0.21-2.97)	0.091
No	192 (63.58%)	110 (36.42%)	1	1	
Status of the pregnancy					
Wanted	444 (61.07%)	283 (38.93%)	0.28 (0.18, 0.97)	0.45 (0.31, 2.03)	0.338
Unwanted	62 (84.93%)	11 (15.07%)	1	1	

more likely to be satisfied with delivery service than those with diploma and above educational status. This finding is in agreement with the study conducted in Arba Minch, Ethiopia, Tanzania, Ghana, and Zambia [21–24]. Higher satisfaction in low literacy setting might attribute to expectation difference that more educated mothers could have higher expectation since they are aware of the care standards and client rights than less educated mothers.

Mothers from rural residence were AOR = 2.63 (95% CI (1.43, 5.80)) times more likely to be satisfied by the overall delivery service provided as compared to mothers from urban residence. This finding is substantiated by other studies conducted in Addis Abeba, Ethiopia, Tshwane, South Africa, and Brazil, where mothers coming from rural residence were more satisfied than those from urban residence [25–27]. This might be due to the difference in media exposure; mothers from rural residence might have poor media exposure regarding delivery service and have less service expectations compared to their urban counterpart.

The other most important predictor of client satisfaction in this study was mother's perceived measure taken to assure her piracy. Those mothers who regarded measure taken to assure their privacy as "good" were AOR = 3.56 (95% CI (1.25, 7.41)) times more likely to be satisfied than their counterpart. Similar finding was suggested by studies conducted in Southern Ethiopia, Northwest Ethiopia, Malawi, and Zambia [25, 28–30]. This could be explained as privacy is a key requirement for a women in the delivery process. A sense of shame is attached to it; hence, inadequate privacy during the procedure increases women's discomfort and diminishes their satisfaction levels.

Mothers who fully attended all the WHO-recommended ANC visits were AOR = 6.23 (95% CI (3.42, 12.87)) times more likely to be satisfied by the overall delivery service provided than those who did not attend ANC. This finding is similar with study conducted in Gamo Gofa Zone, Ethiopia [21]. This might be for the fact that ANC users get the necessary preventive care and are less likely to encounter pregnancy complications. Moreover, mothers who had attended ANC would have prepared for labor and delivery and may not expect everything from the health facility.

5. Conclusion

The overall satisfaction of mothers with childbirth care in public health centers of Bench-Maji Zone is low when compared with other studies. Mothers' educational status, residency, measure taken to assure privacy, and ANC attendance were significantly associated with mothers' satisfaction with overall delivery service provided. Thus, the Ethiopian Federal Ministry of Health and other relevant stakeholders working on enhancing maternal health service should focus on these determinates to improve maternal satisfaction with childbirth care and ultimately reduce maternal mortality and morbidity in the area.

Abbreviation

AOR: Adjusted odd ratio
ANC: Antenatal care
CI: Confidence intervals
SBA: Skilled birth assistance
SPSS: Statistical Package for Social Scientists
WHO: World Health Organization.

Authors' Contributions

SH initiated the study, developed the tool, supervised the data collection process, and carried out the statistical analysis, interpret the result, and wrote the final paper and manuscript based on the journal criteria. AG and ES made considerable contributions to interpretation of the results and reviewing the manuscript.

Acknowledgments

The authors would like to thank Mizan-Tepi University for technical support and ethical approval, study participants, and data collectors.

References

[1] A. Donabedian, "The quality of care. How can it be assessed?," *Archives of Pathology & Laboratory Medicine 1997*, vol. 121, no. 11, pp. 1145–1150, 1988.

[2] Health Strategy Implementation Project, "Measurement of patient satisfaction guidelines measurement of patient satisfaction. Irish Society for Quality and Saftey in Health Care," p. 37, 2003, September 2019, https://www.lenus.ie/handle/10147/43559/.

[3] I. H. Reerink and R. Sauerborn, "Quality of primary health care in developing countries: recent experiences and future directions," *International Journal for Quality in Health Care*, vol. 8, no. 2, pp. 131–139, 1996.

[4] Z. Dettrick, S. Firth, and E. Jimenez Soto, "Do strategies to improve quality of maternal and child health care in lower and middle income countries lead to improved outcomes? A review of the evidence," *Plos One*, vol. 8, no. 12, article e83070, 2013.

[5] "WHO j skilled attendants at birthWHOSeptember 2019, https://www.who.int/gho/maternal_health/mortality/maternal_mortality_text/en/.

[6] W. R. Alliance, *Respectful maternity care: the universal rights of childbearing women*, White Ribbon Alliance, Washington, DC, 2012.

[7] World Health Organization (WHO), *Making Pregnancy Safer: The Critical Role of the Skilled Attendant: A Joint Statement by WHO, ICM, FIGO*, World Health Organization (WHO), Geneva, Switzerland, 2004.

[8] F. Chemir, F. Alemseged, and D. Workneh, "Satisfaction with focused antenatal care service and associated factors among pregnant women attending focused antenatal care at health centers in Jimma town, Jimma zone, South West Ethiopia; a facility based cross-sectional study triangulated with qualitative study," *BMC Research Notes*, vol. 7, no. 1, article 164, 2014.

[9] I. Hildingsson, J. E. Thomas, R. E. Olofsson, and A. Nystedt, "Still Behind the Glass Wall? Swedish Fathers' Satisfaction With Postnatal Care," *Journal of Obstetric, Gynecologic, & Neonatal Nursing*, vol. 38, no. 3, pp. 280–289, 2009.

[10] B. Parker, *Unhappy consciousness: recognition and reification in Victorian fiction*, Columbia University, 2014.

[11] Mizan-Tepi University Teaching HospitalJuly 2018, https://www.mizantepiuniversity.net/about-us.html.

[12] R. A. Mesfin Tafa, "Maternal satisfaction with the delivery services in Assela Hospital, Arsi zone, Oromia region, Ethiopia,2013," *Gynecology & Obstetrics*, vol. 4, no. 12, 2014.

[13] B. Yohannes, M. Tarekegn, and W. Paulos, "Mothers' Utilization of antenatal care and their satisfaction with delivery services in selected public health facilities of Wolaita Zone, Southern Ethiopia," *International Journal of Scientific & Technology Research*, vol. 2, no. 2, 2013.

[14] K. Bitew, M. Ayichiluhm, and K. Yimam, "Maternal satisfaction on delivery service and its associated factors among mothers who gave birth in public health facilities of Debre Markos Town, Northwest Ethiopia," *BioMed Research International*, vol. 2015, Article ID 460767, 6 pages, 2015.

[15] B. Haile Tadesse, "Mothers' satisfaction with institutional delivery service in public health facilities of Omo Nada district, Jimma zone," *Clinical Medicine Research*, vol. 6, no. 1, p. 23, 2017.

[16] K. T. Gashaye, A. T. Tsegaye, G. Shiferaw, A. G. Worku, and S. M. Abebe, "Client satisfaction with existing labor and delivery care and associated factors among mothers who gave birth in university of Gondar teaching hospital; Northwest Ethiopia: Institution based cross-sectional study," *PLoS One*, vol. 14, no. 2, article e0210693, 2019.

[17] E. S. Bazant and M. A. Koenig, "Women's satisfaction with delivery care in Nairobi's informal settlements," *International Journal for Quality in Health Care*, vol. 21, no. 2, pp. 79–86, 2009.

[18] U. Senarath, D. N. Fernando, and I. Rodrigo, "Factors determining client satisfaction with hospital-based perinatal care in Sri Lanka," *Tropical Medicine & International Health*, vol. 11, no. 9, pp. 1442–1451, 2006.

[19] A. Hasan, "Patient satisfaction with MCH services among mothers attending the MCH training institute in Dhaka, Bangladesh," Masters thesis. Mahidol University, Faculty of Graduate Studies, 2007.

[20] A. George, "Quality of reproductive care in private hospitals in Andhra Pradesh. Women's perception," *Economic and Political Weekly*, vol. 37, pp. 1686–1692, 2002.

[21] Z. Dewana, T. Fikadu, A. G/ Mariam, and M. Abdulahi, "Client perspective assessment of women's satisfaction towards labour and delivery care service in public health facilities at Arba Minch town and the surrounding district, Gamo Gofa zone, south Ethiopia," *Reproductive Health*, vol. 13, no. 1, article 11, 2016.

[22] O. T. Oladapo and M. O. Osiberu, "Do sociodemographic characteristics of pregnant women determine their perception of antenatal care quality?," *Maternal and Child Health Journal*, vol. 13, no. 4, pp. 505–511, 2009.

[23] P. Das, M. Basu, T. Tikadar, G. C. Biswas, P. Mridha, and R. Pal, "Client satisfaction on maternal and child health services in rural Bengal," *Indian Journal of Community Medicine*, vol. 35, no. 4, pp. 478–481, 2010.

[24] D. P. Urassa, A. Carlstedt, L. Nystrom, S. N. Massawe, and G. Lindmark, "Quality assessment of the antenatal program for anaemia in rural Tanzania," *International Journal for Quality in Health Care*, vol. 14, no. 6, pp. 441–448, 2002.

[25] T. Melese, Y. Gebrehiwot, D. Bisetegne, and D. Habte, "Assessment of client satisfaction in labor and delivery services at a maternity referral hospital in Ethiopia," *Pan African Medical Journal*, vol. 17, 2014.

[26] S. J. Oosthuizen, A. M. Bergh, R. C. Pattinson, and J. Grimbeek, "It does matter where you come from: mothers' experiences of childbirth in midwife obstetric units, Tshwane, South Africa," *Reproductive Health*, vol. 14, no. 1, article 151, 2017.

[27] J. Gamble, D. K. Creedy, and B. Teakle, "Women's expectations of maternity services: A community-based survey," *Women and Birth*, vol. 20, no. 3, pp. 115–120, 2007.

[28] Z. B. Mengesha, G. A. Biks, T. A. Ayele, G. A. Tessema, and D. N. Koye, "Determinants of skilled attendance for delivery in Northwest Ethiopia: a community based nested case control study," *BMC Public Health*, vol. 13, no. 1, article 130, 2013.

[29] N. MacKeith, O. J. M. Chinganya, Y. Ahmed, and S. F. Murray, "Zambian women's experiences of urban maternity care: results from a community survey in Lusaka," *African Journal of Reproductive Health*, vol. 7, no. 1, pp. 92–102, 2003.

[30] J. Changole, C. Bandawe, B. Makanani et al., "Patients' satisfaction with reproductive health services at Gogo Chatinkha maternity unit, queen Elizabeth central hospital, Blantyre, Malawi," *Malawi Medical Journal*, vol. 22, no. 1, pp. 5–9, 2010.

Assessment of Knowledge, Attitude and Practice of Sunlight Exposure of Infants among Mothers Attending in Governmental Health Facilities in Farta District, South Gondar Zone, North West Ethiopia, 2018

Haileyesus Gedamu [1] **and Yilkal Tafere** [2]

[1]*Nursing Department, Bahir Dar University, Bahir Dar, Ethiopia*
[2]*Public Health Department, Debretabor University, Debretabor, Ethiopia*

Correspondence should be addressed to Haileyesus Gedamu; haileyesusg5@gmail.com

Academic Editor: Hind A. Beydoun

Background. Sunlight exposure serves an important purpose in human bodies. It promotes good health and plays a major role in the production of the very essential vitamin, vitamin D. Vitamin D is important for the growth of healthy, normal bones. Research conducted in different areas suggested that daily exposure to sunshine remains the cheapest, safest, and most effective method of preventing rickets. *Objective.* To assess knowledge, attitude, and practice of infants to sunlight exposure among lactating women in Farta district, in 2018. *Method.* Institution based cross sectional study design was conducted among mothers attending the selected health center. Systematic sampling method was used to select individual respondents. Data were entered and analyzed by using SPSS version 20. *Result.* Among 357 respondents identified for the study, 95% ($n = 339$) was responding to the interview. Of the total respondents, 49.9%, 46%, and 45.7% of them had poor knowledge, unfavorable attitude, and poor practice about sunlight exposure, respectively. *Conclusion and recommendation.* The results of this study showed that almost half of the mothers had inadequate knowledge, attitude, and inadequate practice about sunlight exposure. Therefore, mothers need to be educated about the importance of sunlight exposure.

1. Introduction

Regular sunlight exposure increases the serotonin levels in the body, making it more active and alert. The most important advantage of exposure to sunlight is the ability to boost your body's vitamin D supply [1]. Exposing a child to sunlight through window panes for 10 min twice a day protects mild neonatal jaundice [2]. When people are exposed to sunlight in the morning, their nocturnal melatonin production occurs sooner, and they enter into sleep more easily at night. Melatonin production also shows a seasonal variation relative to the availability of light, with the hormone produced for a longer period in the winter than in the summer. Even if exposure of children to sunlight is important for the development, exposure to high sunlight is a risk factor in the development of skin cancers [3, 4].

Studies suggest that achieving and maintaining an adequate vitamin D blood serum level, as determined by a 25-hydroxyvitamin D (25(OH)D) blood test, is essential to the prevention and treatment of autoimmune diseases such as multiple sclerosis and type 1 diabetes. Additionally, vitamin D appears to play a protective role in cardiovascular health, various types of cancer, Autism, depression, schizophrenia, and respiratory conditions such as cystic fibrosis [5].

Recent knowledge suggests that the risk of some chronic diseases could be reduced if vitamin D intake and sun exposure of the population were increased. In some developed countries, the prevalence of rickets in the general population diminished after the emergence of dietary supplementation. However, in such countries, vitamin D deficiency rickets has re-emerged in recent years, particularly among groups with limited exposure to UVB-containing sunshine [6].

Previous studies indicate that insufficient exposure of sunshine was an important cause of rickets in children [7–10]. Studies indicate that regular exposure to sunshine is the most effective way of preventing the disease [8, 11, 13]. Health education has a vital role on behavioral change regarding infant's exposure to sunshine. Hence in the early 1960s, it was adopted as the main strategy to prevent rickets [13]. Evidence of world health organization indicate that worldwide one billion people have vitamin D deficiency [14]. A risk of rickets is dominant in children who live in crowded houses, which have no sun light [15].

Evidence shows that many people have low vitamin D levels and also there is a well-documented relationship between low vitamin D levels and poor bone health [16]. Beside these, studies in Gaza strip in 2010 among 340 cases and controls show only 65% have sunlight exposure. The prevalence of rickets and its determinant factor were educational status, occupation, number of deliveries, health education, and exclusive breastfeeding (EBF) [17].

Nutritional rickets are gaining the attention of public health professionals and individual clinicians worldwide as the disease remains an endemic problem in many developing countries and has re-emerged in a number of developed countries [18].

In middle east vitamin D deficiency and rickets continue to be a public health problem despite all year sunshine. In some parts of Asia, such as the northern parts of China (including Tibet), Mongolia, and Afghanistan rickets appears to be mainly due to vitamin D deficiency associated with the high latitude, cold winters, and limited skin exposure [19].

Vitamin D deficiency and nutritional rickets are still health problems in developing countries. Despite Turkey being in a geographical location with abundant sun light exposure, vitamin D deficiency continues to be a major health problem. Yearly incidence rates of vitamin D deficiency revealed in Turkey vary from 1.67% to 19%. Thus, sunning for bone development is still being advised [20]. In spite of adequate sunshine, vitamin D deficiency (nutritional) rickets has remained a common problem in the tropics and sub-tropics, including some of the most populated countries such as China, India, Nigeria, Egypt, Iran, and Turkey [21].

In Ethiopia, its prevalence was in the order of 30% in the 1950s and does not seem to have changed over the years. The main cause of nutritional rickets in Ethiopian children is lack of exposure to sunshine and not adequate intake of vitamin D. Lack of awareness and traditional beliefs are major causes for not exposing infants to sunshine [22].

A retrospective study in jimma university specialized hospital revealed that the prevalence of rickets was 10.5% [23]. In a research conducted in Addis Ababa town, four in ten children who had visited health institutions had rickets and the problem was higher in infants [24]. Other study conducted in jimma hospital showed that nearly one in ten children have rickets [25].

2. Methods

2.1. Study Design. Institutional based cross-sectional study design was conducted.

2.2. Study Area and Period. The survey was done from February 15, up to March 25, 2018, in Farta district, Amhara regional state. Farta district is located in the northwest part of Ethiopia and about 667 km from Addis Ababa and 99 km from Bahir Dar. The area is found at the altitude, which ranges from 2000 to 2500 meters above sea level and it consists of four major agro-ecological zones: 25% low land, 45% medium highland, 24% highland, and 6% gorge. The annual temperature ranges between 9 and 25 degree Celsius and the rainfall varies from 1250 mm in the lowlands to 1500 mm in the highland areas during summer.

2.3. Source Population. All lactating women whose child's age was less than 1 year and attended all health institutions of the Farta district for health care and immunization.

2.4 .Study Population. All lactating women whose child's age was less than 1 year and attended selected health institutions of the Farta district for health care and immunization during the study period.

2.5. Inclusion and Exclusion Criteria. Inclusion criteria—All women who were lactating with a child less than 1 year.

Exclusion criteria—Mothers who were unable to communicate were excluded.

2.6. Sample Size Determination and Sample Selection. To determine the sample sizes required existence of estimated prevalence rates is compulsory's the prevalence of knowledge, attitude, and practice of sunlight exposure was 38.8% of Jimma university specialized hospital with an absolute precisions of ±5% and a statistical confidence of 95% [24].

The sample size is computed using the following formula.

$$n = \frac{Z^2 p(1-p)}{d^2}, \quad (1)$$

where, n = sample size; z = statistical certainty chosen; p = estimated prevalence level to be investigated; $q = 1 - p$; d = precision desired

$$n = \frac{(1.96 \times 1.96)(.388 \times .612)}{0.05 \times 0.05} = 365. \quad (2)$$

The total number of infants in Farta district is 4973. Since this figure is below 10,000.

Use the following adjustment formula for the sample size:

$$n = \frac{n}{(1 + n/N)}, \quad (3)$$

where,

n = sample size for population of size above 10,000
N = number of infants in Farta district. Therefore,

$$n = \frac{365}{(1 + 365/4973)}. \quad (4)$$

$$n = 340. \quad (5)$$

Taking 5% [17] non response rate the final sample size was **357.**

Table 1: Socio demographic characteristics of respondents whose child age was less than 12 months in Farta district, Northwest Ethiopia, 2018.

Item	Category	Number	%
Age of mother mean = 28.8, SD = 6.2	<19 years	11	3.1
	20–29 years	176	52
	30–39 years	91	26.8
	40–49 years	61	18
Age of child in months mean = 5.99, SD = 3.25	<4	132	38.8
	5–8	113	33.4
	9–12	94	27.8
Gender of child	M	184	54.3
	F	155	44.7
Number of children	1	72	21.2
	2–5	218	64.3
	6–10	49	14.5
Religion of the mother	Orthodox	332	98
	Muslim	5	1.6
	Protestant	2	.4
Marital status	Single	0	.6
	Married	323	95.2
	Windowed	4	1.2
	Divorced	12	3.5
Educational status of the mother	Unable to read & write	241	71.1
	Able to read & write	54	15.9
	Primary school(1–8)	32	9.4
	Secondary school and above	12	3.5
Husband educational status	Unable to read & write	195	60.5
	Able to read & write	54	16.7
	Primary school(1–8)	49	15.2
	Secondary school and above	25	7.7
Monthly income	<500	102	30
	500–1000	143	42.3
	>1000	94	27.7
Maternal occupation	Farmer	288	85
	Civil servant	4	1.2
	Merchant	5	1.5
	Daily laborer	6	1.8
	House wife	36	10.6
Husband occupation	Farmer	275	85.2
	Civil servant	12	3.7
	Merchant	15	4.6
	Daily laborer	9	2.8
	Other	12	3.7
Mass media	Yes	190	55.9
	No	149	44.1
Type of mass media	Radio	161	84.9
	Television	26	15.1

2.7. Sampling Technique and Procedure. The sampling method employed in this study was a systematic sampling method. That means proportional numbers of mothers were included into the sample from each selected health facility to make up a total sample size. Each study participant was selected using the systematic sampling technique in which every second client was interviewed in each health facility.

Table 2: Obstetric history of women whose child age was less than 12 months in Farta woreda, Northwest Ethiopia, 2018.

Item	Category	Number	%
ANC visit	Yes	306	90.3
	No	33	9.7
Number of visit	One	26	8.6
	Two	97	31.7
	Three	70	22.9
	Four and above	113	37
Place of delivery	Home	54	15.9
	Health post	40	11.8
	Health center	180	53
	Hospital	65	19.2
PNC visit	Yes	188	55.4
	No	151	44.6
Number of visit	One	79	42
	Two	29	15.4
	Three	60	32
	Four	20	10.6

Proportional allocation of the study subjects of the four health facilities were as follows:

$$n \text{ in health facility} = \frac{N \text{ in a health facility} * \text{nt}}{N \text{ total}}$$

where,

n in health facility = proportion of mothers with infants in a given health facility

nt = Total sample size

N in a health facility = Number of mothers with infants in a given health facility

N total = Total number of mothers with infants in all health facilities.

2.8. Variable of the Study

2.8.1. Dependent Variables. Knowledge, attitude, and practice of sunlight exposure of infant.

2.8.2. Independent Variable. Age, occupation, income, educational status, no. of sibling and culture, place of delivery, antenatal care, and postnatal care.

2.9. Data Collection Procedures. A semi structured pre-tested questionnaire was prepared and translated into Amharic by an expert to ensure its consistency. A pretest study was also carried out in other health center to gain some useful feedbacks.

2.10. Data Quality Control. To ensure quality data collection, one day training was provided to data collector to make sure good interviewing techniques. The training was focused on how to complete the questionnaire, proper interview techniques, and proper asking. Through the data collection

TABLE 3: Knowledge of respondents on sunlight exposure of infant in Farta district, Northwest Ethiopia, 2018.

Item	Category	Number	%
Mentioned as they knew the importance of sunlight exposure	Yes	183	53.98
	No	156	46.02
Number of day of sunlight exposure per week	Every day	84	46
	2	39	11.4
	3–4	48	26
	5–6	12	5
Starting day of sunlight exposure	Within 5 days	17	9.3
	5–10 days	20	8.3
	10–15 days	91	37.9
	After 15 days	55	46.7
Time of sunlight exposure	Before 16:00 h	134	73.2
	16:00–19:00 h	38	3.3
	19:00–22:00 h	11	.8
Duration of sunlight exposure	<15 min	49	26.7
	15–20	40	21.9
	20 min–1 h	54	29.5
	Above 1 h	35	19.1
Information on sunlight exposure	Yes	183	53.98
	No	156	46
Source of information on sunlight exposure	Mass media	12	5
	Health professional	100	54.6
	Neighbor	68	36.6
	Parents	3	1.1

process, the researcher was closely supervised and checked for consistency and reliability of the data collected by interviewers.

2.11. Data Processing and Analysis. Data entry formats were designed by defining the variables and labeling values for categorical variables. Specifically coding of the questions and data entry format was prepared and made ready before the data was collected. The data were entered and analyzed using computerized SPSS version 20 software. The raw data were edited and checked to control entry. Table and figures were used to present the finding.

2.12. Ethical Clearance. Ethical clearance was first obtained from the research and publication office of Bahir Dar University. Ethical permission was also secured from, regional health bureau, South Gondar zonal health department & Farta district health office. Participation in the study was voluntary, and data were collected after obtaining permission from each participant.

3. Results

3.1. Socio Demographic Characteristics. Among the 357 mothers identified in the study, 339 (95%) responded to the interview, nearly all 323 (95.3%) were married. More than half, 176 (52%) of the women were in the age group 20–29. Almost all, 332 (98%) of respondents were orthodox and majority, 132 (38.8%) of child's age were under 4 months. More than two-thirds, 241 (71.1%) of maternal educational status were illiterate. More than half, 312 (91.9%) of their occupations were farmer. Almost all (70%) of respondents incomes were above five hundred Birr (Table 1).

3.2 Obstetrical History of Mothers' about Sunlight Exposure of Their Infant. Most, 306 (90.3%) of respondents had ANC follow up and the remaining 33 (9.7%) had no follow up. Among respondents who had ANC follow up, 113 (37%) of having four and above visit, only low proportion, 26 (8.6%) of women had one time visit. More than half, 180 (53%) of the mothers delivered at the health center. One hundred eighty eight (55.4%) of respondents had PNC follow up .Among respondents who had PNC follow up 79 (42%) of 188 respondents have a 1st PNC visit and 60 (32%) had three visits (Table 2).

3.3 Level of Mothers' Knowledge about Sunlight Exposure of Their Infants. Nearly half (49.9%) of the respondents had knowledge of sunlight exposure to their infant. Of 183 respondents, 84 (46%) had knowledge of sunlight exposure every day and 39 (11.4%) two times per week. Nearly three quarters, 134 (73.2%) of 183 respondents had knowledge of sunlight exposure to infants before four hours and the remaining, 7 (2.2%) after four hours. Similarly, more than three quarters, 68 (29.8%) of 183 respondents had knowledge of sunlight exposure of infant in less than 30 min and the remaining, 29 (11.9%) for more than 30 min. More than half, 183 (53.98%) of respondents had information about sunlight exposure of infant and most of

TABLE 4: Practice of respondents on sunlight exposure of infant in Farta woreda, Northwest Ethiopia, 2018.

Item	Category	Number	%
Do you expose your child for sunlight	Yes	176	51.98
	No	163	48.02
Number of day of sunlight exposure per week	Every day	80	45.7
	2	28	15.9
	3–4	43	24.4
	5–6	25	10.6
Starting day of sunlight exposure	Within 5 days	17	7.2
	5–10 days	20	8.5
	10–15 days	91	38.7
	After 15 days	107	45.5
Time of sunlight exposure	Before 4 h	129	73
	4–7 h	38	21.5
	7–10 h	9	5.5
Duration of sunlight exposure	<15 min	59	33.5
	15–20	38	21.5
	20 min–1 h	69	38.5
	Above 1 h	10	5.7
Do you cover the infants body when you exposed	Yes	169	75
	No	56	25
Reason for you cover	To prevent skin damage	44	19.3
	To prevent from evil eye	98	55.7
	Other	27	25
Reason of respondents for not exposing	Fear of blackness	4	2.4
	Lack of knowledge	76	46.6
	Fear of evil eye	59	36.2
	Fear of pneumonia	5	3.1
	Lack of time	5	3.1

the respondents, 120 (54.6%) had got the information from a health professional (Table 3).

3.4. Practice of Respondents on Sunlight Exposure of Infant. Less than half of the participants (45.7%) were exposed their infants to sunlight. Only, 37 (15.7%) of 176 respondents started to expose their child to sunlight before 10 days and the remaining, 198 (84.3%) were after 10 days. Out of 176 respondents, about 80 (45.7%) participants exposed their child to sunlight every day and the remaining 96 (54.3%) were 5 up to 6 times a week and less. Most of, 169 (75%) of respondents covered their infant's body when they exposed (Table 4).

3.5. Attitude of Respondent on Sunlight Exposure of Infant. Of the total respondents, 46% agreed with an advantage of sunlight exposure of their infants. More than half, 176 (51.98%) of respondents were happy when they exposed/if they exposed their child to sunlight and the remaining, 163 (48%) felt anxiety and other. About 156 (46%) of respondents perceived consequences after they exposed or if they exposed their child to sunlight were to become strong and the remaining, 183 (54%) were to be healthy, helps to sleep, and others (Table 5).

TABLE 5 : Attitude of respondents on sunlight exposure of infant in Farta Woreda, Northwest Ethiopia, 2018.

Item	Category	Number	%
Sunlight exposure is Advantageous	Agree	139	41
	Disagree	155	45.7
	Strongly agree	17	10.98
	Strongly disagree	28	2.3
Feeling of respondents while they expose their child	Happy	176	51.98
	Anxiety	80	23.6
	Angry	3	.9
	Other	80	23.6
Perceived consequence of respondents on sunlight exposure of infant	To become healthy	60	17.7
	To become strong	156	46
	Helps to sleep	3	.9
	Exposes my child to cold/pneumonia	94	27.7
	Others	26	7.7
Thought that sunlight exposure cause skin cancer	Yes	203	60
	No	136	40
Thought that sunlight exposure cause nappy rash	Yes	237	70
	No	102	30

4. Discussion

The aim of our study was to assess knowledge, practice, and attitude of sunlight exposure of lactating mothers to their infants in Farta district. Currently the government of Ethiopian gives emphasis to decreasing child morbidity and mortality. Therefore, assessing the knowledge, practice, and attitude of lactating mothers regarding exposing their infants to sunlight is one important aspect in maintaining children's health.

The proportion of respondents who reported that they had the information (knowledge) about sunlight exposure was 53.98%; the same studies done in Turkey and jimma town showed that 86.4% and 100% of mothers had information about sunlight exposure, respectively [20, 12]. Our research was lower than the study done in Turkey and jimma town; the possible reason for this might be different educational status of study participants about sunlight exposure.

Out of the total respondents who responded to the question "is sunlight exposure beneficial?", 75.98% mentioned sunlight exposure was beneficial; our finding was lower than the study done in jimma town which was 99.68% [22]. The reason may be due to mothers in jimma town as mentioned above had 100% information about sunlight exposure and our finding was greater than the study done in sakarya which was 64.1% [21]. The possible reason for this may be mothers in sakarya were educated about harmful effects of sunlight exposure rather than benefits of sunlight exposure because they live in a high temperature region and they had fear of skin cancer. Seventy five percent of the respondents mentioned the most benefit of sunlight exposure was strengthening bone; our finding was similar to the same study done in jimma town which was 64.62% [12]. Regarding the best time to sunlight exposure of infants, 95.7% of the mothers mentioned it was in the morning; this is similar to the same study done in jimma town which was 100% [12].

Regarding the practice of sunlight exposure, 51.98% of mothers exposed their infants to sunlight. This finding is lower than the same study done in sakarya, which was 87.5% of mothers exposed their infants to sunlight [21]. The reason for this difference may be due to the adequate information mothers had in sakarya about sunlight exposure compared to mothers in Farta district. It was also greater than the study done in debre markos town which was 44.6% [28]. The possible explanation for this may be they were found in tropical regions which was increased prevalence of skin cancer; so due to fear of skin cancer, mothers may not have exposed their infants to sunlight.

This study showed that 15.7% of mothers started sunlight exposure of their babies between 0–15 days. This was lower than the study done in jimma town, 42.04% and debre markos town, 23.4% [22, 28]. This study also showed that 51.98% of the mothers exposed their infants to sunlight, but only 40% of mothers exposed their infants to sunlight daily and the rest of the mothers exposed their infants sometimes. This result was lower than the study done in jimma town which was 92.16% of mothers exposed daily [12]. The reason for this difference may be the community had more information and maybe there was a health education program for mothers in jimma.

In our study, 73.2% of mothers exposed their infants to sunlight in the range of time from 8 to 10 AM in the morning and 21.9% of participants exposed their infants with time duration of 15–20 min. It was lower than the study done in debre markos [28].

About 36.5% of respondents had feared to expose their infants to sunlight. Among these 15.2, % of participants not exposed their infants to sunlight due to fear of the evil eye. This finding was higher than the study done in debre markos town which was 11.9% [28]. The possible explanation for this difference may be due to cultural differences between the two populations and differences in a study setting in Farta district; the majority of respondents were residing in rural areas, whereas in the study done in debre markose participants were residing in urban areas, which may have contributed to the observed difference.

For the current study, feeling of lactating women while they exposed their children, 53.98% were happy, 0.3% angry, 18.4% feel anxiety and 4.8% were other which was higher than with ethio-swedish children's hospitals. Respondents perceived consequences while they exposed their child to sunlight, 17.7% were makes healthy, 75% were made strong, 0.9 were helped to sleep, 27.7% were exposé the infant to cold (pneumonia), and 1.8 other which was higher than the result of ethio-swedish children's hospital [7].

However, this study does have some inherent limitations. Though there are wide ranges of factors which affect rickets among mothers attending governmental health institutions, only knowledge, attitude, and practice about sunlight exposure were addressed in this study. Hence, taking into consideration factors from the different contributors like calcium deficiency would have been important.

5. Conclusion

According to our study, participants had not good knowledge, practice, and attitude regarding sunlight exposure of infants. Therefore, health education focusing on the importance of sunlight exposure is important to improve knowledge, practice, and attitude of mother's sunlight exposure of their infants.

Authors' Contributions

All authors participated in proposal conception and designing the proposal, data collection and analysis, and wrote the manuscript. Finally, the paper was approved by all authors.

Acknowledgments

We would like to express our deepest appreciation and heartfelt thanks to Bahir Dar University for giving the chance of doing this project. We also thank the Farta district health officer and community for their cooperation and their valuable information for this work. Last but not the least, we would like to express our heartfelt thanks to all data collectors and supervisor for their valuable contribution.

References

[1] M. F. Holick, "Vitamin D and sunlight: strategies for cancer prevention and other health benefits," *Clinical Journal of the American Society of Nephrology*, vol. 3, no. 5, pp. 1548–1554, 2008.

[2] Medicine, "Newborn Jaundice," http://www.emedicinehealth.com/articles/10101-6.

[3] M. N. Mead, "Benefits of sunlight: a bright spot for human health," *Environmental Health Perspective*, vol. 116, no. 4, 2008.

[4] J. K. Robinson, A. W. Rademaker, J. A. Sylvester, and B. Cook, "Summer sun exposure: knowledge, attitudes, and behaviors of midwest adolescents," *Preventive Medicine*, vol. 26, no. 3, pp. 364–372, 1997.

[5] OpinionBug.com, "Vitamin D Deficiency: A Silent Epidemic among African Americans," April 20, 2013.

[6] O. Gillie, "Sunlight robbery: a critique of public health policy on vitamin D in the UK," *Molecular Nutrition & Food Research*, vol. 54, no. 8, pp. 1148–1163, 2010.

[7] U. S. Interdepartmental Commission and on Nutrition for National Defense, "Ethiopian nutrition survey, section VIII," Washington D. C, pp. 61–65, 1959.

[8] V. H. Ekbote, A. V. Khadilkar, M. Z. Mughal et al., "Sunlight exposure and development of rickets in Indian toddlers," *The Indian Journal of Pediatrics*, vol. 77, no. 1, pp. 61–65, 2010.

[9] T. W. Mariam and G. Sterky, "Severe rickets in infancy and childhood in Ethiopia," *The Journal of Pediatrics*, vol. 82, no. 5, pp. 876–878, 1973.

[10] B. Hojer, M. Gebre-medhin, G. Sterky, R. Zetierstorm, and K. Daniel, "Combined vitamin D deficiency rickets and protein-energy malnutrition in Ethiopian infants," *Journal of Tropical Pediatrics*, vol. 23, no. 2, pp. 73–79, 1977.

[11] S. Lulseged, "Severe rickets in a children's hospital in addis ababa," *Ethiopian Medical Journal*, vol. 28, no. 4, pp. 175–181, 1990.

[12] T. Getaneh, A. Assefa, and Z. Tadesse, "The knowledge and practice of exposure to sunlight in jimma town, south western Ethiopia," *Ethiopian Journal of Health Development*, pp. 29–32, 1998.

[13] S. Lulseged and G. Fitwi, "Vitamin D deficiency rickets: socio-demographic and clinical risk factors in children seen at a referral hospital in addis ababa," *East African Medical Journal*, vol. 76, no. 8, pp. 457–461, 1999.

[14] M. F. Holick and T. C. Chen, "Vitamin D deficiency: a worldwide problem with health consequences," *The American Journal of Clinical Nutrition*, vol. 87, no. 4, pp. 1080S–1086S, 2008.

[15] V. Redy, M. Parkin, and T. Waterston, "Nutritional Rickets: diseases of children in the subtropics & Tropics," *Edward Arnold*, pp. 376–379, 1991.

[16] P. H. Hart, "Vitamin D supplementation, moderate sun exposure, and control of immune diseases," *Discovery Medicine*, vol. 13, no. 73, pp. 397–404, 2012.

[17] E. Daniel, M. Rashed, E. Robert, and H. Abdullah, "Vitamin D sates of infants in northeastern rural Bangladesh," *Journal of Health, Popular and Nutrition*, vol. 28, no. 5, pp. 458–465, 2010.

[18] M. Maged, "Risk factors associated with nutritional rickets among children aged 2 to 36 months old in the gaza strip," *International Journal of Food, Nutrition and Public Health*, vol. 3, no. 1, pp. 36–41, 2010.

[19] M. John, "Vitamin D and calcium deficiency rickets in infants and children: a global," *Indian Journal of Medical Research*, vol. 8, no. 3, pp. 245–249, 2008.

[20] A. Nihal, M. Tuncay, T. Pinar, and G. Sulemina, "Parents' knowledge and behavior concerning sunning their babies," *BMC Pediatrics*, vol. 27, no. 6, pp. 4–9, 2006.

[21] A. Zubaida, B. Nabi, Y. Fadia, and M. Abde, "Study of risk factors of rickets in children," *World Applied Science Journal*, vol. 17, no. 11, pp. 1386–1393, 2012.

[22] C. Kenenisa, H. Ewnetu, and H. Sime, "Retrospective analysis of the prevalence of rickets and associated factors among children Admitted to the pediatric ward in jimma university specialized hospital," *Journal of pediatrics & Neonatal Care*, vol. 1, no. 7, pp. 30–36, 2014.

[23] S. Lulseged and C. Deste, "Behavioral intention and factors influencing intention of Ethiopian mothers to expose infants to sunshine," *Ethiopian Journal of Health Development*, vol. 16, no. 1, pp. 31–40, 2002.

[24] A. Aust-Kettis, K. B. Bjornesjo, E. Mannheimer, T. Cvibah, P. Clark, and M. Debele, "Rickets in Ethiopia," *Ethiopia Medical Journal*, vol. 3, pp. 109–21, 1965.

[25] B. Tefera, G. Abebe, and L. Worku, "Micronutrient deficiency in jimma university," *Ethiopia Medical Journal*, pp. 31–33, 2005.

[26] J. B. Lebrun, M. E. Moffatt, and R. J. Mundy, "Vitamin D deficiency in a Manitoba community," *Children World Applied Science Journal*, vol. 9, no. 1, pp. 23–26, 2006.

[27] M. Eshetu, "Analysis of pediatric admissions to jimma hospital pediatrics ward: a three year retrospective study," *Bulletin of Jimma Institute of Health Sciences*, vol. 4, pp. 1–11, 1994.

[28] A. Abebe, M. Rajalakshmi, and G. Tenaw, "Assessment of practice and factors affecting sunlight exposure of infants among mothers attending governmental health facilities in debre markos town, east gojjam, Ethiopia, 2015," *American Journal of Nursing Science*, vol. 5, no. 1, pp. 30–36, 2016.

15

Disclosure of Intimate Partner Violence and Associated Factors among Victimized Women, Ethiopia, 2018: A Community-Based Study

Liyew Agenagnew,[1] **Bosena Tebeje**,[2] **and Ruth Tilahun**[3]

[1]*Department of Psychiatry, Faculty of Medical Sciences, Institute of Health, Jimma University, Jimma, Ethiopia*
[2]*School of Nursing, Faculty of Health Sciences, Institute of Health, Jimma University, Jimma, Ethiopia*
[3]*Department of Midwifery, College of Health Sciences and Medicine, Dilla University, Dilla, Ethiopia*

Correspondence should be addressed to Liyew Agenagnew; liyew2003@gmail.com

Academic Editor: Hind A. Beydoun

Background. Disclosure is a vital step in the process of finding a lasting solution and breaking the abuse chain in a victim woman by the intimate partner. *Objectives.* This study is aimed at assessing the disclosure of intimate partner violence and associated factors among victim women in Dilla town, Gedeo Zone, South Ethiopia, 2018. *Methods.* A community-based cross-sectional study design triangulated with the qualitative method was employed. Data were collected from 280 women victims of intimate partner violence using pretested, structured, and interviewer-administered questionnaires. SPSS version 20.0 software was used for analysis. Binary logistic regression and a multivariate logistic regression model were fitted to assess the association between the independent and dependent variables. Qualitative data were collected through in-depth interviews and categorized into themes and triangulated with the quantitative result. *Results.* Half of the respondents (51%) disclosed intimate partner violence. Partner alcohol use (AOR = 1.99; 95% CI:1.18, 3.34), women experiencing a single type of intimate partner violence (AOR = 0.38, 95% CI: 0.17, 0.79), women having strong social support (AOR = 2.52; 95% CI:1.44, 4.41), and women whose partners' having primary (AOR = 2.04; 95% CI:1.07, 3.9) and secondary education (AOR = 2.16; 95% CI: 1.07, 4.33) were significantly associated with the disclosure of intimate partner violence as the qualitative result shows most of the women prefer their family to disclose and those who kept silent were due to economic dependency, societal norms towards wife beating, arranged marriage, and not getting the chance especially those who went to the hospital. *Conclusion.* Nearly 50% of victims of intimate partner violence women disclose intimate partner violence to others. Thus, it is needed for stakeholders to use their efforts to further increase the disclosure of violence and respect women's rights and equality.

1. Introduction

Intimate partner violence is fundamental to public health challenges and violates women's human rights. It is one of the most common forms of violence in the direction of women and includes bodily, sexual, and emotional abuse and controlling behaviors by the intimate partner [1].

Approximately 1 in 3 women worldwide have experienced either bodily and/or sexual intimate partner violence in their lifetime [1, 2].

Most victims of intimate partner, women, keep silent, and only a few women disclosed violence to others, in the world only 20% [3], in America, more than 74% intimate partner violence survivor women stayed with an abuser and does not disclose intimate partner violence [4], 77.9% of Serbian women did not disclose intimate partner violence [5], in Nigeria, only 46% women disclosed intimate partner violence to formal or informal services [6], and in Tanzania, 41% of women do not disclose intimate partner violence [7–9].

Not disclosing intimate partner violence may lead to a host of negative sexual and reproductive health consequences for women, including unintended and unwanted pregnancy, abortion and unsafe abortion, sexually transmitted infections including HIV, pregnancy complications, pelvic inflammatory disease, urinary tract infections and sexual dysfunction, physical and mental injury, and death [10–12].

Most frequently mentioned factors in previous studies as the reason behind not disclosing intimate partner violence to others were economic and sociopolitical discrimination of women, being dependent on partners' income [4, 13], the severity of the violence [14–16], those who are severely violated more likely to disclose their experience to the formal social services [17], stress, accepting violence as normal [14], concerns about bringing bad name to the family, lack of confidence, shame/embarrassment/fear of getting blamed, fear for children's future life, women who were unemployed and pregnant, and lack of encouragement by family members [15, 16, 18–20] and educational status [21, 22].

In Ethiopia, intimate partner violence accounts in one-third of the women [23]; however, victimized (violated) women's disclosure status and factors associated with it were not investigated explicitly especially in women found in a rural area. So this study attempted to assess the magnitude of disclosure of intimate partner violence and factors associated with it, in the rural community of Ethiopia, from March 25 to April 25, 2018, by using both qualitative and quantitative methods, which might be helpful health care providers to screen women for intimate partner violence and aid to disclose it as well it will be helpful for different stakeholders to address and intervene the reasons for not disclosing violence to others despite the fact that they are suffering from it.

2. Methods and Materials

2.1. Study Area and Period. The study was conducted from March 25 to April 25, 2018, in Dilla town administrative center of the Gedeo Zone in the Southern Nation Nationalities and People Region, which is found 360 km away from Addis Ababa and 90 km from the capital city of the region Hawassa. The total area of the town is 135 km^2. Total population is 102,624, among which 50,286 (48.9%) are males and 52,338 (51.1%) are females. The total reproductive age group women are 20,204. The total number of households is 20,944. The dominant ethnic group is Gedeo, and most of the people speak Gedeo-Offa and Amharic languages.

2.2. Study Design. A community-based cross-sectional study design was employed.

2.3. Populations

2.3.1. Source Population. The source population was reproductive age women with the experience of intimate partner violence and residing in Dilla town.

2.3.2. Study Population. The study population was reproductive age women with the experience of intimate partner violence in the selected kebele households (Haroresa, Odaya, and Harsu kebeles) in Dilla town.

2.4. Inclusion Criteria and Exclusion Criteria

2.4.1. Inclusion Criteria. Women whose ages are between 18 and 49 years, have/had an intimate partner, and had intimate partner violence before the data collection period were included in the study.

2.4.2. Exclusion Criteria. Severely ill women that are not able to give information at the time of data collection were excluded from the study.

2.5. Sample Size Determination. The sample size was determined by using a single population proportion formula by considering the following assumptions: $P = 31\%$—prevalence of women disclosing violent experience in North West Ethiopia [7], d = margin of error of 0.05 with 95% confidence interval, and $\alpha = 0.05$ (level of significance) using the formula $n = (Z\alpha/2)^2\, p\,(1-p)/d^2$; then the calculated sample size became 329, Since the source population is below 10,000, correction formulae were used $\mathrm{nf} = n/1 + n/N$, where n = a minimum sample size, N = total number of women that experienced intimate partner violence in the study area (1958), and NF = minimum final sample size; it becomes 282. By adding 10% nonresponse rate, the final total sample size was 310.

For the qualitative part, the sample size was determined by saturation of the information.

2.6. Sampling Technique. For the quantitative part, from the total of nine kebeles found in Dilla town, three kebeles called Haroresa kebele (located in Harowelabu subcity), Odaya kebele (located in Sesa subcity), and Harsu kebele (located in Bedecha subcity) were selected by using the lottery method. In those selected kebeles, there were a total number of 6117 households, i.e., 3295, 1409, and 1413, respectively. We screened women found in those kebeles (10,235) for having intimate partner violence, and we got a total of 1958 women who had a positive reply for intimate partner violence from three kebeles. Then, by using a simple random sampling technique, we selected our study participants by the lottery method from the prepared sampling frame. Data collectors trace the selected participants for interviews with the help of health extension workers who know the kebeles very well using the coded household and women selected from the sampling frame. One house was visited with a maximum of three times, but if data collectors cannot get respondents for the third time, they considered it nonrespondent.

For the qualitative part, a purposeful sampling technique was used. Potential respondents were selected for the in-depth interview. Key informants were selected based on their experience of violence in their lifetime and who can express the required information about the problem clearly. A total of 8 women participated in this study.

2.7. Data Collection Procedures and Instruments. Data was collected through face to face interviews moving from house to house by using 6 female diploma nurses as a data collector after written consent was obtained from the respondents. The data collection process was conducted individually at a convenient location for the respondents.

To assess disclosure of intimate partner violence, a validated tool with 13 items was adapted and used by reviewing different literatures [24, 25]; for other variables, structured questionnaires were used, which were prepared in the English language then translated to the local languages, *Amharic* and *Gedeo-Offa* for data collection purpose. The questionnaires have five parts, involving the sociodemographic and behavioral characteristics (16 items), reproductive health-related (10 items), social support (3 items), and women empowerment (9 items).

Intimate partner violence was assessed by the self-reported experience of one or more acts of any form of violence by a current or former partner including physical, sexual, psychological, and controlling behavior during the last 12 months.

A woman who shares her violent experience by their former or current intimate partner to any other person or any service was taken as having intimate partner violence disclosure.

Test-retest reliability was measured to determine the reliability of the tool, and to measure its internal consistency, Cronbach's alpha was used and it becomes 0.7.

For the qualitative part, semistructured guiding questions with five items were used and data were collected by the principal investigator. The average length of the interview was 30 minutes. The key guiding questions were as follows: (1) Do you know what intimate partner violence is? (2) What are the different types of intimate partner violence? (3) Does anyone of your neighbor or relative share their violent experience to you? (4) Have you ever share your intimate partner violence experience to others? (5) Why you share your violent experience with others? Audiotape recorders and notes were used to document the data at the time of in-depth interviews and key informant discussion.

2.8. Data Quality Control. To assure the data quality, one-day training was given for data collectors and supervision was made at the time of data collection in each kebele; also, data collection tools were translated from English to Amharic and Gedeo-Offa by experts and back-translated to English to check the consistency. Moreover, a pretest was done in Boiti kebele by taking 5% [16] of the total sample size before one week of the actual data collection, and data were checked for completeness and corrective measures were taken immediately.

2.9. Data Processing and Analysis. Data were cleaned and entered using Epi data version 3.1 then exported to SPSS version 20 for analysis. Data were analyzed using SPSS version 20. Descriptive statistics were computed to determine the prevalence of disclosure of intimate partner violence. Binary and multivariate logistic regression analysis was done to see the association between the dependent (disclosure status of intimate partner violence) and independent variables. Binary logistic regression was used to identify variables that are a candidate for multivariate logistic regression analysis at p value < 0.25, and multivariate logistic regression analysis was used to determine the factors that are independently associated with disclosure status of intimate partner violence at p value < 0.05 with a 95% confidence level. Finally, variables with P value < 0.05 were considered statistically significant. Model fitness was assessed through the Hosmer and Lemeshow test ($p = 0.087$).

For the qualitative part, the data was transcribed and translated from Amharic to the English language by the research team and language teachers independently. Texts were thoroughly read repeatedly to identify thematic areas. Their inductive meanings were extracted and described in narratives thematically. Three of the authors have participated in the thematic analysis. Finally, ideas were triangulated with the quantitative result.

2.10. Ethical Considerations. Ethical clearance was obtained from Jimma University Institute of Health Institutional Review Board with approval number IHRPGD/69/19. Written consent was obtained from the study participants, and the data were collected at a private place to assure confidentiality of the participants. Participants have the right to stop the interviews at any time if they were not interested. Participant information was locked in the file cabinet in the personal possession of the researcher only and will be burned after 5 years. For women who experienced intimate partner violence at the time of screening, the linkage was established with the women's affairs office depending on their willingness for further discussion about violence and to find a solution.

3. Results

3.1. Sociodemographic Characteristics of Study Participants. Two hundred eighty victimized women have participated in the quantitative study that yields a response rate of 90%. The mean age of women was 30.4 (SD ± 5.7) years. The majority (41.6%) of women were Gedeo by their ethnicity and Protestant followers by their religion (43.9%) and 88 (31.1%) were housewives, and about 207 (74%) household heads were partners/husbands; 57 (20.4%) of women reported that their partner had other relationships with other women; majority of the participants (183 (65.4%)) reported that their partner drinks alcohol (Table 1).

3.2. Types of Intimate Partner Violence and Social Support. The most common type of intimate partner violence reported was controlling behavior (236 (84.3%)) followed by physical and emotional violence accounted for 209 (74.6%) and 183 (65.3%), respectively, while sexual violence was the least reported (106 (38.9%)) type of intimate partner violence (Table 2).

More than half (239 (85.4%)) of victimized women had strong social support, and the other (41 (14.6%)) had poor and moderate social support.

3.3. Women Empowerment. From the total of 280 victimized women, 107 (62.5%) of them had access to information about intimate partner violence, 193 (68.9%) were able to visit their family, 244 (87.1%) and 223(79.6%) could independently make a decision on their own and children's health, respectively, and more than half of respondents (166 (59%)) could contribute and make the decision on household purchases.

Table 1: Sociodemographic and behavioral characteristics of respondents ($n = 280$).

Variables	Category	Frequency	Percent
Age of women	18-24	41	14.6
	25-33	164	58.6
	34-49	75	26.8
Ethnicity	Gedeo	136	48.6
	Oromo	69	24.6
	Amhara	40	14.3
	Gurage	26	9.3
	Other (Silta, Dawuro)	9	3.2
Religion	Orthodox	87	31.1
	Protestant	123	43.9
	Muslim	42	15
	Catholic	28	10
Women's educational status	No education	28	10
	Primary education	139	49.6
	Secondary education	54	19.3
	Postsecondary	59	21.1
Partner's educational status	No education	10	3.6
	Primary education	118	42.1
	Secondary education	86	30.7
	Postsecondary	66	23.8
Women's occupational status	Housewife	88	31.4
	Daily laborer	48	17.1
	Governmental worker	65	24.9
	Merchant	38	17.4
	Nongovernmental worker	34	9.5
	Others (no job)	7	2.5
Monthly income in Ethiopian birr	<500	13	4.6
	501-1500	130	46.4
	1501-2500	101	36.1
	>2501	36	12.9
Partner alcohol use status	Yes	183	65.4
	No	97	34.6
Marital duration	<10 years	202	72.1
	>11	78	27.8

3.4. Reproductive Health-Related Characteristics. From the total of 280 victimized women, majority (171 (61.1%), 151(53.9%)) got married and had their first sexual intercourse after the age of 18, majority (182 (65%)) had 1-4 children, and more than one-third (104 (37.1%)) of women were pregnant during the last 12 months.

3.5. Disclosure of Intimate Partner Violence. More than half of victimized women (144 (51.4%)) disclosed their experience of violence by their intimate partner to someone (local elders, family, police, and religious fathers), and most of them (107 (73.8%)) disclosed their intimate partner violence experience to their family (Table 2).

Table 2: Frequency distribution on types of intimate partner violence and its disclosure to whom the disclosure was made among study participants ($n = 280$).

Variable	Frequency	Percent (%)
Types of intimate partner violence ($n = 280$)	280	41.0
(1) Controlling behavior	236	84.3
(2) Physical violence	209	74.6
(3) Emotional violence	183	65.3
(4) Sexual violence	109	38.9
(5) Multiple types of intimate partner violence	239	85.5
Disclosure of intimate partner violence	144	51.4
(1) Family	107	73.8
(2) Husband's family	91	62.8
(3) Friends	76	52.8
(4) Neighbors	81	56.3
(5) Religious leader	44	30.3
(6) Health care provider	12	8.3
(7) Police	23	15.9
(8) Lawyer	8	5.5
(9) Community-based organization	17	11.9
(10) Women affair	30	20.7
(11) Local elders	40	28

From the total victimized women, 136 (48.6%) do not disclose their violent experience by their intimate partner to others due to the following reasons: feeling of embarrassment/shame (72%), do not know where to go (45.2%), not wanting others to be involved (39.5%), and afraid they may not believe me (36.7%) (Figure 1).

3.6. Factors Associated with Disclosure of Intimate Partner Violence. All variables were assessed independently with the dependent variable in the bivariate logistic regression analysis, and those variables having a p value < 0.25 were candidates for multivariate logistic regression analysis (Table 3). Then, from the multivariate logistic regression analysis at p value < 0.05, partner alcohol use (p value = 0.012), partners' educational status (p value = 0.014), social support ($p < 0.01$), the total number of intimate partner violence experienced (p value = 0.003) were significantly associated with disclosure of intimate partner violence.

The Hosmer and Lemeshow goodness of fit test ($p = 0.087$) provides evidence of model fitness with the predicators.

Women whose partners drink alcohol are nearly 2 times more likely to disclose their experience to others (AOR = 1.99, 95% CI: 1.18, 3.34) as compared to those whose partners do not drink alcohol.

Women who experienced only one type of violence were 62% less likely to disclose their violent experience compared to those who experienced multiple types of

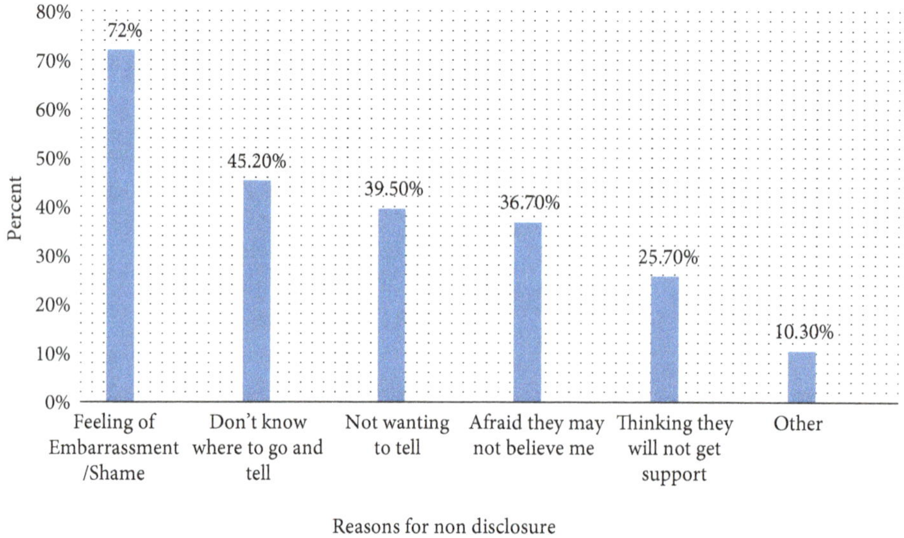

FIGURE 1: Reasons for not disclosing intimate partner violence among violated women in Dilla town, Ethiopia ($n = 136$). *Other—fear of revenge: 10 (7.3%); warned not to tell to any one: 4 (3%).

violence (AOR = 0.38, 95% CI: 0.19, 0.79). Likewise, women who have strong social support were 2.5 times more likely to disclose their violent experience to others as compared to those who have poor social support (AOR = 2.52, 95% CI: 1.44, 4.41).

Women whose husband attain primary and secondary education were two times more likely to disclose their violent experience to others as compared to those women whose husbands attain more than secondary education (AOR = 2; 95% CI:1.07, 3.90) and (AOR = 2; 95% CI:1.07, 4.33), respectively (Table 3).

3.7. Qualitative Part

3.7.1. Reasons for Not Disclosing Intimate Partners' Violence. Taking intimate partner violence as normal, waiting for others to let them talk about their intimate partner violence, and economic dependency on the intimate partner were the main reasons for not disclosing their experience of violence for others as most key informants were saying.

Key informant one reported, "…my mother told me that it is a part of marriage and I go back to my life and nowadays I start taking his behavior normal".

Key informant two also reported, "One day he kicked me severely and I bleed on my left leg and went to the hospital and expecting an opportunity to be asked my experience and waiting for them to ask me about the cause and the offender but they didn't, they only treat the bleeding leg and sent me back, after that time I decided to live my life as it is with a hope that he will be changed".

Key informant three stated, "he was the one who covered almost everything for my mother's medical fee, and school fee since I was grade 8, so how could I leave this man…all of my expenses have been covered by him".

Fear of interference of the third party was one of the reasons for not disclosing intimate partners' violence evidenced by key informants had said.

3.7.2. For Whom They Disclosed Intimate Partners' Violence. Most respondents disclosed their intimate partner violence to their family, supported by the key informants saying.

As key informants, one and three reported, "when they faced intimate partner violence they run away to their family and told their mother…".

3.7.3. Reasons for Intimate Partners' Violence. Women whose partners drink alcohol and having poor social support were the main reasons mentioned by the key informants.

Key informants one and four reported, "…he nagged me, kick me especially things worsen when he drinks alcohol and he became drunk…".

Key informant five said, "since I have good relations with my neighbors…… I get more comfort when they told me their experience …. If they were not on my side things would become worsen".

4. Discussion

This study determines the disclosure of intimate partner violence and associated factors, which is very helpful clinically for health care providers to identify the reasons behind not disclosing violence and to address it before any complication happened by screening women for intimate partner violence routinely. A total of 280 victimized women were involved in the study. The current study revealed that physical violence was the predominant next to controlling behavior and 85% of violated women were reported to be victims of multiple forms of intimate partner violence. It is much higher as compared with the study done in Southeast Nigeria that indicated 58% of violated women experienced multiple forms of intimate partner violence [12].

This study also showed 51.4% (95% CI: 44.7%-57.5%) of violated women disclosed their intimate partner violence experience to others, which is higher than the study done in Lagos, Nigeria, that found out 46% of violated women

Table 3: Bivariate and multivariate logistic regression analysis on factors associated with disclosure of intimate partner violence among victim women, in Dilla town, Ethiopia ($N = 280$).

Variable	Category	Disclosure status Yes	No	COR (95% CI)	p value	AOR (95% CI)
Women's educational status	No education	14 (50%)	14 (50%)	1.27 (0.51, 3.12)	0.006	0.847 (0.3, 2.5)
	Primary education	74 (53.2%)	65 (46.8%)	1.44 (0.78, 2.67)		0.88 (0.4, 1.9)
	Secondary education	30 (55.6%)	24 (44.4%)	1.59 (0.75, 3.34)		1.01 (0.43, 2.34)
	Postsecondary education	26 (44.1%)	33 (55.9%)	1		1
Husband/partner educational status	No education	6 (60%)	4 (40.0%)	2.62 (0.67, 10.2)	0.046	2.1 (0.51, 8.54)
	Primary education	64 (54.2%)	54 (45.8%)	2.07 (1.12, 3.85)		2.04 (1.07, 3.9)*
	Secondary education	50 (58.1%)	36 (41.9%)	2.43 (1.26, 4.70)		2.16 (1.07, 4.33)*
	Postsecondary education	24 (36.4%)	42 (63.6%)	1		1
Husband alcohol use	Yes	105 (57.4%)	78 (42.6%)	2.0 (1.35, 4.06)	0.002	2 (1.18, 3.34)*
	No	39 (40.2%)	58 (59.8%)	1		1
Total number. Of intimate partner violence types(IPV)	≥2 types of IPV	109 (45.6%)	130 (54.4%)	1		1
	1 type of IPV	27 (65.9%)	14 (34.1%)	0.43 (0.22, 0.87)	0.023	0.38 (0.17, 0.79)*
Physical violence	Yes	103 (56.3%)	80 (43.7%)	1		1
	No	41 (42.3%)	56 (57.7%)	1.76 (1.07, 2.09)	0.075	1.58 (0.9, 2.87)
Emotional violence	Yes	114 (54.5%)	95 (45.5%)	1		1
	No	30 (42.3%)	41 (57.7%)	1.64 (0.95, 2.82)	0.026	1.35 (0.7, 2.58)
Social support	Strong	109 (55.1%)	89 (44.9%)	2.50 (1.42, 4.42)	0.001	2.52 (1.44, 4.41)**
	Poor and moderate	27 (32.9%)	55 (67.1%)	1		1
Age at first marriage	≥18 years old	50 (45.9%)	59 (54.1%)	0.7 (0.43, 1.12)	0.225	0.95 (0.82, 1.11)
	≥18 years old	94 (55.0%)	77 (45.0%)	1		1
Age at first sexual intercourse	<18 years old	58 (45.0%)	71 (55.0%)	0.62 (0.38, 0.99)	0.046	0.62 (0.38, 1.01)
	≥18 years old	86 (57.0%)	65 (43.0%)	1		1
Able to visit family	Yes	102 (52.8%)	91 (47.2%)	1.75 (1.04, 2.92)	0.034	0.73 (0.42, 1.13)
	No	34 (39.1%)	53 (60.9%)	1		1
Contribute to the household purchase	Yes	87 (52.1%)	80 (47.9%)	1		1
	No	49 (43.4%)	64 (56.6%)	1.42 (0.88, 2.3)	0.152	1.19 (0.49, 2.91)
A decision on household purchase	Yes	79 (47.6%)	87 (52.4%)	1		1
	No	65 (57.0%)	49 (43.0%)	0.68 (0.42, 1.11)	0.122	0.82 (0.34, 1.95)

AOR: adjusted odds ratio; COR: crude odds ratio; CI: confidence interval, 1: Reference. **Statistically significant at $p < 0.01$; $^{*}p < 0.05$.

disclosed their experience to others [6]. This is also higher as compared with other studies done in Tanzania (40%) [8], Dhaka slums (21%) [26], Nigeria (28%) [6, 12], and Northwest Ethiopia (31%) [13].

The higher proportion of women disclosure in this study area might be due to the difference in gender norms and the presence of conservative cultures that support wife beating which put the women ashamed to disclose their violent experience to others that they rather accept it as part of their life; meanwhile, most of the studies were done in town, whereas this study was done in rural areas.

The majority (73%) of the women disclosed their experience of violence to their family, which is in agreement with the World Health Organization multicountry study [9] and a cross-sectional study done in Nigeria [6, 12, 24], where most women disclose their experience to their family; this might be due to fear of revenge, not wanting to get the perpetrator into trouble, the feeling that the situation was not worth reporting and to keep the situation more private [5, 24]. These outcomes further substantiate the position of the extended circle of relatives in arbitrating intimate partner conflicts, which include violence.

As this study indicates, only 8% of victim women disclosed their violent experience to health care providers that is inconsistent with a study done in Serbia, which suggests 25.7% of victim women disclosed their violent experience to health caregivers [5]. This is probably because of a lack of screening devices, cognizance, and time constraint. From the qualitative part, although individuals wanted to reveal, the findings indicate that possibilities for possible disclosure in healthcare settings are no longer an alternative because most women in the study said they have been in no way asked about intimate partner violence occurrences.

The outcomes on the motives for disclosing propose that encouragement from own family and friends and worry of the impact of the violence on children are the maximum vital triggers for a female to disclose after experiencing intimate partner violence. This is consistent with the findings coming from the WHO multicountry study which states to take a look at women and domestic violence [19]. However, women refraining from disclosing intimate partner violence to the formal institutions could also be an illustration that they lack acceptance as true with or facts on those establishments or that such institutions lack interest in domestic violence [27].

This finding is in line with a look at that accomplished in the United States of America [27] and Dhaka slums [26]. Being embarrassed, having desire to get privacy, and wanting not to contain others on personal lifestyles, fearing of revenge, taking it as a minor incident, preserving it as non-public, and losing belief at the police were the motives raised for no longer disclosing intimate partner violence [27]. This finding also is in keeping with research carried out in south-east Nigeria [12] and Nepal [28]. Meanwhile, encouragement from own family, fear of the impact on children, and severity of the violence are the factors recognized for the motives for disclosure of their violent experience. This is likewise in keeping with different studies performed in deferent countries like Ethiopia [13], Nigeria [24], Nepal [28], and Serbia [5].

Economical dependency turned into an additionally different aspect which hindered women from disclosing their violence to others that is supported by the quantitative result that about half of the respondents have been housewives and the maximum of the choice had been made by their husbands, so a woman may also take her home like a jail so she only does what she was told to by her husband. In such conditions, women regularly fail to disclose to others to sought assistance. This finding is in line with the different studies done in Tanzania [29] and Dhaka slum [26].

This study also showed women whose husbands attained primary and secondary education are more likely to disclose their experience as compared to those who attain more than secondary education [21, 22]. It might be because women, a wife of an educated man, are more likely to keep a secret, to keep his dignity to the level expected by society as an educated, respected, and well-conducted man.

The study also found that woman whose husband drinks alcohol is positively and significantly associated with the disclosure of intimate partner experience to others; this might be due to the fact when they consume alcohol, they may have been more likely to become aggressive and the severity of violence sustained from the drunken perpetrator and this finding is in agreement with a study done in Indonesia [15] and Colombia [25].

Women who have strong social support are more likely to disclose their violent experiences to others compared to those who got poor and moderate social support. This finding is in line with previous studies [30] with the United States of America [27, 31]; however, it is inconsistent with some studies that recognized seeking friend support can trigger negative consequences. Possible clarification is that some friends responded to disclosures and requests for help with negative reactions inclusive of judgment, disbelief, fear, anger, or blaming. These responses, in turn, can cause shame, embarrassment, fear, self-isolation, and a reluctance to disclose abuse at the part of intimate partner violence [4]. This in line with the qualitative finding which reveals fear of interference of the third party was one of the reason; this could be due to the fact that the woman become prejudgmental or the third parties were judgmental; this can display how much the society accepted male dominance in family life so that a woman in violent relation would not volunteer in disclosing her experience of intimate partner violence.

The woman reported being victimized with more than one type of intimate partner violence was more likely to disclose their violent experience to others as compared to those who were a victim of one type of violence. This may be due to the severity of the violence which is in line with a study done worldwide [32, 33].

Women may hide the information as a result of the issue being family secrecy, recall bias, and social desirability bias; not including all screened women for intimate partner violence and not getting 30 women in their home for interview were the limitations of this study.

5. Conclusions

Out of ten victim women, five disclosed their experience to others. Very few women disclose their condition to formal sectors such as women's affairs, health care providers, and police because of embarrassment about the condition; otherwise, the majority disclosed their condition to their family. This showed that the problem is still hidden due to family secrecy. So policymakers, gender offices, and woman's associations should develop strategies that increase women's autonomy and gender equality, involve men and educate them on the gender issue, and encourage them to engage in interspousal communication and on intimate partner violence disclosure; health care providers may help women to reduce subsequent health risks and prevent further violence by early detection of a problem which leads early management and prevents further complications.

Finally, the authors recommend for future researchers to better have men participate in the study especially on the qualitative part and to conduct further interventional research by involving all stakeholders.

Consent

Written consent was obtained from the study participants. Confidentiality and privacy were maintained during data collection, analysis, and reporting.

Authors' Contributions

LA, BT, and RT have contributed to the design, data collection, data analysis, manuscript write up and development, edition, and revision of the final manuscript. All authors read and approved the final manuscript.

Acknowledgments

We would like to thank Jimma University for the financial support, and we are also very grateful to Dilla City Administration for providing important information. Lastly, we would like to extend our deepest gratitude to the study participants.

References

[1] World Health Organization & Pan American Health Organization, "Understanding and addressing violence against women: intimate partner violence," 2012, https://apps.who.int/iris/handle/10665/77432.

[2] Women U nations, *Handbook for Legislation on Violence against Women*, United Nations New York, 2010.

[3] Nations U, *Transforming our World: The 2030 Agenda for Sustainable Development*, United Nations, 2015.

[4] K. M. Sylaska and K. M. Edwards, "Disclosure of intimate partner violence to informal social support network members : a review of the literature," *Trauma, Violence, & Abuse*, vol. 15, no. 1, pp. 3–21, 2013.

[5] B. Djikanović, S. Lo Fo Wong, H. A. Jansen et al., "Help-seeking behavior of Serbian women who experienced intimate partner violence," *Family Practice*, vol. 29, pp. 189–195, 2011.

[6] L. E. E. Okenwa, S. Lawoko, and B. Jansson, "Factors associated with disclosure of intimate partner violence among women in Lagos, Nigeria," *Journal of Injury and Violence Research*, vol. 1, no. 1, pp. 37–47, 2009.

[7] R. M. Laisser, L. Nyström, G. Lindmark, H. I. Lugina, and M. Emmelin, "Screening of women for intimate partner violence: a pilot intervention at an outpatient department in Tanzania," *Global Health Action*, vol. 4, no. 1, p. 7288, 2011.

[8] V. Katiti, G. N. Sigalla, J. Rogathi, R. Manongi, and D. Mushi, "Factors influencing disclosure among women experiencing intimate partner violence during pregnancy in Moshi Municipality, Tanzania," *BMC Public Health*, vol. 16, no. 1, 2016.

[9] C. García-Moreno, H. A. F. M. Jansen, M. Ellsberg, L. Heise, and C. Watts, *WHO Multi-Country Study on Women's Health and Domestic Violence against Women*, World Health Organization, Geneva, Switzerland, 2005.

[10] C. Watts and S. Mayhew, "Reproductive health services and intimate partner violence : shaping a pragmatic response in sub-Saharan Africa," *International Family Planning Perspectives*, vol. 30, no. 4, pp. 207–213, 2004.

[11] T. Riddell, M. Ford-Gilboe, and B. Leipert, "Strategies used by rural women to stop, avoid, or escape from intimate partner violence," *Health Care for Women International*, vol. 30, no. 1-2, pp. 134–159, 2008.

[12] F. C. Anolue, O. I. Uzoma, and O. I. Uzoma, "Intimate partner violence : prevalence, contributing factors, and spectrum among married couples in Southeast Nigeria," *International Journal of Reproduction, Contraception, Obstetrics and Gynecology*, vol. 6, no. 9, pp. 3748–3753, 2017.

[13] A. Semahegn, M. A. Tefera Belachew, and G. Tesfaye, "Women's response towards domestic violence and influencing factors among married women in Fagitalekoma District, North-Western Ethiopia: a cross-sectional study," *EC Gynaecology*, vol. 6, no. 4, pp. 103–112, 2017.

[14] E. N. Hayati, U. Högberg, M. Hakimi, M. C. Ellsberg, and M. Emmelin, "Behind the silence of harmony : risk factors for physical and sexual violence among women in rural Indonesia," *BMC Women's Health*, vol. 11, no. 1, p. 52, 2011.

[15] E. N. Hayati, *Domestic violence against women in rural Indonesia Searching for multilevel prevention*, Umeå University, Sweden, 2013.

[16] L. Michau, D. Naker, and S. Sauve, *Mobilising communities to prevent domestic violence: a resource guide for organisations in East and Southern Africa*, Raising Voices, Kampala, Uganda, 2003.

[17] I. P. Violence and D. Countries, *Estimating the Costs and Impacts of Intimate Partner Violence in Developing Countries a Methodological Resource Guide*, International Center for Research on Women, Kampala, Uganda, 2006.

[18] A. Semahegn and B. Mengistie, "Domestic violence against women and associated factors in Ethiopia; systematic review," *Reproductive Health*, vol. 12, no. 1, p. 78, 2015.

[19] T. Abramsky, C. H. Watts, C. Garcia-Moreno et al., "What factors are associated with recent intimate partner violence? Findings from the WHO multi-country study on women's health and domestic violence," *BMC Public Health*, vol. 11, no. 1, p. 109, 2011.

[20] C. O. Shire, G. P. Shire, and S. Shire, *Preventing and addressing violence against women and children: Strategic Plan*, Geelong Region Alliance, 2015.

[21] Z. N. Azene, H. Y. Yeshita, and F. A. Mekonnen, "Intimate partner violence and associated factors among pregnant women attending antenatal care service in Debre Markos town health facilities, Northwest Ethiopia," *PLoS One*, vol. 14, no. 7, article e0218722, 2019.

[22] B. H. Gebrezgi, M. B. Badi, E. A. Cherkose, and N. B. Weldehaweria, "Factors associated with intimate partner physical violence among women attending antenatal care in Shire Endaselassie town, Tigray, northern Ethiopia : a cross-sectional study, July 2015," *Reproductive Health*, vol. 14, no. 1, p. 76, 2017.

[23] K. Yitbarek, M. Woldie, and G. Abraham, "Time for action: intimate partner violence troubles one third of Ethiopian women," *PLoS One*, vol. 14, no. 5, article e0216962, 2019.

[24] A. O. Ayodapo, O. O. Sekoni, and M. C. Asuzu, "pattern of intimate partner violence disclosure among pregnant women attending ante-natal clinic in Oyo East Local Government, Nigeria," *South African Family Practice*, vol. 59, no. 2, pp. 67–71, 2017.

[25] A. M. Gomez, "Sexual violence as a predictor of unintended pregnancy, contraceptive use, and unmet need Among Female Youth in Colombia," *Journal of Women's Health*, vol. 20, no. 9, pp. 1349–1356, 2011.

[26] K. Parvin, N. Sultana, and R. T. Naved, "Disclosure and help seeking behavior of women exposed to physical spousal violence in Dhaka slums," *BMC Public Health*, vol. 16, no. 1, 2016.

[27] T. Srinivas and A. P. DePrince, "Links between the police response and women's psychological outcomes following intimate partner violence," *Violence and Victims*, vol. 30, no. 1, pp. 32–48, 2015.

[28] P. Silwal, *Violence during Pregnancy among Young Married Women in Nepal*, University of Connecticut, 2012, https://opencommons.uconn.edu/gs_theses/264.

[29] S. Vyas and J. Mbwambo, "Physical partner violence, women's economic status and help-seeking behaviour in Dar es Salaam and Mbeya, Tanzania," *Global Health Action*, vol. 10, no. 1, article 1290426, 2017.

[30] M. R. Yoshioka, L. Gilbert, N. El-bassel, and M. Baig-Amin, "Social support and disclosure of abuse : comparing South

Asian, African American, and Hispanic Battered battered Women women 1," *Journal of Family Violence*, vol. 18, no. 3, 2008.

[31] A. S. Reina, B. J. Lohman, and M. M. Maldonado, "He said they'd deport mevol. 29, no. 4, pp. 593–615.

[32] A. L. Heise and M. Hossain, *Measuring intimate partner violence*, Tech Brief, 2017.

[33] Organization WH, *Putting Women First*, World Health Organization, Geneva, Switzerland, 2001.

16

Histological Pattern of Endometrial Biopsies in Women with Abnormal Uterine Bleeding in a Hospital in North Central Nigeria

Ifeyinwa Mary Asuzu[1] **and Olaejirinde Olaniyi Olaofe**[2]

[1] *Department of Pathology and Forensic Medicine, University of Abuja, Abuja 902101, Nigeria*
[2] *Department of Morbid Anatomy & Forensic Medicine, Obafemi Awolowo University, Ile-Ife 220282, Nigeria*

Correspondence should be addressed to Olaejirinde Olaniyi Olaofe; rindeolaofe@yahoo.com

Academic Editor: Samir Hamamah

The study is a retrospective cross-sectional study carried out in the Department of Pathology of Premier Hospital, Abuja, on specimens received over a one-year period. Four hundred and eighty-six samples of endometrial biopsies and curettings from women presenting with abnormal uterine bleeding sent to the histopathology laboratory were analyzed. The most common biopsies were those of product of conception which accounted for 304 cases (62.6%). Most of the cases of endometrial hyperplasia were typical. Endometritis and chorioamnionitis were the inflammatory conditions seen. Twenty-three women had molar pregnancies. The most common cause of abnormal uterine bleeding in this population is retained products of conception. There may be need to retrain some of the staff involved in the management of pregnancy related complications. There is need to further evaluate pregnancy related complications to ascertain the causes and circumstances responsible for them so as to appropriately direct interventional protocols.

1. Introduction

Endometrial biopsies are obtained for a number of reasons that include abnormal uterine bleeding in certain age groups, incomplete abortions, or suspected neoplasia and the endometrium may be sampled prior to certain procedures to treat infertility to determine the phase of the cycle to guide further tests or treatments [1].

The protocol to handle any endometrial sampling material is guided by the clinical indication for the specimen submission which may be for evaluation of infertility or preparation for In Vitro Fertilization (IVF), evaluation of abnormal uterine bleeding, and follow-up of a previous cytological or histological diagnosis [2].

The endometrium may be examined as part of a hysterectomy specimen and may be the site of a primary or secondary neoplastic process.

Cases of DUB may have structural or functional causes depending greatly on the age of the patient and clinical history [1].

Some studies showed infertility as the most common indication for endometrial biopsy and secretory phase endometrium as the commonest morphologic pattern encountered [3].

A low prevalence of tuberculous endometritis and endometrial carcinoma was also noted in similar studies [3].

Other studies reported endometrial hyperplasia as the most common morphological pattern encountered as well as a good number of endometritis cases though it was not said if endometrial culture was carried out in these cases [4]. Endometrial hyperplasia which is an intraepithelial nonneoplastic proliferative lesion was said to peak around the perimenopausal and menopausal period [5] with variable incidence in other studies [6, 7].

Lesions like endometrial polyps were found among other causes to be the most common structural cause of abnormal uterine bleeding and were of particular importance in patients being considered for IVF [8].

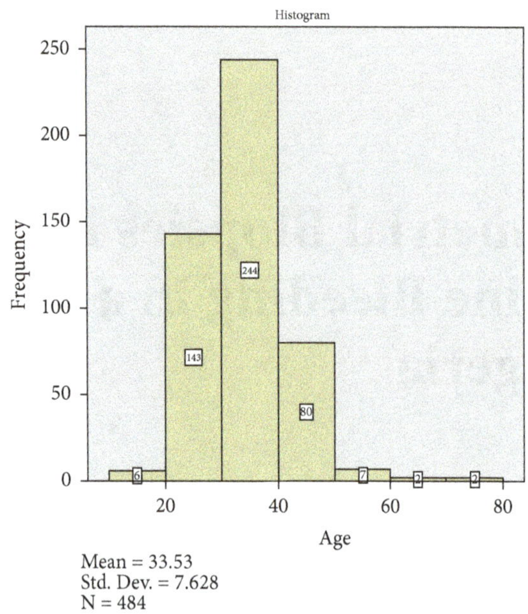

FIGURE 1: Age distribution of the study population. The age group of 30-40 years account for the highest number of cases.

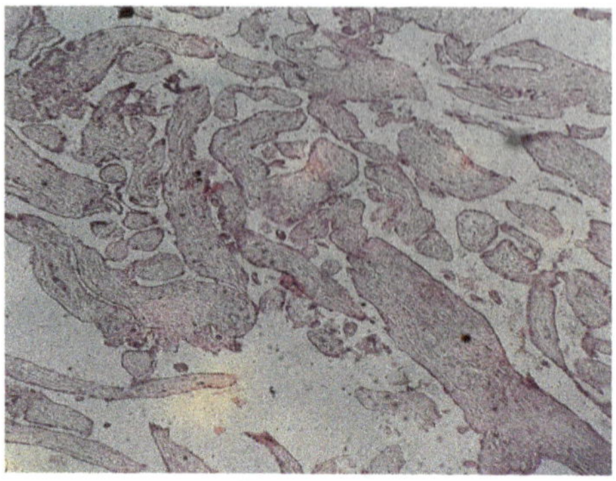

FIGURE 2: Products of conception (MVA). Chorionic villi in a 32-year-old woman who presented with bleeding per vaginam of 8 hours' duration.

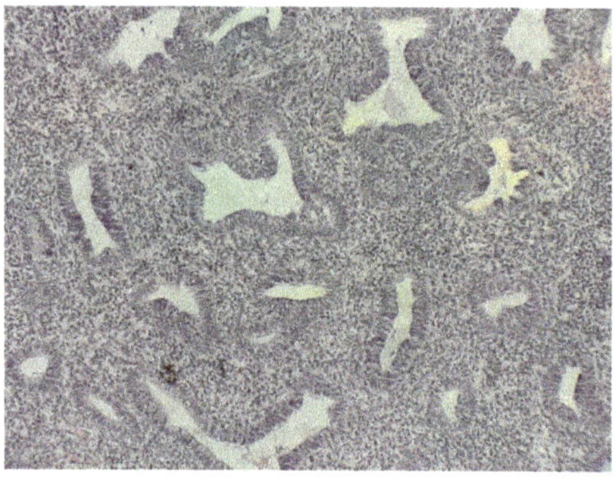

FIGURE 3: Simple typical hyperplasia. Typical hyperplastic glands in a 42-year-old woman who presented with bleeding per vaginam (intermenstrual).

Varied morphological patterns have been reported in various parts of our country and the world usually from tertiary health care centres which may serve as regional reference centres and results from these studies may project abnormally high number of cases. We aim to document findings from a one-year review of cases seen in a community group private practice that caters to both primary health concerns and some degree of specialized care.

2. Materials and Methods

The study is a retrospective cross-sectional study carried out in the Department of Pathology of Premier Hospital, Abuja, on specimens received over a one-year period (June 2016- July 2017).

Four hundred and eighty-six samples of endometrial biopsies and curettings from women presenting with abnormal uterine bleeding sent to the histopathology laboratory were analyzed. Samples were fixed in 10% formal saline and routinely processed and stained with H&E. Histopathological evaluation was done under light microscope and consensus diagnosis was reached by two general pathologists.

Patients were categorized into reproductive age groups (18-40 yrs), perimenopausal (41-50), and postmenopausal (>50yrs).

3. Results and Discussion

A total of 486 endometrial biopsies were seen in Premier Hospital, Abuja, during the study period. The mean age of the patients was 33.53 yrs (SD=7.6). The age distribution of the study population is shown in Figure 1.

The most common biopsies were those of product of conception which accounted for 304 cases (62.6%). A typical case with products of conception is shown in Figure 2. The next most common sample received was that of endometrial hyperplasia (49 cases, 10%). This was closely followed by endometrial polyp which accounted for 48 cases (9.9%). These are shown in Table 1.

The mean age of cases of endometrial hyperplasia was 38.3 years with a range of 22-62 years. Most of the cases of endometrial hyperplasia were typical (41cases). Majority (61%) of the typical endometrial hyperplasia fall in the age group of 18-40 years, while 13 cases (31.7%) were found in the range of 41-50 years. A case of simple typical hyperplasia is shown in Figure 3. Each of the age groups, 18-40 and 41-50 years, account for 4 cases of atypical endometrial hyperplasia.

Most of the cases of endometrial polyp are found in the age group of 30-50 years which accounted for 41 cases (85.4%). Only 3 cases of endometrial polyp were found in women above 50 years of age. These are presented as a chart in Figure 4.

Endometritis and chorioamnionitis were the inflammatory conditions seen. Only four cases of chorioamnionitis were seen. Three of these were in the age group of 18-40 years. Of the seven cases of endometritis seen in this study, one was

TABLE 1: List of various diagnosis and the corresponding age groups.

	18-40 (years)	41-50 (years)	>50 (years)
	INFLAMMATORY LESIONS		
Acute endometritis	3 (75%)	1 (25%)	0 (0%)
Chronic endometritis	3 (100%)	0 (0%)	0 (0%)
Chorioamnionitis	3 (75%)	1 (25%)	0 (0%)
	PROLIFERATIVE NON-NEOPLASTIC LESIONS		
Atypical Hyperplasia-	4 (50%)	4 (50%)	0 (0%)
Typical Hyperplasia	26 (63.4%)	13 (31.7%)	2 (4.9%)
Endometrial polyp	24 (50.0%)	21 (43.8%)	3 (6.3%)
	NEOPLASTIC LESIONS		
Leiomyoma	0 (0%)	2 (100%)	0 (0%)
Partial mole	10 (100%)	0 (0%)	0 (0%)
Complete mole	12 (92.3%)	1 (7.7%)	0 (0%)
Endometroid carcinoma	0 (0%)	0 (0%)	2 (100%)
	NORMAL ENDOMETRIUM		
Proliferative phase	17 (73.9%)	6 (26.1%)	0 (0%)
Secretory phase endometrium	13 (75%)	2 (25.0%)	1 (0%)
	OTHERS		
Products of conception	286 (94.1%)	18 (5.9%)	0 (0%)
Calcified endometrial tissue	2 (100%)	0 (0%)	0 (0%)
Osseous metaplasia	2 (100%)	0 (0%)	0 (0%)
Stromo-glandular dissociation	1 (33.3%)	2 (66.7%)	0 (0%)
Inconclusive	0 (0%)	1 (100.0%)	0 (0%)
TOTAL	406 (83.5%)	72 (14.8%)	8 (1.6%)

a case of tuberculosis seen in a 31-year-old woman with a clinical diagnosis of molar pregnancy.

Two cases of endometrial carcinoma were seen during the study period. The oldest was a 70-year-old woman while the youngest was 60 years old. They both presented with postmenopausal bleeding.

Calcified endometrial tissue was seen in two women aged 38 and 32 years. The two cases were associated with the presence of foreign body in the uterus.

Twenty-three women had molar pregnancies. Ten of these were partial moles which were all found in women in the age group of 18-40 years. This age group also accounted for 12 cases of complete mole. Only one complete mole was seen in the age range of 41-50 years. The mean age of patients with partial mole was 30.3 years, while that of complete mole was 29.8 years. There was no significant association between the types of mole and the age groups ($p=0.37$). A case of complete hydatidiform mole is shown in Figure 5.

There were two cases of osseous metaplasia, all in the age group of 18-40 years. They were associated with the presence of foreign body within the uterus. A case of osseous metaplasia is seen in Figure 6.

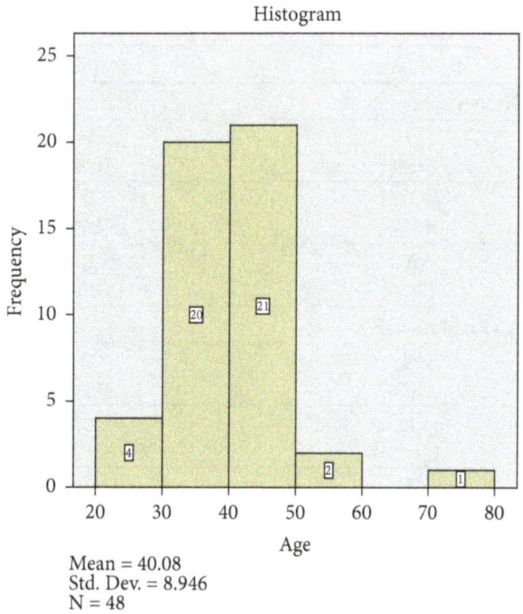

FIGURE 4: Histogram of cases of endometrial polyp. It shows the preponderance of cases of endometrial polyp in the age group of 30-50 years.

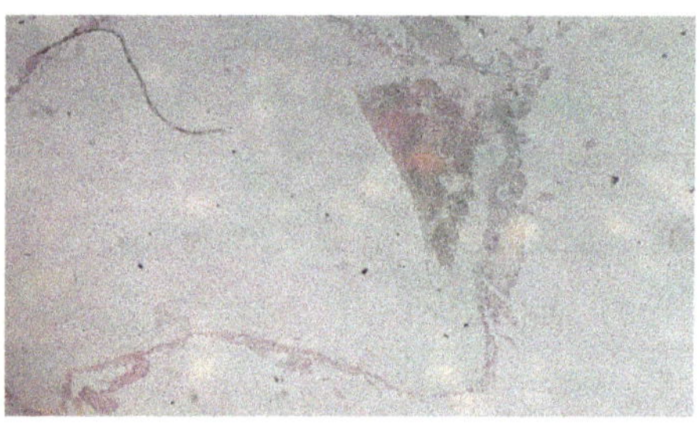

FIGURE 5: Hydropic villus in complete hydatidiform mole. A histologic section of hydropic villus in a 36-year-old woman presenting with vaginal bleeding and passage of grape-like vesicles per vaginam.

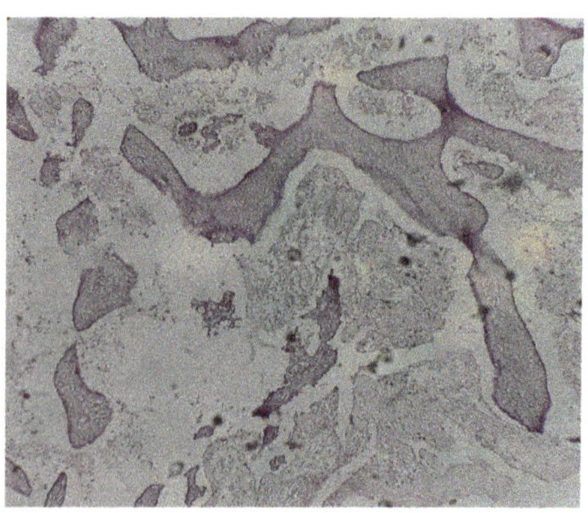

FIGURE 6: Osseous metaplasia. A histologic section of osseous metaplasia in a 29-year-old woman with primary infertility and history of missed abortion.

Submucous leiomyoma was seen in two cases. The older and the younger patients were 44 and 41 years, respectively. They presented with abnormal vaginal bleeding.

Normal endometrium was found in 39 cases. Twenty-three was in proliferative phase and 16 in secretory phase. Most of these cases with normal biopsies were being managed for infertility.

4. Discussion

The study population mainly comprises of women with reproductive health conditions as the hospital is partly specialized in treatment of infertility. Expectedly, the vast majority of the patients fall within the main reproductive years 20-50 age group (467 cases). This is similar to report from a study by Ojo *et al.* from a tertiary center in the same region and studies in a tertiary center in India [1, 3].

The most common cause of abnormal uterine bleeding in this population is retained products of conception similar to reports from India [1] and Ilorin, Nigeria [3], and at variance with studies by Khan *et al.* (5.8%) [4]. This may be attributable to the relatively poor maternal health care in Nigeria, with dwindling resource allocation to health care. Many publications have identified the relatively high incidence of retained products of conception in Nigeria [3]. This can contribute to anaemia and morbidity in women [9]. It may be noteworthy to mention that many minor obstetric procedures are carried out by poorly trained paramedical staff and traditional birth attendants. There may be need to retrain some of these staff in management of such pregnancy related complications. There is also need to further evaluate these cases to ascertain the causes and circumstances responsible for them so as to appropriately direct interventional protocols. S vaidya *et al.* found normal endometrium to be the most common morphological correlate [10].

Endometrial polyp was found in the same frequency in patients above and below 40 years of age. Clinicians should be aware of this fact and should have a high index of suspicion of endometrial polyp in women older and younger than 40 years of age. The high prevalence of endometrial polyps in the patients in this study may not be unrelated to the fact that a number of them may have been on hormonals used for management of infertility. It is important to note that the relatively skewed age distribution may contribute to this finding.

About 39 cases had normal endometrium at either the proliferative or the secretory phases. This accounts for 8% of the cases and were cases of dysfunctional uterine bleeding (DUB). This is at variance with reports from Ilorin which revealed a high frequency of secretory phase endometrium (20.3%) [3] and studies from elsewhere in the world [11, 12]. Gynaecologists should endeavour to thoroughly investigate all cases and not be in a hurry to make diagnosis of DUB. Our study has shown presence of various pathologies in over 90% of cases.

Molar pregnancy was found in 23 cases (4.7%). This is similar to findings in Ilorin (1.5%) [3], due to the relative rarity of the lesion. Most of the patients were below 40 years of age. This is not surprising as the entity is associated with gestation in most cases. Although relatively uncommon, molar gestation should be suspected in all cases of abnormal uterine bleeding especially if there are markedly elevated serum human chorionic gonadotrophins.

Inflammatory conditions were found in 11 cases. Similar frequencies have been reported in Ilorin and some studies from Asia [3, 4, 10, 12], areas with similar socioeconomic conditions. Interestingly, one was a case of tuberculous endometritis. Tuberculosis though said to be endemic in Nigeria is relatively under control especially with the very successful directly observed therapy. It is also important to highlight the fact that the rarity of tuberculous endometritis could be explained by the rapid decline in incidence of disseminated tuberculosis in the country. The study centre is an urban area and may not explain findings in relatively rural settings. However, gynaecologists should be aware that disseminated tuberculosis can result in chronic endometritis with resultant abnormal uterine bleeding. This further reinforces the fact that exhaustive investigations should be carried out on every case of unusual uterine bleeding.

As has been shown in various reports, endometrial carcinoma was found in postmenopausal women [1, 3, 10]. Only two cases were seen in this study similar to reports from comparative studies [1, 3, 10, 11]. This low frequency can be attributed to the fact that the study population mainly consists of women of reproductive age.

5. Conclusions

The most common cause of abnormal uterine bleeding in this population is retained products of conception. There may be need to retrain some of the staff involved in the management of pregnancy related complications. There is need to further evaluate pregnancy related complications to ascertain the causes and circumstances responsible for them so as to appropriately direct interventional protocols. Although relatively uncommon, molar gestation should be suspected in all cases of abnormal uterine bleeding especially if there are markedly elevated serum human chorionic gonadotrophins.

Disclosure

The research was funded by the authors.

References

[1] R. Rena Deka, "Tanma Saikia, Amitabh Handique, Basanta Sonowal. Histopathologic spectrum of Endometrial changes in Women presenting with abnormal uterine bleeding with reference to endometrial malignancies: A two Years Hospital Based Study," *Annals of Applied Bio-Sciences*, vol. 3, no. 2, pp. 152–156, 2016.

[2] G. Steven Silverberg, "The Endometrium. Pathologic Principles and Pitfalls," *Arch Pathol Lab Med*, vol. 131, pp. 372–382, 2007.

[3] B. Ojo, P. Aboyeji, M. Buhari, and M. Abdulraman, "Endometrial pathology in a teaching hospital in North Central Nigeria: a histopathological survey," *Nigerian Journal of Health and Biomedical Sciences*, vol. 4, no. 2, 2006.

[4] R. Khan, R. Sherwan, and S. Rena, "Clinicopathologic pattern in women with DUB," *Iran J Pathol*, vol. 11, no. 1, 2016.

[5] S. D. Reed, K. M. Newton, W. L. Clinton et al., "Incidence of endometrial hyperplasia," *American Journal of Obstetrics & Gynecology*, vol. 200, no. 6, pp. 678–e6, 2009.

[6] LS. Abdullah and NS. Bondaji, "Histopathologic pattern of endometrial sampling performed for abnormal uterine bleeding," *Bahrain Med Bull*, vol. 33, no. 4, pp. 1–6.

[7] S. Dexon, R. Labastide, and A. Anon, "Hysteroscopy in abnormal uterine bleeding," in *In Segler Am. Linde hysteroscopy: Principles and Practice*, pp. 121–134, JB Lippincott, Philadelphia, 1984.

[8] O. G. Eryilmaz, C. Gulerman, E. Sarikaya, H. Yesilyurt, F. Karsli, and N. Cicek, "Appropriate interval between endometrial polyp resection and the proceeding IVF start," *Archives of Gynecology and Obstetrics*, vol. 285, no. 6, pp. 1753–1757, 2012.

[9] M. Mahapatra and P. Mishra, "Clinicopathological evaluation of abnormal uterine bleeding," *Journal of Health Research and Reviews*, vol. 2, no. 2, p. 45, 2015.

[10] F. Deeba, Shaista, and B. Khan, "Histological Pattern Of Endometrial Samples In Postmenopausal Women With Abnormal Uterine Bleeding," *Journal of Ayub Medical College*, vol. 28, no. 4, pp. 721–724, 2016.

[11] P. Kaur, A. Kaur, A. K. Suri, and H. Sidhu, "A two year histopathological study of endometrial biopsies in a teaching hospital in Northern India," *Indian Journal of Pathology and Oncology*, vol. 3, no. 3, p. 508, 2016.

[12] S. Vaidya, M. Lakhey, S. Amatya Vaidya et al., "Histopathological pattern of abnormal uterine bleeding in endometrial biopsies," *Nepal Medical College Journal*, vol. 15, no. 1, pp. 74–77, 2013.

17

Intimate Partner Violence in Pregnancy: Knowledge and Experiences of Pregnant Women and Controlling Behavior of Male Partners in Sokoto, Northwest Nigeria

Oche Mansur Oche, Habibullah Adamu, Aisha Abubakar, Munira Sahabi Aliyu, and Abubakar Shehu Dogondaji

Department of Community Health, Usmanu Danfodiyo University, Sokoto, Nigeria

Correspondence should be addressed to Oche Mansur Oche; ochedr@hotmail.com

Academic Editor: Hind A. Beydoun

Background. Violence against women perpetrated by an intimate partner is an important public health issue. In recent years, attention has focused also on intimate partner violence (IPV) during pregnancy due to its prevalence, adverse health consequences, and intervention potentials. *Aim.* To determine the knowledge, experiences, and factors influencing IPV, including the controlling behaviors of male partners of pregnant women attending an antenatal clinic (ANC) of a tertiary health facility in Sokoto. *Materials and method.* A descriptive cross-sectional study was conducted among 260 pregnant women attending ANC in a tertiary health facility in the Sokoto metropolis. They were selected using a systematic sampling technique, and a set of pretested questionnaire items was used for data collection. Data were analysed using IBM SPSS version 20. *Results.* The respondents' ages ranged from 19 to 40 years with a mean of 29.09 ± 4.99 years, and up to 83.5% of them were in a monogamous setting. Three-quarters of them were Muslims mostly from urban areas (72.1%), and 36.4% had a university or HND degree. Majority of them responded correctly to questions on IPV; overall, up to 99.2% of them had good knowledge of IPV. About 33% of the respondents have experienced IPV while pregnant and up to 61.7% of them said they did nothing because of fear. Some of the controlling behaviors of male partners included always asking for permission before seeing friends and family members and also controlling their finances. Factors associated with IPV include tribe, place of residence, and partner consuming alcohol. *Conclusion.* Majority of the respondents had good knowledge of IPV with about one-third of them ever experiencing it. Respondent's partners were mostly jealous and exhibited some form of controlling behaviors. Physical violence was the most prevalent form, and most of the victims did nothing about it. Government and women's right groups should push for the implementation of tougher punitive measures against perpetrators of IPV.

1. Introduction

Violence against women is a major public health and human rights concern, with intimate partner violence and sexual violence being among the most pervasive forms of violence against women [1]. Although women can be violent in relationships with men, the most common perpetrators of violence against women are male intimate partners or ex-partners [2]. Until recently, most governments have considered violence against women (particularly "domestic" violence by a husband or other intimate partner) to be a relatively minor social problem [3]. In recent times, however, violence against women is recognized as a global concern [3, 4]. Intimate partner violence (IPV) is defined as threatened, attempted, or completed physical or sexual violence or emotional abuse by a current or former intimate partner. It describes the physical, sexual, or psychological harm by a current or former intimate partner or spouse, and this type of violence can also occur among heterosexual or same-sex couples [4]. The World Health Organization (WHO) defines intimate partner violence as an act of coercion, physical abuse, or threat of violence in an intimate relationship [5].

According to WHO, IPV is the most common form of violence against women. Violence by an intimate partner is manifested by physical, sexual, or emotional abusive acts as well as controlling behaviors; although violence occurs in different forms and settings including the workplace, school, and community, violence at home by intimate partner violence is considered as the most prevalent form [6]. The act of physical violence includes slapping, kicking, pushing, and beating, as well as forced sexual intercourse and other forms of sexual coercion. Psychological abuse involves insults, belittling, constant humiliation, threats of harm, or controlling behaviors that consist of isolating a person from friends and families; monitoring their movements; and restricting access to financial resources, employment, education, or medical care [7].

Studies conducted in sub-Saharan African and Asian countries showed an IPV rate ranging from 28% in Madagascar, 74% in Ethiopia, and 57% in India to 87% in Jordan [8]. In a multicountry study conducted in 10 different countries, a rate ranging from 18.5 to 75.8% was reported; domestic violence by an intimate partner alone had a rate of 15.5 to 70.9%, while violence by nonpartners ranged between 5.1 and 64.6% [5]. In Nigeria, a study conducted in Lagos, Southwest Nigeria, on the prevalence and predictors of intimate partner violence exposure showed a one-year prevalence of 29%, with significant proportions reporting psychological (23%), physical (9%), and sexual (8%) abuse, while in Oyo, a study showed that there was a 31.1% prevalence of wife beating among women of reproductive age [9, 10]. In Northern Nigeria, studies conducted among pregnant women in Zaria and Jos showed 28% and 63.2% of the respondents, respectively, experienced some form of abuse [11, 12].

Intimate partner violence in pregnancy has been identified among the leading causes of maternal mortality in some developed countries like the United States and the United Kingdom [13]. Pregnancy-related IPV has been reported to be associated with high perinatal and neonatal mortality risk among exposed women compared to unexposed pregnant women [14]. Neonatal complications include intrauterine growth retardation, preterm delivery, and low birth weight with extended intensive hospitalization [15–19].

Maternal consequences associated with IPV during pregnancy include abortions, miscarriages, preeclampsia, gestational diabetes, and placental abruption [20].

Although the prevalence of IPV is quite high in Nigeria, far fewer cases are reported. This is probably because of the influence of religion and culture especially in many parts of Africa, where culture may allow couples to solve their problem by the use of violence, since most cases of violence against an intimate partner are not seen as wrong. Nigeria still remains patriarchal in nature, where men are regarded as "gods" of the household, controlling every affair, including the women's right to reproductive capabilities [21]. Incidents are therefore, underreported because doing so is viewed as causing indignity to the husband and being disrespectful of family members and elders whose roles include arbitrating in such matters. As a result of this, the true magnitude of the problem is relatively unknown and unexamined [22–24].

Despite increasing research on the prevalence and health effects of IPV during pregnancy from numerous countries around the globe, several gaps in knowledge still exist especially in low- and middle-income countries including Nigeria [25]. Though several studies have been conducted on IPV globally, in Nigeria there is still dearth of information on IPV; most of the studies conducted looked at IPV among women generally, but not much studies had been carried out among pregnant women in Sokoto State despite its effect on the health of the mothers and their babies. Systematic reviews were conducted on domestic violence, which included studies done in different parts of the world; however, studies among pregnant women were not included in the review. The findings showed that relatively few studies and publications emerged from Africa compared to North America and Europe [26]. Furthermore, there are differences in cultural and religious patterns in the different zones in the country; even in the northern part of the country, there are differences in what people regard as IPV [27].

This study, therefore, is aimed at examining the knowledge of IPV, controlling behaviors of male partners, and experiences of intimate partner violence among women attending an antenatal clinic at the Usmanu Danfodiyo University Teaching Hospital, Sokoto.

2. Materials and Method

The study was conducted at the Usmanu Danfodiyo University Teaching Hospital (UDUTH), Sokoto between June and August, 2018. Being a tertiary institution, the hospital provides specialized health care service to Sokoto State, the entire northwestern region of the country, and the neighboring Niger Republic. With a bed capacity of 850, UDUTH has staff strengths of over 1705, which includes doctors, nurses, pharmacists, medical laboratory scientists, and physiotherapists spread across all departments providing curative, preventive, and rehabilitative services. Antenatal clinic service is provided on all the weekdays with an average daily attendance of 250 pregnant women.

The study employed a descriptive cross-sectional study design, and all pregnant women presenting at the ANC clinic for booking or routine antenatal care and must have had a previous pregnancy (inclusion criteria) constituted the study population. Respondents were recruited into the study using the formula for estimating sample size in a population less than 10,000 [28].

After adjusting for a nonresponse rate of 10%, a total of 260 respondents were recruited into the study.

A systematic sampling technique was used to select the study participants after calculating the sampling interval as follows:

$$\begin{aligned}\text{Sampling interval } (k) &= \text{number of pregnant women per booking clinic},\\ \text{Sample size} &= \frac{100}{264},\\ K &= \frac{1}{3}.\end{aligned} \tag{1}$$

Based on the above sampling interval, the systematic sampling technique was carried out as follows:

(i) The first participant was selected using simple random sampling carried out among the first three pregnant women that came for booking

(ii) Thereafter, every third pregnant woman that came to the ANC clinic for booking was enrolled in the study until the required sample size was obtained. This was continued every day until the desired sample size was obtained

A set of pretested semistructured interviewer-administered questionnaire items was administered on the respondents which sought information on respondents' sociodemographic characteristics, their knowledge of IPV, the controlling behavior of partners during pregnancy, the experiences of respondents, and factors influencing IPV during pregnancy.

Data collection using the instrument described above was done with the help of three medical students who were trained by the researchers on the objectives of the study, general principles of research ethics, interpersonal communication, and techniques of data collection.

The data from the questionnaire was manually checked for completeness and entered into IBM SPSS version 20 for electronic data cleaning and analysis. Each correct response to a knowledge variable was awarded a score of one mark, and a zero mark was awarded to each incorrect response. The knowledge scores were added up, converted to percentage, and graded as either good knowledge (score of ≥50%) or poor knowledge (<50%). Continuous variables were summarized as mean and standard deviation, and categorical variables were summarized and presented as frequencies and percentages. This was followed by inferential statistics (bivariate analysis), which were used to identify the major determinants of IPV during pregnancy. The level of statistical significance was set at 5% ($p < 0.05$).

Permission for the study was obtained from the ethics and research committee of UDUTH. Participants were informed of the objectives of the study and were assured of the confidentiality of the information volunteered. Informed verbal consent was also obtained from all the respondents.

3. Results

The respondents' ages ranged from 19 to 40 years with a mean age of 29.09 ± 4.99 years, and up to 83.5% of them were in a monogamous setting. Up to three-quarters of them were Muslims mostly from urban areas (190 (72.1%)), and 92 (36.4%) had a university or HND and 96 (36.9%) belonged to the upper socioeconomic class (SEC); for their partners, 170 (65.4%) were in the upper SEC (Table 1).

Majority of the respondents (239 (92.3%)) were aware of what intimate partner violence is, and a greater proportion of them (102 (39.2%)) heard it from the media. Majority of them responded correctly to questions on IPV; overall, up to 258 (99.2%) of them had good knowledge of IPV (Table 2 and Figure 1).

About one-third of the respondents (84 (32.3%)) said they have to seek for their partners' permission before seeing friends and family, and partners controlled and monitored all their movements (69 (26.5%)) and controlled their finances (28 (10.6%)) (Figure 2).

The lifetime prevalence of IPV in pregnancy was 30.4% ($N = 79$) (Figure 3); a total of 26 (32.9%) of the women experienced IPV in their first pregnancies, while 53 (67.1%) of them occurred during their subsequent pregnancies. About two-thirds of the respondents said the IPV they experienced occurred frequently, and 44 (55.7%) of them said it was less frequent during pregnancy than outside pregnancy. The most common forms of IPV were physical and sexual violence (62.70 and 57.30%, respectively (Figure 4)). Other forms of IPV experienced by respondents include being insulted (78 (30%)), being humiliated (61 (23.5%)), and being forced to have sexual intercourse (39 (15%)) (Table 3).

Regarding the reactions of respondents following the incidences, up to 46 (61.3%) of them admitted doing nothing following IPV, mainly because of fear (35 (77.8%)). Majority of the respondents (236 (90.8%)) believed that IPV is associated with drugs and alcohol consumption, while 249 (95.8%) of them were of the opinion that it is associated with exposure to violence between parents (Table 4).

Regarding factors associated with IPV during pregnancy, up to 31 (62.0%) of those who are of the Yoruba tribe had experienced IPV, whereas only 25 (14.8%) among the Hausa tribe experienced it; the relationship was statistically significant ($X^2 = 71.280$, $p < 0.001$). Similarly, more than half (39 (55.7%)) of those who lived in rural areas experienced IPV as against those living in urban areas and the relationship was statistically significant ($p < 0.001$). Other factors significantly associated with IPV in pregnancy were age ($p = 0.008$), religion ($p < 0.001$), SEC class of both partners, witnessing IPV during childhood ($p < 0.001$), and consumption of alcohol and illicit substances by both partners ($p < 0.001$). Factors such as length of relationship, parity, and knowledge of IPV were not significantly associated with IPV (Table 5).

4. Discussion

Intimate partner violence is a reality that affects people in all walks of life and has remained a problem of public health importance. In this study, the mean age of the respondents was 29.09 ± 4.99 years, which is similar to what was reported in a study on workplace violence and sexual harassment in Ethiopia [29]. The similarity observed in both studies could be attributed to the fact that more than half of the respondents were below 30 years of age; moreover, up to 47.3% of them were within the age group of 20-29 years. More than two-thirds of the respondents in this study were Hausa Muslims, and this could be a reflection of the study area which predominantly comprises of Muslims and people of Hausa ethnicity. However, there is also a notably significant proportion of other tribes including the Yoruba and Igbo

Table 1: Sociodemographic characteristics of respondents.

Variables	Frequency (%)
Age group (years)	
<20	13 (5.0)
20-29	123 (47.3)
30-39	122 (46.9)
40-49	2 (0.8)
Mean	**29.09 ± 4.99**
Marital status	
Married	259 (99.6)
Widowed	1 (0.4)
Type of marriage	
Monogamous	217 (83.5)
Polygamous	43 (16.5)
Religion	
Islam	198 (76.2)
Christianity	61 (23.5)
Others	1 (0.4)
Tribe	
Hausa	169 (65.0)
Yoruba	50 (19.2)
Igbo	21 (8.1)
Fulani	20 (7.7)
Place of residence	
Urban	190 (72.1)
Rural	70 (26.9)
Level of education of wife	
University/HND graduate	92 (36.4)
Diploma/NCE/SSCE	34 (13.1)
Completed primary school/JSS	47 (18.1)
Primary school not completed/	13 (5.0)
Qur'anic school only/none	74 (28.5)
Level of education of husband or partner	
University/HND graduate	140 (53.8)
Diploma/NCE/SSCE	55 (21.2)
Completed primary school/JSS	49 (18.8)
Primary school not completed/	6 (2.3)
Qur'anic school only/none	10 (3.8)
Occupation of wife	
Senior civil servant/professional/manager/ contractor/large scale business	63 (24.2)
Intermediate school civil servant/secondary school teacher	14 (5.4)
Junior secondary school teacher/driver/artisan	53 (20.4)
Petty trader/labourer/messenger	12 (4.6)
Subsistent farmer/student/full-term house wife	118 (45.4)
Occupation of husband/partner	
Senior civil servant/professional/manager/ contractor/large scale business	133 (51.5)
Intermediate school civil servant/ secondary school teacher	39 (15)
Junior secondary school teacher/driver/artisan	42 (16.2)
Petty trader/labourer/messenger	38 (14.6)
Subsistent farmer/student/full-term house wife	7 (2.7)
Wife's SEC	
Upper class	96 (36.9)
Middle class	41 (15.8)
Lower class	123 (47.3)
Husband/partner's SEC	
Upper class	170 (65.4)
Middle class	53 (20.4)
Lower class	37 (14.2)

and this is understandable as this study was conducted in a urban area which is mainly cosmopolitan.

Those who had completed their tertiary education constituted the highest proportion of the respondents (96 (36.4%)), and this is probably because the study was conducted in a teaching hospital located within the metropolis; moreover, most people who belong to the high echelon of society preferred sending their wives to the teaching hospital for ANC where we have an array of specialist gynecologists. The findings were comparable to studies carried out within and outside of Nigeria [2, 11, 30].

Majority of the respondents (92.3%) were aware of what IPV is, and a greater proportion of them 102 (39.2%) heard about it from the media. This high level of awareness observed is not surprising because this study also revealed that up to 99% of the respondents had good knowledge of IPV. Studies conducted in Delta State and Abuja, Nigeria, also made similar observations [31, 32].

Most of the respondents had correct responses to the question regarding forms of violence; however, questions relating to physical violence had more correct responses compared to questions on psychological and sexual violence. The high level of knowledge of the physical form of IPV observed in this study and other studies may likely be attributed to the influence of culture on the perception of what constitutes violence, such that most women especially in Africa only consider the physical form of IPV as violence but do not consider some other forms of IPV as violence. As a result of cultural factors, women tend to believe once you are married, it is the man's right to demand for sex at any time and forcing his spouse to have sexual intercourse is not considered as sexual violence; even the Nigerian law does not clearly state anything regarding issues like marital rape [33–35]. Studies in rural Ethiopia and America on cultural difference in knowledge of violence among Hispanics, African American, and Polish residents also made similar observations where most of the women considered only physical violence as IPV [36, 37]. This underscores the need to educate women on other forms of IPV in a culturally acceptable manner. In terms of overall knowledge of IPV, this study observed that up to 99% of the respondents had

TABLE 2: Knowledge of IPV among pregnant women.

Variables	Frequency (%)
Have you heard of IPV?	
Yes	239 (92.3%)
No	20 (7.7)
Source of information on IPV	
Media	102 (39.2%)
Personal experience	34 (13.1%)
Hospital/health worker	1 (0.4%)
Lecture/seminar	104 (40%)
IPV is a serious public health issue	
Yes	253 (97.3%)
No	7 (2.7%)
Slapping, kicking dragging, beating, choking, pushing, etc., are examples of IPV	
Yes	250 (96.2%)
No	10 (3.8)
Forcing partner to have sex when he/she does not want to	
Yes	227 (87.3%)
No	33 (12.7%)
Forcing partner to do something sexual that he/she finds degrading or humiliating	
Yes	219 (84.2%)
No	41 (15.8%)
Belittling or humiliating a partner in front of other people	
Yes	230 (88.5%)
No	30 (11.5%)
Restricting a partner from contact with family or friends	
Yes	243 (93.5%)
No	17 (6.5%)
Denial of food and other nutritional substance	
Yes	231 (88.8%)
No	29 (11.2)

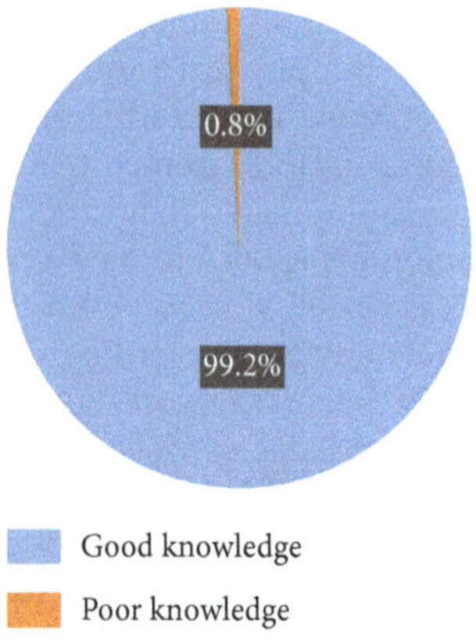

FIGURE 1: Knowledge of intimate partner violence.

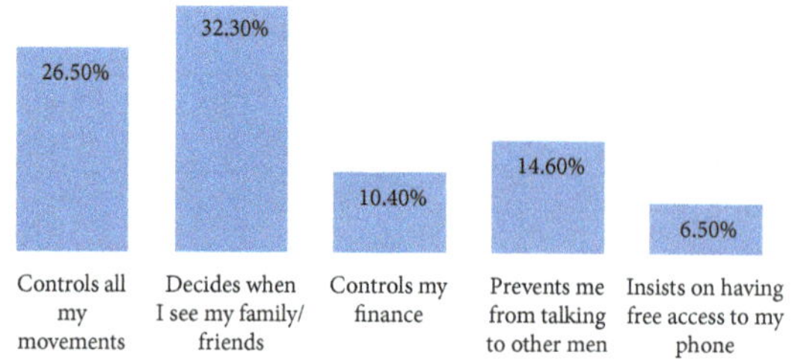

FIGURE 2: Controlling behavior of partner (multiple responses considered).

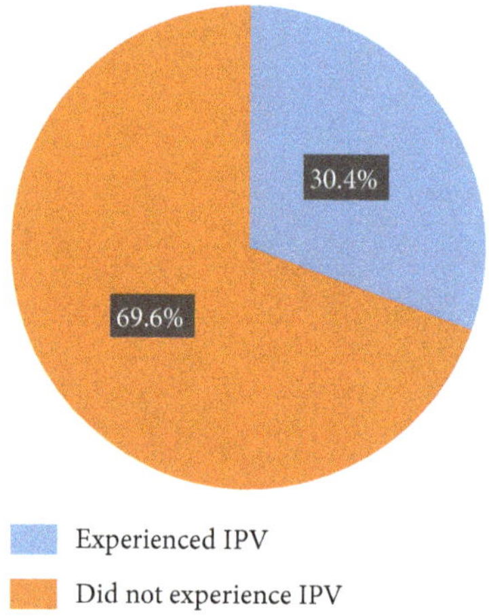

FIGURE 3: Lifetime prevalence of IPV during pregnancy.

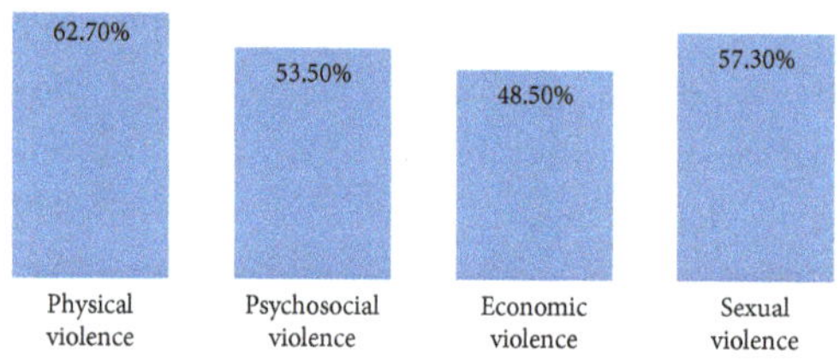

FIGURE 4: Forms of IPV in pregnancy experienced by respondents (multiple responses considered).

good knowledge of IPV and this is much higher than the 72% and 75.7% reported in studies conducted in Jos and Kano Nigeria, respectively [38, 39]. This high proportion of respondents with good knowledge of IPV is not surprising because more than half of the respondents had up to tertiary level education.

Controlling behaviors reported by respondents include having to always ask for permission before seeing friends and family (32.6%) and partners controlling all their movements, including controlling their finances (10.6%). These findings are similar to what was reported in a study involving the use of secondary data from NDHS 2008 but lower than the 43.3% reported in another study conducted in Kano [27, 40]. Controlling behavior by the husband/partner has been shown to be associated with both physical and sexual IPV [41, 42], and it is a reflection of the increased vulnerability to abuse by women residents in societies that validate a male-dominated family structure and social order and

TABLE 3: Experience of women on various forms of IPV during pregnancy.

Variables	Frequency (%)
Have you ever experienced IPV during pregnancy?	
Yes	79 (30.4%)
No	181 (69.6%)
If yes, during which pregnancy was IPV experienced?	
First	26 (32.9%)
Subsequent pregnancies	53 (67.1%)
Was the pregnancy you experienced IPV desired and planned for?	
Yes	217 (83.5%)
No	43 (16.5%)
Number of times you ever experienced IPV during pregnancy?	
Once	13 (16.5%)
Twice	9 (11.4%)
More than twice	5 (6.3%)
Frequently	52 (65.8%)
Magnitude of intimate partner violence during pregnancy compared to outside pregnancy	
More frequent	7 (8.8%)
Less	44 (55.7%)
Same	28 (35.4%)
Type of physical violence experienced during pregnancy	
Pushing, shoving, pulling hair, or slapping	14 (17.8%)
Kick on the abdomen, beating, or choking	58 (73.4%)
Thrown something at, attempted burning	7 (8.8%)
Has your partner ever insulted or made you feel bad?	
Yes	78 (30%)
No	182 (70%)
Did your partner ever belittle or humiliate you before people	
Yes	61(23.5%)
No	199 (76.5%)
Has your partner/husband ever taken your earnings or savings against your will?	
Yes	48 (18.5%)
No	212 (81.5%)
Has your partner ever refused to give you money for household expenses?	
Yes	78 (30%)
No	182 (70%)
Have you ever been forced by your partner to have sexual intercourse by threatening you or withholding certain things?	
Yes	39 (15%)
No	221 (85%)
Do you agree to have scxual intercourse with your partner when you do not want to?	
Yes	110 (42.3%)
No	150 (57.7%)

TABLE 4: Reactions of respondents following their experience of IPV during pregnancy.

Variables	Frequency (%)
If you have experienced IPV during pregnancy, what did you do?	
Nothing	46 (61.3%)
Reported him to relations	19 (25.3%)
Quit relationship	10 (13.3%)
If nothing, why?	
Fear	35 (77.8%)
I forgave him	10 (22.2%)
Did you seek for medical care following the effect of the violence?	
Yes	58 (79.5%)
No	15 (20.5%)
If yes, how were you managed?	
In-patient	29 (50.9%)
Out-patient	28 (49.1%)
If you did not seek for medical care why?	
Due to fear	5 (33.3%)
Lack of finance	3 (20.0%)
Shame	7 (46.7%)
If you have experienced IPV during pregnancy, did anyone try to help you out?	
Yes	40 (51.9%)
No	37 (48.1%)
If yes, who?	
Family	24 (60.0%)
Close friends	16 (40.0%)
IPV is associated with harmful use of drugs and alcohol	
Yes	236 (90.8%)
No	24 (9.2%)
IPV is associated with exposure to violence between parents	
Yes	249 (95.8%)
No	11 (4.2%)
IPV affects the victim's health status and lifestyle	
Yes	250 (96.2%)
No	10 (3.8%)
Do you think IPV during pregnancy should be encouraged by the society?	
Yes	0 (0.0%)
No	260 (100%)

encourage men to exercise control over women. This finding is in support of the feminist theory [43] and is also in favor of the hypothesis that controlling behavior is associated with increased likelihood of violence, most likely acting as a precursor to violence.

Close to one-third of the respondents had experienced IPV at least in one of their pregnancies, with a significant proportion (65.8%) of women reporting frequent exposure

TABLE 5: Factors associated with IPV during pregnancy.

Variables	Ever experienced IPV during pregnancy? Yes	No	Test statistic
Age (years)			
<20 years	0 (0)	13 (100)	$X^2 = 11.105$
20-29 years	47 (38.2)	76 (61.8)	
30-39 years	32 (26.2)	90 (73.8)	$p = 0.008$
40-49 years	0 (0)	2 (100)	
Tribe			
Hausa	25 (14.8)	144 (85.2)	$X^2 = 71.286$
Yoruba	31 (62.0)	19 (38.0)	
Igbo	6 (28.6)	15 (71.4)	$p < 0.001$
Fulani	17 (85.0)	3 (15.0)	
Religion			
Islam	39 (19.7)	159 (80.3)	$X^2 = 45.44$
Christianity	39 (63.9)	22 (36.1)	$p < 0.001$
Others	1 (100)	0 (0)	
Place of residence			
Urban	40 (21.1)	150 (78.9)	$X^2 = 29.055$
Rural	39 (55.7)	31 (44.3)	$p < 0.001$
Wife's SEC			
Upper class	5 (5.2)	91 (94.8)	$X^2 = 47.49$
Middle class	15 (36.6)	26 (63.4)	$p < 0.001$
Lower class	59 (48.0)	64 (52.0)	
Husband/partner's SEC			
Upper class	36 (21.2)	134 (78.8)	$X^2 = 19.709$
Middle class	25 (47.2)	28 (52.8)	$p < 0.001$
Lower class	18 (48.6)	19 (51.4)	
Parity			
Primi	5 (14.3)	30 (85.7)	$X^2 = 5.054$
Multipara	58 (32.4)	121 (67.6)	$p = 0.076$
Grand multipara	16 (34.8)	30 (65.2)	
Length of relationship			
1-5 years	19 (26.4)	53 (73.6)	$X^2 = 3.820$
6-10 years	46 (35.9)	82 (64.1)	$p = 0.149$
>10 years	14 (23.3)	46 (76.7)	
Witnessed IPV during your childhood?			
Yes	30 (88.2)	4 (11.2)	$X^2 = 61.887$
No	49 (21.7)	177 (78.3)	$p < 0.001$
Who chose your partner for you?			
Parents	16 (34.8)	30 (65.2)	$X^2 = 0.511$
Myself	63 (29.4)	151 (70.6)	$p = 0.483$
Who takes the most important decision for your family?			
My partner	16 (100)	0 (0)	$X^2 = 52.342$

TABLE 5: Continued.

Variables	Ever experienced IPV during pregnancy? Yes	No	Test statistic
Both of us	58 (24.3)	181 (75.7)	$p < 0.001$
In-laws	5 (100)	0 (0)	
Do you consume alcohol?			
Yes	8 (88.9)	1 (11.1)	$X^2 = 15.085$
No	71 (28.3)	180 (71.7)	$p < 0.001$
Does your partner consume alcohol?			
Yes	41 (95.3)	2 (4.7)	$X^2 = 102.795$
No	38 (17.5)	179 (82.5)	$p < 0.001$
Do you use illicit drugs/substances?			
Yes	29 (96.7)	1 (3.3)	$X^2 = 71.403$
No	49 (21.4)	180 (78.6)	$p < 0.001$
Does your partner use illicit drugs/substances?			
Yes	6 (85.7)	1 (14.3)	$X^2 = 10.411$
No	73 (28.9)	180 (71.1)	$p = 0.004$
Is your partner very jealous?			
Yes	75 (32.5)	156 (67.5)	$X^2 = 3.894$
No	4 (14.3)	24 (85.7)	$p = 0.052$
Knowledge of IPV			
Good knowledge	2 (100)	0 (0)	$p = 0.091$
Poor knowledge	76 (29.7)	180 (70.3)	(Exact)

by their husband/male partner. This is in tandem with the finding from the study by Sigalla et al. in Tanzania where a prevalence of IPV in pregnancy of 30% was observed [44].

However, the prevalence of IPV recorded in our study is lower than what was reported from similar studies on magnitude and correlates of IPV in Ethiopia [45] and in Southwest Nigeria [46], where the lifetime prevalence of intimate partner violence was 70%. The lower prevalence in this study could probably be due to the fact that this study looked at IPV in pregnancy as against the other studies that looked at lifetime prevalence both in and outside pregnancy. Despite the fact that the prevalence of IPV observed in this study is lower than the lifetime prevalence observed in other studies, it still carries huge public health implications because IPV in pregnancy has been shown to be associated with a higher rate of maternal and foetal outcomes [19, 47–50].

Of the various forms of IPV experienced during pregnancy, physical violence was the most common (62.7%). Studies conducted in Kano and Oyo States reported lower prevalences [40, 51]. However, higher rates of physical violence were also reported in studies conducted in southwest Ethiopia, Tanzania, eastern Nigeria, Bangladesh, Ukraine, and Peru [45, 50–54].

Close to two-thirds of the study subjects opined that they received kicks on the abdomen, beating, and choking whereas a smaller proportion (17.8%) said pushing, shoving, pulling of hair, and slapping were the forms of physical violence that they experienced. Empirical evidence has shown that such kicks to the pregnant abdomen do result in devastating effects on both the mother and the foetus; in a Tanzanian study, 23 and 38% of all women exposed to physical violence during pregnancy suffered blows to the abdomen [50] which may lead to placental damage, rupture of the membrane, and consequently premature uterine contractions [55].

These forms of physical violence were also reported from other studies within and outside Nigeria; for example, in a study conducted in Southwest Nigeria, the major types of physical violence experienced were being slapped (27.2%), being kicked (14.4%), and being hit (13.4%), [56] and in Malawi 20% reported being pushed, shaken, slapped, or punched [57]. A little above half (57.3%) of the respondents experienced sexual violence during pregnancy. A World Health Organization multicountry study observed that the lifetime prevalence of sexual violence by an intimate partner in most sites studied was between 10 and 50% [5]. Sexual violence was reportedly lower compared to physical violence probably because of the fact that issues of sex are still regarded as a taboo and should not be openly discussed [35, 36]. In a similar study carried out in Lima, Peru, the lifetime prevalence of sexual violence was 8.7% [58].

Regarding the action taken by respondents after exposure to IPV, up to 61.3% of them said they did nothing and the reason given by 77.8% of them was that it was because of fear of repercussions. In a study on the disclosure of IPV conducted in Lagos, slightly more than half (54%) of the respondents agreed that they would not disclose their experiences of violence to anyone [59]. Traditionally, women especially in rural areas are often encouraged to stay in abusive relationships without disclosing their experiences to anyone, due to the strong cultural belief that a woman's place is with her husband and also because divorced and separated women are not held in high social esteem compared to women who remain in marriage. This could well be the reasons why most felt reporting was unnecessary and couples should rather handle their own issues as culture and religion advocates that women should learn to endure and be patient in all circumstances. Anecdotal evidence in most parts of Nigeria showed that mothers of victims of IPV would ask them to remain in their husbands' homes saying "after all, we the mothers went through the same experiences in the hands of your fathers".

Regarding factors associated with IPV during pregnancy, this study revealed that the tribe of the respondents was significantly associated with IPV; up to 62% of those who are of the Yoruba tribe had experienced IPV, whereas only 14.8% from among the Hausa tribe experienced it. This is not surprising because according to the NDHS 2013 report, IPV in pregnancy is higher in Southwest Nigeria (where Yoruba is the predominant tribe) than in Northwest Nigeria which has the highest proportion of people of the Hausa tribe in the country [27]. This may not be related to the fact that the sociocultural milieu of Sokoto State, the study area, does not encourage the reporting of incidents of IPV. Also, more than half (55.7%) of those who lived in the rural areas experienced IPV compared to those living in urban areas and this is similar to what was observed in other studies from Southwest Nigeria [23, 46].. However, findings from a study in Southwest Nigeria and Ethiopia were at variance with what was obtained in this study, where those with formal education formed a larger proportion of those experiencing abuse [45, 59]. This variation shows that violence cuts across all groups, and the belief that only women who are uneducated face violence may be exaggerated because there are many other factors that contribute to women's risk of intimate partner violence. Other factors significantly associated with IPV in pregnancy are age, religion, witnessing IPV during childhood, and consumption of alcohol and illicit substances by both partners. Evidence has shown that IPV occurred more among those whose partners consumed alcohol [51]. This suggests that if alcohol consumption by male intimate partners can be well controlled, then the prevalence of IPV may also be reduced significantly. Factors such as length of relationship, parity, and knowledge of IPV were not significantly associated with IPV.

Findings from this study buttresses the fact that the occurrence of IPV is an interplay of different factors which may solely be due to differences in individuals, culture, and the society, as what is obtained in one setting, even though it may be similar, may not apply in another.

5. Conclusion

A very high proportion of the respondents had good knowledge of IPV, and about one-third of them had experienced IPV in pregnancy. A sizeable number of the respondents that experienced IPV did nothing about it, mainly due to fear of what might follow. This fear may not be unrelated to the sociocultural milieu of the study area where religion controls the social lives of the inhabitants especially the womenfolk. Factors associated with IPV include tribe, place of residence, level of education of partners, and alcohol consumption. Increased public awareness on the dangers inherent in IPV should be intensified while governments at all levels and law enforcement agencies should ensure that the perpetrators are made to face the law and stiffer penalties are meted out to perpetrators of IPV, while at the same time encouraging victims of IPV to speak out regardless of length of onset. Women's organizations must be in the vanguard for the fight against IPV and to come up with avenues and measures to break the cycle of silence and to fight for the rights of women, while also rehabilitating victims of such acts.

5.1. Study Limitations. Intimate partner violence is a culturally sensitive issue in this part of the world and victims are afraid of retributions, hence some may inadvertently hoard important information. We tried from the onset to allay their fears and assure them of the confidentiality of any information divulged to the researchers.

References

[1] World Health Organization, "Responding to intimate partner violence and sexual violence against women: WHO clinical and policy guidelines," *NLM classification: HV 6625*, 2013, May 2015, https://www.who.int/iris/bitstream/10665/85240/1/9789241548595_eng.pdf.

[2] World Health Organization, *Understanding and addressing violence against women. Publication No.*, WHO/RHR/12.36, 2012, June 2015, https://www.who.int/iris/bitstream/10665/77432/1/WHO_RHR_12.36_eng.pdf.

[3] E. Abama and M. A. Chris, "Violence against women in Nigeria: how the Millennium Development Goals addresses the challenge," *The Journal of Pan African Studies*, vol. 3, pp. 23–34, 2009.

[4] National Institute of Justice, "Intimate partner violence," 2007, January 13, 2019 https://www.nij.gov/topics/crime/intimatepartner-violence/Pages/welcome.aspx.

[5] C. Garcia-Moreno, H. A. F. M. Jansen, M. Ellsberg, L. Heise, and C. H. Watts, "Prevalence of intimate partner violence: findings from the WHO multi-country study on women's health and domestic violence," *The Lancet*, vol. 368, no. 9543, pp. 1260–1269, 2006.

[6] World Health Organization, "Violence: A Public Health Priority," in *WHO Global Consultation on Violence and Health*, World Health Organization, Geneva, 1996, document WHO/EHA/SPI.POA.2.

[7] E. G. Krug, J. A. Mercy, L. L. Dahlberg, and A. B. Zwi, "The World report on violence and health," *The Lancet*, vol. 360, no. 9339, pp. 1083–1088, 2002.

[8] O. A. Uthman, S. Lawoko, and T. Moradi, "Factors associated with attitudes towards intimate partner violence against women: a comparative analysis of 17 sub-Saharan countries," *BMC International Health and Human Rights*, vol. 9, no. 1, article 14, 2009.

[9] L. E. Okenwa, S. Lawoko, and B. Jansson, "Exposure to intimate partner violence amongst women of reproductive age in Lagos, Nigeria: prevalence and predictors," *Journal of Family Violence*, vol. 24, no. 7, pp. 517–530, 2009.

[10] O. I. Fawole, A. L. Aderonmu, and A. O. Fawole, "Intimate partner abuse: wife beating among civil servants in Ibadan, Nigeria," *African Journal of Reproductive Health*, vol. 9, no. 2, pp. 54–64, 2005.

[11] N. Ameh and M. A. Abdul, "Prevalence of domestic violence amongst pregnant women in Zaria, Nigeria," *Annals of African Medicine*, vol. 3, no. 1, pp. 4–6, 2004.

[12] A. Gyuse and A. P. Ushie, "Pattern of domestic violence among pregnant women in Jos, Nigeria," *South African Family Practice*, vol. 51, no. 4, pp. 343–345, 2009.

[13] G. Lewis, "Statistics: incidence and prevalence of domestic violence," 2007, https://www.wewillspeakout.org/wp-content/uploads/2013/03/domestic-violence.

[14] E. I. Mbadugha, "Intimate partner violence and sexual violence against women: any end in sight?," *International journal of Medicine and Biomedical Research*, vol. 5, no. 1, pp. 9–18, 2016.

[15] N. Linos, N. Slopen, S. V. Subramanian, L. Berkman, and I. Kawachi, "Influence of community social norms on spousal violence: a population-based multilevel study of Nigerian women," *American Journal of Public Health*, vol. 103, no. 1, pp. 148–155, 2013.

[16] A. Bandura, *Social Learning Theory*, General Learning Press, New York, NY, 1977, http://www.asecib.ase.ro/mps/Bandura_SocialLearningTheory.pdf.

[17] M. A. A. Nunes, S. Camey, C. P. Ferri, P. Manzolli, C. N. Manenti, and M. I. Schmidt, "Violence during pregnancy and newborn outcomes: a cohort study in a disadvantaged population in Brazil," *The European Journal of Public Health*, vol. 21, no. 1, pp. 92–97, 2011.

[18] S. E. Sanchez, A. V. Alva, G. Diez Chang et al., "Risk of spontaneous preterm birth in relation to maternal exposure to intimate partner violence during pregnancy in Peru," *Maternal and Child Health Journal*, vol. 17, no. 3, pp. 485–492, 2013.

[19] D. K. Kaye, F. M. Mirembe, G. Bantebya, A. Johansson, and A. M. Ekstrom, "Domestic violence during pregnancy and risk of low birthweight and maternal complications: a prospective cohort study at Mulago Hospital, Uganda," *Tropical Medicine and International Health*, vol. 11, no. 10, pp. 1576–1584, 2006.

[20] K. M. Devries, S. Kishor, H. Johnson et al., "Intimate partner violence during pregnancy: analysis of prevalence data from 19 countries," *Reproductive Health Matters*, vol. 18, no. 36, pp. 158–170, 2010.

[21] S. Ahmed, M. A. Koenig, and R. Stephenson, "Effects of domestic violence on perinatal and early-childhood mortality: evidence from North India," *American Journal of Public Health*, vol. 96, no. 8, pp. 1423–1428, 2006.

[22] R. M. Laisser, L. Nyström, H. I. Lugina, and M. Emmelin, "Community perceptions of intimate partner violence - a qualitative study from urban Tanzania," *BMC women's Health*, vol. 11, no. 1, article 13, 2011.

[23] A. O. Fatusi and O. I. Alatise, "Intimate partner violence in Ile-Ife, Nigeria: women's experiences and men's perspectives," *Gender and Behaviour*, vol. 4, no. 2, pp. 764–781, 2007.

[24] M. Rani, S. Bonu, and N. Diop-Sidibe, "An empirical investigation of attitudes towards wife-beating among men and women in seven sub-Saharan African countries," *African Journal of Reproductive Health*, vol. 8, no. 3, pp. 116–136, 2004.

[25] World Health Organization, *Understanding and Addressing Violence against Women: Intimate Partner Violence during Pregnancy*, World Health Organization, 2012, WHO_RHR_11_.35_eng.pdf.

[26] S. Alhabib, U. Nur, and R. Jones, "Domestic violence against women: systematic review of prevalence studies," *Journal of Family Violence*, vol. 25, no. 4, pp. 369–382, 2010.

[27] National Population Commission-NPC/Nigeria and ICF, *Nigeria Demographic and Health Survey 2018*, NPC and ICF, Abuja, Nigeria and Rockville, MD, USA, 2019.

[28] M. O. Araoye, *Research Methodology with Statistics for Health and Social Sciences*, Nathadex Publishers, Ilorin, 2004.

[29] J. Marsh, S. Patel, B. Gelaye et al., "Prevalence of workplace abuse and sexual harassment among female faculty and staff," *Journal of Occupational Health*, vol. 51, no. 4, pp. 314–322, 2009.

[30] L. Heise, "Violence against women: global organizing for change," in *Future Interventions with Battered Women and their Families*, J. L. Edleson and Z. C. Eisikovits, Eds., pp. 7–33, CA, Sage Publications, Thousand Oaks, 1996.

[31] V. Awusi, V. Okeleke, and B. Ayanwu, "Prevalence of domestic violence during pregnancy in Oleh, a suburban Isoko commu-

nity, Delta State, Nigeria," *Benin Journal of Postgraduate Medicine*, vol. 11, no. 1, 2009.

[32] E. R. Efetie and H. A. Salami, "Domestic violence on pregnant women in Abuja, Nigeria," *Journal of Obstetrics and Gynaecology*, vol. 27, no. 4, pp. 379–382, 2007.

[33] K. A. Oyediran and U. C. Isiugo-Abanihe, "Perceptions of Nigerian women on domestic violence: evidence from 2003 Nigeria Demographic and Health Survey," *African Journal of Reproductive Health*, vol. 9, no. 2, pp. 38–53, 2005.

[34] O. Ogunsiji, L. Wilkes, D. Jackson, and K. Peters, "Suffering and smiling: West African immigrant women's experience of intimate partner violence," *Journal of Clinical Nursing*, vol. 21, no. 11-12, pp. 1659–1665, 2012.

[35] E. Robson, "Wife seclusion and the spatial praxis of gender ideology in Nigerian Hausaland," *Gender, Place & Culture*, vol. 7, no. 2, pp. 179–199, 2000.

[36] W. Shanko, M. Wolday, N. Assefa, and A. R. Aro, "Domestic violence against women in Kersa, Oromia region, eastern Ethiopia," *Eastern Mediterranean Health Journal*, vol. 19, no. 1, pp. 18–23, 2013.

[37] K. Wytrykowska, "Cultural Differences in Knowledge and Reporting of Domestic Violence, [*M. S. thesis*]," Criminal Justice submitted to Central Connecticut State University, 2011.

[38] E. Ochai, "Knowledge and attitude of women towards intimate partner violence: a study of women in Tudun Wada community in Jos," *Injury Prevention*, vol. 16, article A229, Supplement 1, 2010.

[39] A. Salaudeen, T. M. Akande, O. I. Musa, J. O. Bamidele, and F. A. Oluwole, "Assessment of violence against women in Kano metropolis, Nigeria," *The Nigerian Postgraduate Medical Journal*, vol. 17, no. 3, pp. 218–222, 2010.

[40] T. S. Tanimu, S. Yohanna, and S. Y. Omeiza, "The pattern and correlates of intimate partner violence among women in Kano, Nigeria," *African Journal of Primary Health Care and Family Medicine*, vol. 8, no. 1, pp. e1–e6, 2016.

[41] A. J. Gage and P. L. Hutchinson, "Power, control and intimate partner sexual violence in Haiti," *Archives of Sexual Behavior*, vol. 35, no. 1, pp. 11–24, 2006.

[42] G. Krantz and N. D. Vung, "2The role of controlling behaviour in intimate partner violence and its health effects: a population based study from rural Vietnam," *BMC Public Health*, vol. 9, no. 1, article 143, Article ID 1546, 2009.

[43] T. K. Shackelford and A. T. Goetz, "Men's sexual coercion in intimate relationships: development and initial validation of the sexual coercion in intimate relationships scale," *Violence and Victims*, vol. 19, no. 5, pp. 541–556, 2004.

[44] G. N. Sigalla, D. Mushi, D. W. Meyrowitsch et al., "Intimate partner violence during pregnancy and its association with preterm birth and low birth weight in Tanzania: a prospective cohort study," *PLoS One*, vol. 12, no. 2, article e0172540, 2017.

[45] K. Deribe, B. K. Beyene, A. Tolla, P. Memiah, S. Biadgilign, and A. Amberbir, "Magnitude and correlates of intimate partner violence against women and its outcome in Southwest Ethiopia," *PloS One*, vol. 7, no. 4, article e36189, 2012.

[46] M. O. Balogun, E. T. Owoaje, and O. I. Fawole, "Intimate partner violence in southwestern Nigeria: are there rural-urban differences?," *Women & Health*, vol. 52, no. 7, pp. 627–645, 2012.

[47] B. Parker, J. McFarlane, and K. Soeken, "Abuse during pregnancy: effects on maternal complications and birth weight in adult and teenage women," *Obstetrics and Gynecology*, vol. 84, no. 3, pp. 323–328, 1994.

[48] H. Blencowe, S. Cousens, M. Z. Oestergaard et al., "National, regional, and worldwide estimates of preterm birth rates in the year 2010 with time trends since 1990 for selected countries: a systematic analysis and implications," *The Lancet*, vol. 379, pp. 2162–2172, 2012.

[49] B. Mahenge, S. Likindikoki, H. Stöckl, and J. Mbwambo, "Intimate partner violence during pregnancy and associated mental health symptoms among pregnant women in Tanzania: a cross-sectional study," *BJOG: An International Journal of Obstetrics & Gynaecology*, vol. 120, no. 8, pp. 940–947, 2013.

[50] H. Stockl, C. Watts, and J. K. Kilonzo Mbwambo, "Physical violence by a partner during pregnancy in Tanzania: prevalence and risk factors," *Reproductive Health Matters*, vol. 18, no. 36, pp. 171–180, 2010.

[51] O. Yusuf, O. Arulogun, O. Oladepo, and F. Olowokeere, "Physical violence among intimate partners in Nigeria: a multi level analysis," *Journal of Public Health and Epidemiology*, vol. 3, no. 5, pp. 240–247, 2011.

[52] A. L. Ilika, "Women's perception of partner violence in a rural Igbo community," *African Journal of Reproductive Health*, vol. 9, no. 3, pp. 77–88, 2005.

[53] M. J. Hindin, S. A. Kishor, and L. Donna, *Intimate partner violence among couples in 10 DHS countries: predictors and health outcomes*, Macro International Inc., Calverton, MD, 2008.

[54] L. Ismayilova and N. El-Bassel, "Prevalence and correlates of intimate partner violence by type and severity: population-based studies in Azerbaijan, Moldova, and Ukraine," *Journal of Interpersonal Violence*, vol. 28, no. 12, pp. 2521–2556, 2013.

[55] J. Campbell, S. Torres, J. Ryan et al., "Physical and nonphysical partner abuse and other risk factors for low birth weight among full term and preterm Babies: A Multiethnic Case-Control Study," *American Journal of Epidemiology*, vol. 150, no. 7, pp. 714–726, 1999.

[56] E. Owoaje and F. Olaolorun, "Women at risk of physical intimate partner violence: a crosssectional analysis of a low-income community in Southwest Nigeria," *Journal of Reproductive Health*, vol. 16, no. 1, pp. 43–51, 2012.

[57] S. Bazargan-Hejazi, S. Medeiros, R. Mohammadi, J. Lin, and K. Dalal, "Patterns of intimate partner violence: a study of female victims in Malawi," *Journal of Injury and Violence Research*, vol. 5, no. 1, pp. 38–50, 2013.

[58] M. T. Perales, S. M. Cripe, N. Lam, S. E. Sanchez, E. Sanchez, and M. A. Williams, "Prevalence, types, and pattern of intimate partner violence among pregnant women in Lima, Peru," *Violence Against Women*, vol. 15, no. 2, pp. 224–250, 2009.

[59] L. E. E. Okenwa, S. Lawoko, and B. Jansson, "Factors associated with disclosure of intimate partner violence among women in Lagos, Nigeria," *Journal of Injury and Violence Research*, vol. 1, no. 1, pp. 37–47, 2009.

18

Epidemiology of High Fertility Status among Women of Reproductive Age in Wonago District, Gedeo Zone, Southern Ethiopia: A Community-Based Cross-Sectional Study

Medhin Girmay Reda,[1] Girma Tenkolu Bune,[2] and Mohammed Feyisso Shaka[2]

[1]*College of Medicine and Health Sciences, Adigrat University, Adigrat, Ethiopia*
[2]*School of Public Health, College of Health Sciences and Medicine, Dilla University, Dilla, Ethiopia*

Correspondence should be addressed to Mohammed Feyisso Shaka; mamfys8@gmail.com

Academic Editor: Robert Gaspar

Background. High fertility remains one of the most important public health issues hampering the health and welfare of mothers and the survival of their children in developing nations. In Ethiopia, the high fertility rate has been seen for a long historical period with some pocket areas of high fertility still showing poor improvement. Hence, this study was aimed at determining the magnitude of high fertility status (number of children ever born alive ≥ 5) and associated factors among women of the reproductive age group in Wonago district. *Methods.* A community-based cross-sectional study was conducted on randomly selected 512 women in Wonago district. Data were collected using a pretested structured interviewer administered questionnaire. Data was entered into EpiData version 3.1 and then analyzed by SPSS version 25. Logistic regression was used to analyze the data, and the adjusted odds ratio with the 95% confidence interval was computed, and a significant association was declared at p value ≤ 0.05. *Result.* This study revealed that 354 (69.1%) of the respondents have high fertility. High fertility is independently associated with residing in rural area [AOR = 4.88, 95% CI: 3.21, 7.86], desire for children [AOR = 6.97, 95% CI: 3.24, 11.40], history of under-five child mortality [AOR =5.32, 95% CI: 2.59, 8.43], poor knowledge of contraception [AOR = 2.67, 95% CI: 1.66, 4.04], and low wealth tertile [AOR = 2.21, 95% CI: 1.51, 3.58]. On the other hand, women with age at first birth above 18 years [AOR = 0.34, 95% CI: 0.17, 0.68] and those with birth interval ≥ 24 months [AOR = 0, 26, 95% CI: 0.14, 0.49] were less likely to have high fertility. *Conclusion and Recommendation.* The substantial number of women in the study area has high fertility status far away from the country's costed implementation plan of reducing the total fertility rate to 3.0. Considering these, much is needed to be done among poor, rural residents, who have not yet attained their desired number of children, and on enhancing the knowledge of mothers towards contraceptive methods.

1. Introduction

Based on the demographic concept, fertility is the product or output of reproduction and not the ability to have children. This is to mean that fertility is the actual reproductive performance of a couple [1]. The population's fertility is measured by children ever born, and it shows how many children a certain age cohort of women who have completed childbearing actually produced during their childbearing years [2]. It is one of the three principal components of population dynamics that determines the size and structure of the population of a country [3]. High fertility is defined as five or more births per woman over the reproductive period. It affects health of children and their mothers, detracts from human capital investment, slows economic growth, and exacerbates environmental threats [4].

World population has increased by 2 billion people over the past 25 years, from 5.3 billion in 1990 to 7.3 billion in 2015, and globally, the total fertility rate is 2.5 children per woman Africa has the highest rate of population growth among the main areas of high fertility where the population growth rate is growing at 2.55% annually in 2015 [5].

The United Nations (UN) has projected the median world population for the year 2100 to be 11 billion, and the median projected for Mid-African Countries (MAC) is more than 3.97 billion [6, 7]. High and slowly decreasing fertility resulted in the remarkable increase in the projected population of the great majority of the sub-Saharan (and hence Mid-African Countries) African countries [8]. The fertility decline in this region started nearly 20 years later compared to the rest of the developing countries [5] and, once begun, is estimated to have been one-fourth as fast as in Asia and Latin America at the equivalent demographic stage [9].

Uncontrolled fertility has adverse influences on socioeconomic, demographic, and environmental development of a country [10]. Women with five or more pregnancies have a significantly higher risk of dying due to maternal causes, and there is also poor child survival for women from countries with high fertility [4]. For instance, for every 100,000 births in African countries with high fertility, 640 women die due to related complications of pregnancy and childbirth [11].

Sub-Saharan African countries particularly have population growth rates that are outpacing their economic growth. Fertility still remains far above the replacement level in a significant number of countries. Each African mother is replacing herself with nearly two daughters with replacement level fertility of 2.1, which leads to fast population growth [12].

Though there is a significant decrement in fertility in the world since the previous decades, it is still unacceptably high in most of the Sub-Saharan African countries. Despite the substantial decline in the total fertility rate in Ethiopia, the country is still characterized by high fertility and very young population structure. In addition, the pattern of decline in fertility is not evenly shared among different societal characteristics and geographical areas [13]. There is a fall in fertility in some regions of the country while some are showing no change and others still have shown an increment in the total fertility rate [14].

In Ethiopia, the high and persistent fertility rate has been seen for a long period. The TFR has slightly declined from 5.5 in 2000 to 5.4 children per woman in 2005 to 4.8 children per woman in 2011 and to 4.6 children per woman in 2016. Even though a declining trend is shown, like many African countries, the fertility rate of Ethiopia is still high as compared to developed nations [15–17].

In Ethiopia, the levels of maternal mortality and morbidity are also among the highest in the world. Unspaced birth with low maternal health service access seriously affects the health of mothers and children [18, 19]. Recent estimates showed that the country still experiences higher rates of maternal mortality, under-five mortality, and infant mortality of 412 deaths/100,000, 67 deaths/1000 live births, and 48 deaths/1000 live births, respectively [19].

From the Ethiopian population, about 83.5% of people live in rural areas, whereas the high fertility and rapid population growth rate especially in the rural area is unacceptably high with the total fertility rate of above 6 children per woman. Having many children is still considered to be a prestige and gift of God in most Ethiopian rural communities [20]. Particularly, Wonago woreda which is the study area for this study has 864 persons/sq. km in 1999, and currently, the carrying capacity of the land has reached a climax point where about 1300 persons live per square kilometers [21].

Taking into consideration these realities and scenarios, this study was aimed at visualizing the current fertility status and factors contributing to uncontrolled high fertility in the study area. This is important to forward the implication of current activities of the government for the achievement of the desired fertility status, particularly the achievement of the costed implementation plan of reducing total fertility of Ethiopian women to 3.0. Moreover, this study will bring about the where and how to focus on such pocket areas of high fertility.

2. Methodology

2.1. Study Design, Setting, and Study Period. A community-based cross-sectional study was conducted among women of reproductive age residing in Wonago district, Gedeo zone, Southern Ethiopia, located 377 km to the south of Addis Ababa. The district is well known for being the most densely populated area in the country and having the highest total fertility rate. The district has 21 kebeles (the smallest local administrative classification in Ethiopia), of which 17 kebeles are rural administration and 4 are semiurban. The dominant ethnic group in the study area is the Gedeo ethnic group. This study was conducted from 05 December 2017 to 18 January 2018.

2.2. Population. The study population was all women of the reproductive age group from 25 to 49 years. This group of women was taken for this particular study by considering the fact that women in the study area who have given birth at an early age have the possibility of delivering four and above children before they celebrate their twenty-fifth birthday. In this study, women with the number of children ever born alive greater than four were considered having high fertility.

2.3. Sample Size and Sampling Technique. The sample size of this study was calculated using the formula for estimation of single population proportion based on the proportion of women with a high fertility rate (p) 28% [22], 95% level of confidence with $Z_{\alpha/2}$ of 1.96, and margin of error (d) of 0.05. With this, the calculated sample size was

$$n = \frac{(Z_{\alpha/2})^2 p(1-p)}{d^2} = \frac{(1.96)^2 \times 0.28\,(1-0.28)}{(0.05)^2} = \frac{0.7745}{0.0025} = 309.7 \approx 310. \quad (1)$$

Considering the design effect (DEFF) of 1.5, the sample size becomes 310 ∗ 1.5 = 465. Finally, by adding the 10% nonresponse rate to increase the precision by reducing the sampling error, the final sample size was 512.

To select the study participants, the study area was stratified into semiurban and rural, after which two [2] kebeles from semiurban and five [5] kebeles from rural were selected by simple random sampling technique. In each selected kebele, a list of women of reproductive age in the selected age range (25-49 years) and their full addresses was generated by conducting census. From this sampling frame, the final study units were selected from the list of the sampling frame based on probability proportional to size allocation using simple random sampling technique (SRS).

2.4. Data Collection Procedure and Data Analysis. A validated structured tool adapted from the survey tools developed by EDHS Survey [19] and World Fertility Survey [23] was used. The tool was also modified after reviewing different published literatures in English version, and a pretest was conducted to customize the objectives of the study and local contexts.

The questionnaire prepared originally in English was then translated to Amharic and the local language (Gedeo-uffa). To check for consistency of the meaning of each question, the questionnaire was further back translated from the local language to Amharic and English by different translators. The data was collected by trained diploma-holder health professionals who are fluent in Gedeo-uffa (local language) and Amharic. Before data collection, the data collectors were trained thoroughly. The principal investigator strictly supervised the overall activities of data collection.

For data analysis, the data was entered into the EpiData version 3.1 statistical software package and later exported into SPSS version 25 [24]. Descriptive analysis was conducted, and logistic regression was done to assess the determinants of high fertility. As a rule of thumb, variables with p value less than 0.25 on bivariate analysis were further included in the multivariable analysis model. The adjusted odds ratio with their corresponding confidence interval was used as a measure of association, and p values < 0.05 were taken as statistically significant.

The model goodness of fit was tested by the Hosmer and Lemeshow test. Multicollinearity was checked at the cutoff point of VIF > 10 to test if the independent variables were related.

2.5. Measurements

2.5.1. Fertility Status. The outcome variable was fertility status measured by the number of children ever born (CEB) alive. It is categorized as low fertility when CEB alive is <5 and high fertility when CEB alive is ≥ 5. The cutoff point of 5 is taken because the medical and obstetric risk for mothers with the number of CEB greater or equal to 5 is significantly higher compared with that of less than five [25]. It is also based on the population policy of Ethiopia which is aimed at achieving less than five children per woman by the end of 2015.

2.5.2. Children Ever Born (CEB). CEB represents the number of all children ever born alive to a particular woman in her lifetime fertility experience by the time of the survey.

2.5.3. Knowledge about Contraception. Maternal knowledge towards contraception was assessed by asking six knowledge-related questions. A score of 1 was given if the mother answered the given questions correctly and 0 if not. The sum of each question was computed. Taking into account the distribution of the sum score which was normally distributed, the mean was used to categorize the overall score of each participant into two groups: greater than the mean as good knowledge and less than or equal to the mean as poor knowledge.

2.5.4. Estimation of the Household Wealth Index. Household wealth status was estimated by principal component analysis based on fourteen household variables (source of food, presence of own farmland, type of toilet facility, presence of kitchen, electricity, radio/tape, motorcycle, cotton/-sponge/spring mattress, roof of house with corrugated iron sheet, wall type of household, sleeping bed, presence of own animals, and number of cows, oxen, horses/mules/donkeys, goats/sheep, beehives, and hens) that measure household assets. SPSS version 25 software was used to perform principal component analysis (PCA). Household wealth status was estimated with 3 components that explained a total variance of 62.5% and measure of sampling adequacy of 0.72. Finally, wealth status can be categorized into three groups and ranked as low, middle, and high as it was given by the factor analysis result.

2.6. Ethical Consideration. Ethical clearance was obtained from Dilla University College of Health Sciences and Medicine Institutional Review Board. Verbal consent was obtained from each study participant after detailed explanation of the main purpose of the study.

3. Result

3.1. Sociodemographic and Socioeconomic Characteristics of the Respondents. Wide ranges of variables which can potentially affect fertility status were included in the analysis. The mean age of mothers was 35 years (SD = 5.7), and one-third of the mothers (168, 32.8%) were within the age range of 35-39 years. Majority of the study participants are Gedeo in ethnicity (405, 79.1%). Most of the children's parents (433, 84.5%) were married and live together. The residence of 383 (74.8%) mothers is rural setting, and more than half of the mothers (311, 60.7%) were illiterate. Occupationally, 268 (52.5%) mothers were housewives. About 210 (41%) of the participants in the study area were in the lowest wealth tertile (Table 1).

3.2. Reproductive Characteristics of the Respondents. Three hundred fifty-four (69.1%) of mothers were found to have "high fertility." About 17.8% of the participants' husbands in the study area have two or more wives. One hundred fifty-six (30.5%) of the women in the study area have ever aborted or had still birth, and 186 (36.3%) had history of under-five child mortality. The mean number of children ever born (CEB) alive for women (age 25-49 years) in this study is 6.00 with (SD = 2.1), and the parity ranges from 1 to 12. The mean age at first childbirth for the participated women is 17 years with (SD = 1.9) (Table 2).

Table 1: Sociodemographic characteristics of women of reproductive age (25-49 years) in Wonago district, Southern Ethiopia, January 2018 ($n = 512$).

Variables	Variable level	No. (%)
Current age category in years	25-29	88 (17.2%)
	30-34	75 (14.6%)
	35-39	168 (32.8%)
	40-44	111 (21.7%)
	45-49	70 (13.7%)
	Mean ± SD	35 ± 5.7
Residency	Urban	129 (25.2%)
	Rural	383 (74.8%)
Ethnicity	Gedeo	405 (79.1%)
	Oromo	65 (12.7%)
	Silte	16 (3.1%)
	Amhara	26 (5.1%)
Marital status	Married/living together	433 (84.5%)
	Divorced	50 (9.8%)
	Widowed	29 (5.7%)
Mother's educational status	Illiterate	311 (60.7%)
	Primary education	99 (19.3%)
	Secondary & above education	102 (19.9%)
Father's educational level	Illiterate	113 (22.1%)
	Primary education	197 (38.5%)
	Secondary & above education	202 (39.5%)
Occupation of mother	Housewife	268 (52.3%)
	Farmer	152 (29.7%)
	Government employee	30 (5.9%)
	Merchant	62 (12.1%)
Wealth index	Low	210 (41.0%)
	Middle	104 (20.3%)
	High	198 (38.7%)

SD: standard deviation.

Table 2: Reproductive characteristics of the study participants in Wonago district, Gedeo zone, January 2018 ($n = 512$).

Variables	Variable level	No. (%)
Fertility status	High fertility	354 (69.1%)
	Low fertility	158 (30.9%)
Currently have children	<5	201 (39.3%)
	≥5	311 (60.7%)
Ever aborted or still birth	No	356 (69.5%)
	Yes	156 (30.5)
Under-five child mortality	Yes	186 (36.3%)
	No	326 (63.7%)
Age at marriage	<18 years	286 (55.9%)
	18 and above	226 (44.1%)
	Mean ± SD	16 ± 2.5
Age at first birth	<18	277 (54.1%)
	18 and above	235 (45.9%)
	Mean ± SD	17 ± 1.9
Age at last birth	≤30	202 (39.5%)
	31 and above	310 (60.5%)
	Mean ± SD	32 ± 4.6
Two or more wives	Yes	91 (17.8%)
	No	421 (82.2%)
Average birth interval	<2 years	322 (62.9%)
	≥2 years	190 (37.1%)
	Mean ± SD	2 ± 0.5
Duration of breastfeeding	<12 months	93 (18.2%)
	12-24 months	206 (40.2%)
	>24 months	213 (41.6%)
	Mean ± SD	24 ± 6.7
Delayed sexual contact after delivery	<2 months	270 (52.7%)
	≥2 months	242 (47.3%)

SD: standard deviation.

3.3. Mother's Knowledge about Contraceptive Methods. Interviewers collected information regarding knowledge of contraceptive methods, and the result revealed that 397 (77.5%) of women have commendable knowledge about contraceptive methods and 115 (22.5%) of women did have poor knowledge of contraceptive methods.

3.4. Factors Associated with High Fertility Status of Participants. After controlling for the effects of possible confounders, current age category, place of residence, mother's education, wealth index, age at first birth, birth interval, knowledge of contraceptive, desire for children, and history of under-five mortality were significantly associated with fertility status (Table 3). As it is literally expected, women in the older age group were more likely to have more children compared to younger women.

Regarding the place of residence, women living in rural areas were about 5 times (AOR = 4.88, 95% CI: 3.21, 7.86) more likely to have high fertility as compared to those living in semiurban settings. Women who have given their first birth at 18 years and above are 65.9% (AOR = 0.34, 95% CI: 0.17, 0.68) more likely to have high fertility compared to women who have given their first birth before 18 years. Similarly, women with average birth spacing ≥ 2 years were about 74% (AOR = 0.26, 95% CI: 0.14, 0.49) less likely to have high fertility compared to those who have a shorter birth interval (less than 2 years).

Women who have poor knowledge of contraceptive methods were nearly 3 times (AOR = 2.67, 95% CI: 1.66, 4.04) more likely to have higher fertility as compared to those who have good knowledge. Mothers within the low wealth tertile were also 2 times (AOR = 2.21, 95% CI: 1.51, 3.58) more likely to have higher fertility as compared to those

Table 3: A multivariable analysis of factors associated with fertility status in Wonago district, Southern Ethiopia, January 2018.

Exposure variables	High (354) No. (%)	Low (158) No. (%)	Crude OR (95% CI)	Adjusted OR (95% CI)
Current age category				
25-34 years	117 (53.2%)	103 (46.8%)	1.00	1.00
35-44 years	166 (82.2%)	36 (17.8%)	4.06 (2.59-6.35)	2.94 (1.41-6.10)
45 and above	71 (78.9%)	19 (21.1%)	3.29 (1.90-5.83)	3.39 (1.04- 6.05)
Residency				
Rural	75 (19.6%)	308 (80.4%)	7.41 (4.76-11.50)	4.88 (3.21-7.86)
Urban	83 (64.3%)	46 (35.7%)	1.00	1.00
Age at first birth				
<18 years	230 (83.0%)	47 (17.0%)	1.00	1.00
18 and above	124 (52.8%)	111 (47.2%)	0.23 (0.15-0.34)	0.34 (0.17-0.68)
Wealth index				
Low	152 (72.4%)	58 (27.6%)	2.29 (1.18-5.30)	3.62 (1.86-7.06)
Middle	90 (85.7%)	15 (14.3%)	1.97 (2.19-3.28)	3.03 (1.21-7.58)
High	112 (56.9%)	85 (43.1%)	1.00	1.00
Knowledge of contraceptive				
Poor knowledge	98 (85.2%)	17 (14.8%)	3.18 (1.82-5.53)	3.13 (1.31-7.46)
Good knowledge	256 (64.5%)	141 (35.5%)	1.00	1.00
Birth interval				
<2 years	233 (72.4%)	89 (27.6%)	1.00	1.00
≥2 years	121 (63.7%)	69 (36.3%)	0.67 (0.46-0.98)	0.26 (0.14-0.49)
Desire for children/before birth				
<5	38 (40.9%)	55 (59.1%)	1.00	1.00
≥5	58 (59.2%)	40 (40.8%)	2.10 (1.18-3.74)	3.53 (1.60-7.79)
As God given	258 (80.4%)	63 (19.6%)	5.93 (3.61-9.64)	6.97 (3.24-11.40)
Under-five child mortality				
No	183 (56.1%)	143 (43.9%)	1.00	1.00
Yes	171 (91.9%)	15 (8.1%)	8.91 (5.03-11.77)	5.32 (2.59-8.43)

Variables included in the model are as follows: current age, mother's education, residency, wealth index, age at marriage, age at last birth, age at first birth, birth interval, want for more children, desire for children/before birth, ever aborted/still birth, contraceptive use, knowledge of contraception, and history of under-5 mortality.

with high wealth tertile. Women who express their desired number of children as God given were nearly 7 times (AOR = 6.97, 95% CI: 3.24, 11.40) more likely to have high fertility than those who desire to have less than five children. On the other hand, women with history of under-five child mortality were 5 times (AOR = 5.32, 95% CI: 2.59, 8.43) more likely to have higher fertility than women who did not have history of under-five child mortality (Table 3).

4. Discussion

The intention of this study was to determine the magnitude and factors associated with high fertility among women of the reproductive age group aged 25-49 years. The finding revealed that 69% (95% CI: 65%-73%) of the 512 respondents had high fertility. This figure is also significantly higher compared to other findings from studies conducted in different parts of Ethiopia, which include a study from Enderta district (51%) [26] and Butajira district (28%) [22]. The main underlying reason for this variation may be the lower mean age at first birth in this study which is smaller than the other observed studies.

Different sociodemographic characteristics have been indicated to be associated with high fertility in these studies. Regarding the household wealth tertile, women within the lower wealth tertile were more likely to have high fertility than those within the high wealth tertile. This could be due to poor access to media and health care services including family planning and low educational status by the poor. This finding is also similar to the facts in EDHS 2016 [19] and findings from Gilgel Gibe Field Research Center of Jimma University [10], in which fertility status has a strong association with wealth quintiles.

Residency also showed a strong association to high fertility in the current study. The fertility levels in the urban and rural areas tend to be different; women who live in the rural area have more children as compared to those living in the urban area. It is generally true that women residing in the urban area stay longer in school, thereby delaying the time for marital engagement. Moreover, the demand for human power in agrarian living condition and the notion of considering the family with a large number of children as a blessed family in the rural area in the district may drive couples to have an increased number of children. This is consistent with previous studies done in the case of Butajira [27], Ghana [28], and Nepal [29]. In a similar context, high fertility was significantly higher among women whose means of subsistence is farming than those living in urban areas that are mainly characterized by trade, access to media, general health knowledge, and better health service information.

Early childbearing is a leading sociodemographic characteristic that indicates the exposure of women to teenage pregnancy. In the area of the current study, early marriage is found to be a common phenomenon as also suggested by the result showing that more than half of the women that participated in this study had their first birth before 18 years of age. Women who gave their first birth at the age of 18 year and above were more likely to have fewer children than those who gave their first birth at an earlier age. For women with their first pregnancy at an earlier age, the period of fertility is obviously longer, resulting in higher fertility. This phenomenon is particularly serious in this study area where a large number of the women have poor knowledge of contraceptive methods. This finding is similar with previous studies done in Kersa district [30], Enderta district [26], Nigeria [31], Nambia [32], and Ghana [28]. However, the issue of early childbearing is considerably alarming in the current study area than the findings from those areas.

Another interesting factor in this study was a desire for compensation or replacement for loss of under-five children. In this study, women who have history of under-five mortality have higher probability of having a large number of children. This finding is consistent with previous studies done in Kersa district [30], Enderta district [26], Gilgel Gibe Field Research Center of Jimma University [10], Butajira [27], Nigeria [33], Nepal [29], and Kenya [34]. This can be explained by the fact that death of the child may create a fear of loss of more children to women resulting in having an unintended higher number of children.

Knowledge of contraception is found to be another determinant factor where women with poor knowledge on contraception were at higher risk of having higher fertility as compared to those who have good knowledge. Similar studies have been found in other parts of the country including Addis Ababa [35], Bale Zone, and South East Ethiopia [36]. As this result indicates, one of the main reasons for higher fertility in the study area may be emanated from the poor knowledge of contraceptive methods which implies that the women could also have a higher unmet need for family planning.

Women of the reproductive age group having an average birth interval of less than 2 years were at higher risk of having high fertility as compared to those with a birth interval more than or equal to two years. This finding is also consistent with a study conducted in Arbaminch district [37] and in Dodota woreda, Arsi zone [38].

This study considered a wide range of fertility variables to see high fertility differentials among women in the study, and it used a reasonable sample of respondents selected with probable sampling technique. However, there are some important limitations in using the finding of this study. As the study is quantitative in nature, there are some hidden factors that need to be addressed by qualitative study. Though the assessment was carefully done to reduce the recall bias, estimation of some sociodemographic variables like age at first birth might have been mistaken.

5. Conclusion and Recommendation

The finding of this study implies that fertility status in the study area was alarmingly high, contesting the effort of the country to achieve the lower total fertility rate as planned on the costed implementation plan of 2020. Moreover, the finding implies that the women in the study area have a substantial unmet need for family planning that needs public health attention. Among the impressive factors influencing fertility status were the following: loss of under-five children, low wealth tertile, residing in rural areas, age at first birth, desire for children, and poor knowledge of contraception. Targeted works on knowledge about contraception, the negative effect of early childbearing/marriage, and correcting the desire for children among women in the study area are urgent public health concerns needing due consideration.

Abbreviations

BCC: Behavior change communication
CEB: Child ever born
CSA: Central Statistical Agency
EDHS: Ethiopian Demographic and Health Survey
HAD: Health Development Army
HEW: Health extension worker
IEC: Information education communication
MPH/RH: Masters of Public Health/Reproductive Health
OR: Odds ratio
SNNP: Southern Nations Nationalities and Peoples
SPSS: Statistical Package for the Social Sciences
TFR: Total fertility rate.

Consent

Written consent was obtained from the participants. Data was collected after assuring confidentiality (anonymity and not writing the address) and receiving consent of the mother.

Disclosure

The funding body had no role in the design of the study, data collection, analysis, and interpretation and in writing the manuscript.

Authors' Contributions

The contributions of the authors involved in this study are as follows: Medhin Girmay (MG): conceptualization, data curation, analysis, result writing, editing, investigation, methodology, project administration, resources, software, and supervision; Girma Tenkolu Bune (GT): conceptualization, data curation, analysis, result writing, editing, investigation, methodology, project administration, resources, software, and supervision; and Mohammed Feyisso Shaka (MF): conceptualization, data curation, analysis, result writing, editing, investigation, methodology, project administration, resources, software, and supervision.

Acknowledgments

We would like to express our thanks to the Dilla University College of Health Sciences and Medicine NORHED/SE-NUPH project for financial support. We also acknowledge our data collectors and study participants.

References

[1] J. Bongaarts and R. G. Potter, "Natural Fertility and Its Proximate Determinants," in *Fertility, Biology, and Behavior*, pp. 21–51, Academic Press, New York, 1st edition, 1983.

[2] O. Frank, *The demography of fertility and infertility*, World Health Organization, Geneva, 2017.

[3] P. Gerland, A. Biddlecom, and V. Kantorová, "Patterns of fertility decline and the impact of alternative scenarios of future fertility change in sub-Saharan Africa," *Population and Development Review*, vol. 43, pp. 21–38, 2017.

[4] S. Chowdhury, *Determinants and consequences of high fertility : a synopsis of the evidence*, World Bank, 2010.

[5] United Nations Department of Economic and Social Affairs Population Division, *World Fertility Patterns 2015 - Data Booklet (ST/ESA/SER. A/370)*, United Nations, 2015.

[6] United Nations, *World population prospects: Methodology of the United Nations population estimates and projections*, United Nations, New York, 2015, https://esa.un.org/unpd/wpp/.

[7] P. Gerland, A. E. Raftery, H. ev ikova et al., "World population stabilization unlikely this century," *Science*, vol. 346, no. 6206, pp. 234–237, 2014.

[8] K. Andreev, V. Kantorova, and J. Bongaarts, *Demographic components of future population growth*, Population Division, Dept. of Economic and Social Affairs, United Nations, New York, New York, 2013.

[9] J. Bongaarts and J. Casterline, "Fertility transition: is sub-Saharan Africa different?," *Population and Development Review*, vol. 38, Supplement 1, pp. 153–168, 2013.

[10] D. Jara, T. Dejene, and M. Taha, "Determinants of high fertility status among married women in Gilgel Gibe Field Research Center of Jimma University, Oromia, Ethiopia: a case control study," *Public Health Research*, vol. 3, no. 2, pp. 9–17, 2013.

[11] K. Johnson, "Changes in the direct and indirect determinants of fertility in sub-Saharan Africa," *DHS Analytical Studies*, vol. 23, 2011.

[12] United Nations, Department of Economic and Social Affairs PD, *World Population Prospects: The 2015 Revision, Key Findings and Advance Tables (ESA/P/WP.241)*, United Nations, 2015.

[13] A. Hailemariam, "Implementation of the population policy of Ethiopia: achievements and challenges," *Population Horizons*, vol. 13, no. 1, pp. 19–30, 2016.

[14] H. Teklu, A. Sebhatu, and T. Gebreselassie, "Components of fertility change in Ethiopia. Further analysis of the 2000, 2005 and 2011 demographic and health surveys," in *DHS Further Analysis Reports*, p. 80, ICF International, Calverton, 2013.

[15] United Nations Department of Economic and Social Affairs Population Division, *World Fertility Patterns 2015 - Data Booklet*, 2015.

[16] K. Johnson, N. Abderrahim, and S. O. Rutstein, *Changes in the direct and indirect determinants of fertility in sub-Saharan Africa, DHS analytical studies 23: United States Agency for International Development*, ICF Macro Calverton, Maryland, USA, 2011.

[17] Central Statistical Authority [Ethiopia] and ORC Macro, *Ethiopia Demographic and Health Survey 2000*, Central Statistical Authority and ORC Macro, Addis Ababa and Calverton, 2001.

[18] T. Laelago, Y. Habtu, and S. Yohannes, "Proximate determinants of fertility in Ethiopia; an application of revised Bongaarts model," *Reproductive Health*, vol. 16, no. 1, p. 13, 2019.

[19] Central statistical agency (CSA) [Ethiopia] and ICF, *Ethiopia demographic health survey*, CSA and ICF, Addis Ababa, and Rockville, 2016.

[20] D. G. Ayele, "Determinants of fertility in Ethiopia," *African Health Sciences*, vol. 15, no. 2, pp. 546–551, 2015.

[21] A. Legesse, B. Teferi, and A. Baudouin, "Indigenous agroforestry knowledge transmission and young people's participation in agroforestry practices: The case of Wonago Woreda, Gedeo Zone, Southern Ethiopia," *Acta Geographica-Trondheim: Serie A*, no. 26, 2013.

[22] W. Mekonnen and A. Worku, "Determinants of low family planning use and high unmet need in Butajira District, South Central Ethiopia," *Reproductive Health*, vol. 8, no. 1, p. 37, 2011.

[23] G. Rodriguez and T. Croft, "Extracting and reshaping world fertility survey data in Stata," *Demographic Research*, vol. 36, pp. 893–904, 2017.

[24] Z. Bursac, C. H. Gauss, D. K. Williams, and D. W. Hosmer, "Purposeful selection of variables in logistic regression," *Source Code for Biology and Medicine*, vol. 3, no. 1, p. 17, 2008.

[25] Y. Fitaw, Y. Berhane, and A. Worku, "Differentials of fertility in Rural Butajira," *Ethiopian Journal of Health Development*, vol. 17, no. 1, 2003.

[26] G. Atsbaha, D. Hailu, H. Berhe, A. G. Slassie, D. Yemane, and W. Terefe, "Determinants of high fertility among ever married women in Enderta district, Tigray Region, Northern Ethiopia," *Journal of Health & Medical Informatics*, vol. 7, no. 5, 2016.

[27] W. Mekonnen and A. Worku, "Determinants of fertility in rural Ethiopia: the case of Butajira Demographic Surveillance System (DSS)," *BMC Public Health*, vol. 11, no. 1, p. 782, 2011.

[28] E. E. Ameyaw, *Proximate Determinants of Fertility in Ghana*, University of Ghana, 2014, http://ugspace.ug.edu.gh.

[29] R. Adhikari, "Demographic, socio-economic, and cultural factors affecting fertility differentials in Nepal," *BMC Pregnancy and Childbirth*, vol. 10, no. 1, p. 19, 2010.

[30] N. Kassa, Y. Berhane, and A. Worku, "Predictors of unintended pregnancy in Kersa, eastern Ethiopia, 2010," *Reproductive Health*, vol. 9, no. 1, p. 1, 2012.

[31] O. O. Alaba, O. E. Olubusoye, and J. O. Olaomi, "Spatial patterns and determinants of fertility levels among women of childbearing age in Nigeria," *South African Family Practice*, vol. 59, no. 4, pp. 143–147, 2017.

[32] N. Indongo and L. Pazvakawambwa, "Determinants of fertility in Namibia," vol. 16, pp. 50–57, 2012.

[33] L. D. G. Ibisomi, "Fertility transition in Nigeria: exploring the role of desired number of children," *African Population Studies*, vol. 23, no. 2, 2008.

[34] S. W. Mungai, *Explaining high fertility in the north eastern region of Kenya*, University of Nairobi, 2015.

[35] K. Yosef, *Determinants of fertility in Ethiopia: Application of Binary Logistic Regression*, L LAMBERT Acad Publ, 2013.

[36] S. S. Belda, M. T. Haile, A. T. Melku, and A. K. Tololu, "Modern contraceptive utilization and associated factors among married pastoralist women in Bale eco-region, Bale Zone, South East Ethiopia," *BMC Health Services Research*, vol. 17, no. 1, 2017.

[37] D. Hailu and T. Gulte, "Determinants of short interbirth interval among reproductive age mothers in Arba Minch District, Ethiopia," *International Journal of Reproductive Medicine*, vol. 2016, Article ID 6072437, 17 pages, 2016.

[38] T. Nigus, N. Tesfaw, A. Gizachew, G. M. Kassa, and A. Alemu, "Skilled delivery service utilization and associated factors among mothers who gave birth in the last two years in Northwest Ethiopia," *BMC Reproductive Health*, vol. 9, no. 33, 2012.

Physical Violence and Associated Factors among Housemaids Living in Debre-Tabor Town, Northwest Ethiopia: Does Employer Alcohol Intake Increase Housemaid Violence?

Kefyalew Amogne Azanaw,[1] Abebaw Addis Gelagay,[2] Ayenew Molla Lakew,[3] and Destaw Fetene Teshome[3]

[1]*Department of Nursing, Debre Tabor Health Science College, Ethiopia*
[2]*Department of Reproductive and Child Health, College of Medicine and Health Sciences, University of Gondar, Gondar, Ethiopia*
[3]*Department of Epidemiology and Biostatistics, College of Medicine and Health Sciences, University of Gondar, Gondar, Ethiopia*

Correspondence should be addressed to Ayenew Molla Lakew; mayenew15@gmail.com

Academic Editor: Stefania A. Nottola

Background. Violence against women and girls continues to be a global epidemic, including Ethiopia. Housemaids are a neglected segment of the population, and there are no sufficient findings in our country. This study aimed to assess the magnitude of physical violence and associated factors among housemaids aged 15 years and above living in Debre Tabor town, northwest Ethiopia. *Methods.* A community-based cross-sectional study was conducted in Debre Tabor town, northwest Ethiopia from April 1 to 30, 2018. A total of 634 housemaids were selected using cluster sampling method. Data were entered into Epi info version 7.2.2.6 and analyzed with SPSS version 20 using descriptive and analytic statistics. Binary logistic regression analysis was carried out to identify independent significant factors. Adjusted odds ratio (AOR) with 95% confidence interval (CI) was used to report the strength of associations. *Results.* From 634 housemaids that participated in the study, 235 (37.1%, 95% CI: 33.1–41.0) of them experienced at least one type of physical violence in their lifetime. Housemaids who previously lived in rural areas ($AOR = 2.82$, 95% CI: 1.61, 4.94), had high working experience ($AOR = 2.17$, 95% CI: 1.27, 3.71), not having parents ($AOR = 2.02$, 95% CI: 1.18, 3.46), being divorced ($AOR = 2.23$, 95% CI: 1.31, 4.20), employer alcohol consumption ($AOR = 4.97$, 95% CI: 2.81, 8.79), and presence of extended family with employers ($AOR = 2.26$, 95% CI: 1.42, 3.59) were independently associated with the probability of housemaid physical violence. *Conclusion.* High prevalence of housemaid physical violence has been reported. Socio-demographic characteristics of both employers and employees and the behavioral characteristics of employers contributed to physical violence. It is important to give special attention to housemaids who came from rural areas and do not have parents. It is also important to make work experience of housemaids as short as possible.

1. Introduction

According to the World Health Organization (WHO) definition, violence against women is any act of Gender-Based Violence (GBV) that results in, or is likely to result in, physical, sexual, or psychological harm or suffering to women, including threats of such acts, coercion, or arbitrary deprivation of liberty [1]. Universally, all types of violence overlap in a relationship and a significant public health problem, but the level and pattern of violence greatly vary between setting, culture, and segment of the population [2]. Ethiopia is one of the countries where the highest prevalence of both physical and sexual violence against women by an intimate partner is documented [3].

Most studies conducted on violence against women agreed that lower educational status, abuse of alcohol, khat and smoke, and younger women are more likely to increase the experience of violence against women [4–6].

Globally, 10–69 percent of women suffered from physical violence by their intimate partners [7]. In sub-Saharan Africa, the experience of women with physical and/or sexual violence by their intimate partner ranges from 27–59% [8]. In Ethiopia, the prevalence of housemaid physical violence was 16.3% [6].

Gender-based violence is an insidious human right issue and has public consequences [8]. The impact of violence is beyond physical injuries; it also accounts for disability, depression, physical, and reproductive problems, and risky sexual behavior [9].

Worldwide within its informal nature, domestic workers are still challenged to regulation and policy implementation which leads to limited opportunities for access to social and legal protection [10]. Violence often goes unrecognized and unreported, and also masked in a culture of silence. Due to less reportable nature of violence, reliable information on the prevalence of the various forms of violence remains scarce.

Even though there are studies conducted on violence globally and also in the country of Ethiopia, there is a lack of sufficient information about the magnitude and associated factors of physical violence against housemaids. Housemaids are neglected segment of the population, and there is no sufficient information identified as a priority in the national planning documents in Ethiopia. Thus, this study aimed to assess the magnitude and associated factors of physical violence against housemaids.

The finding of the research will provide valuable information to labor and social affairs, health professionals, and policymakers to plan their resource and implementation.

2. Materials and Methods

A community-based cross-sectional study was conducted in the Debre Tabor town from April 1 to 30, 2018. The town is located 666 km north of Addis Ababa, the capital city of Ethiopia. All housemaids aged 15 years and above who were living in the Debre Tabor town were considered as the source population. The sample size was calculated using the single population proportion formula assuming 16.3% prevalence of physical violence against housemaids [6], 95% confidence level, and 4% margin of error. Considering a 5% nonresponse rate and using the design effect of 2, the total sample size was 626. Since cluster sampling was employed, 634 individuals were finally sampled.

A cluster sampling technique was employed to select the participants. In the study area, there are four Kebeles (the smallest administrative unit) from which 50% of ketenas (also known as villages) were selected using the simple random sampling technique. The sample size was proportionally allocated for each Kebele, and clusters of households were enumerated from selected ketenas. Then, an eligible participant from each household was selected. All housemaids aged 15 years and above who were living for at least 6 months in the town preceding the data collection period were included.

The dependent variable was physical violence, defined as any acts of slapped or thrown something that could hurt, kicked, pushed or shoved her or pulled her hair, dragged her or beaten her up, hit her with his fist or with something else that could hurt her, choked or burnt her on purpose, and threatened to use or actually used a gun, knife or other weapon against her [11]. Socio-demographic and behavioral characteristics of employers (age, educational status, marital status, religion, occupation, family size, khat chewing, and alcohol drinking) and socio-demographic characteristics of housemaids (age, previous resident, marital status, educational status, religion, family life situation, salary, and working experience as a housemaid in current home) were included as independent variables.

A pretested structured interviewer-administered questionnaire, adopted from the WHO multicountry study, was used to collect data. The questionnaire was written in English and then translated to the local language Amharic. The data were collected by eight trained health extension workers and supervised by four master holder individuals. To ensure data quality, training was given for data collectors and supervisors, and a close follow up and supervision were made.

Data were entered into Epi-info version 7.2.2.6 and exported into SPSS version 20 for analysis. Descriptive analysis was done to describe the data, binary logistic regression analysis was used to identify the associated independent factors. The Adjusted Odds Ratio (AOR) with 95% confidence interval (CI) was used to report the strength of associations of variables. Finally, a significant association was declared at a p-value of less than 0.05. The Hosmer and Lemeshow goodness of fit test was also made to check the model fitness. Ethical approval was obtained from the University of Gondar, Institute of Public Health Ethical Review Committee. An official letter was obtained from the Debre Tabor town administration, mayors' office. Verbal informed consent was obtained from participants whose age was 18 years and above. Participants whose age was less than 17 years, verbal assent was obtained from their employers after describing the purpose, benefit, and risk of the study and their right on the decision to participate in the study. Their names were omitted to ensure confidentiality and privacy. The interview was performed at a suitable and secure place. Finally, the questionnaire was cleaned, stored and analyzed at a secured place.

3. Results

3.1. Socio-Demographic Characteristics of Housemaids. A total of 634 housemaids participated in the study with a 100% response rate. Among the participants, 386 (60.9%) were in the age group of 15–19 years with a median age of 18.5 (IQR: 17, 21) years. Of the total participants, 519 (81.9%) previously lived in a rural area, and 574 (90.5%) were single. Concerning work experience, 491 (71.4%) of housemaids had 1–4 years of work experience, only 251 (39.6%) housemaids had both father and mother, and 141 (22.2%) had no parents (Table 1).

3.2. Socio-Demographic Characteristics of Employers. One-fourth, 162 (25.6%), of the employers were in the age group of 30–34 years with a median age of 35 (IQR: 30–40) years. Around half, 325 (51.3%), of the employers had a certificate and above educational level, majority, 538 (84.9%) were married, and 297 (46.8%) were government employees (Table 2).

3.3. Prevalence of Physical Violence. From the participants, 235 (37.1%) (95% CI: 33.1, 41.0) have experienced physical violence during their lifetime while they became housemaids, and 105 (16.6%) (95% CI: 13.7, 19.5) experienced in the last

Table 1: Socio-demographic characteristics of housemaids, Debre Tabor town, Ethiopia, 2018.

Variables		Frequency (%)
Previous residence	Urban	115 (18.1)
	Rural	519 (81.9)
Educational status	No education	317 (50.0)
	Primary education	181 (28.5)
	Secondary above education	136 (21.5)
Age of housemaid	15–19	386 (60.9)
	20–24	164 (25.9)
	25+	84 (13.2)
Housemaid's religion	Orthodox	588 (92.7)
	Protestant	8 (1.3)
	Muslim	38 (6.0)
Marital status of housemaid	Married	34 (5.4)
	Single	574 (90.5)
	Divorced + widowed	26 (4.1)
Salary of housemaid	100–300	282 (44.5)
	301–500	306 (48.3)
	501+	46 (7.3)
Family living situation	Both alive	251 (39.6)
	Only father alive	112 (17.7)
	Only mother alive	130 (20.5)
	Both dead	141 (22.2)
Work experience	[0.5–2) years	212 (33.4)
	[2–4) years	269 (42.2)
	4+ years	153 (24.1)

12 months. For those who experienced lifetime violence, 164 (56.9%) were from their female employers (Figure 1).

3.4. Factors Associated with Housemaid Violence. Housemaid's previous resident, working experience, family living situation, employer's marital status, employer alcohol consumption, and extended family living with employers were independently associated with housemaid physical violence.

Accordingly, the odds of physical violence were almost three folds among housemaids who previously lived in rural areas compared to urban (*AOR* = 2.82, 95% CI: 1.61, 4.94). The housemaid who had neither father nor mother was about two times more likely to experience physical violence compared to those who had both father and mother. Either of the male or female employer is an alcohol user increases the likelihood of housemaid physical violence by five folds (*AOR* = 4.97, 95%CI: 2.81, 8.79) (Table 3).

Table 2: Socio-demographic and behavioral characteristics of employers, Debre Tabor town, Ethiopia 2018.

Variables		Frequency (%)
Age of employer	Below 30	115 (18.1)
	30–34	162 (25.6)
	35–39	112 (17.7)
	40–44	135 (21.3)
	45–49	32 (5.0)
	50 and above	78 (12.3)
Employer's religion	Orthodox	547 (86.3)
	Protestant	22 (3.5)
	Muslim	65 (10.3)
Employer's educational status	Not read and write	53 (8.4)
	Read and write but not formal education	55 (8.7)
	Grade 1–8	63 (9.9)
	Grade 9–12	138 (21.8)
	Certificate and above	325 (51.3)
Employer occupation	Housewife	158 (24.9)
	Government/private employ	297 (46.8)
	Merchant and/driver	168 (26.5)
	Pension	11 (1.7)
Family size	1–3	149 (23.5)
	4–6	425 (67.0)
	7+	60 (9.5)
Marital status of employer	Married	538 (84.9)
	Single	28 (4.4)
	Divorced	37 (5.8)
	Widowed	31 (4.9)
Extended family of employer	Yes	129 (20.3)
	No	505 (79.9)
Khat-chewing	Yes	68 (10.7)
	No	566 (89.3)
Alcohol consumption	Yes	92 (14.5)
	No	542 (85.5)

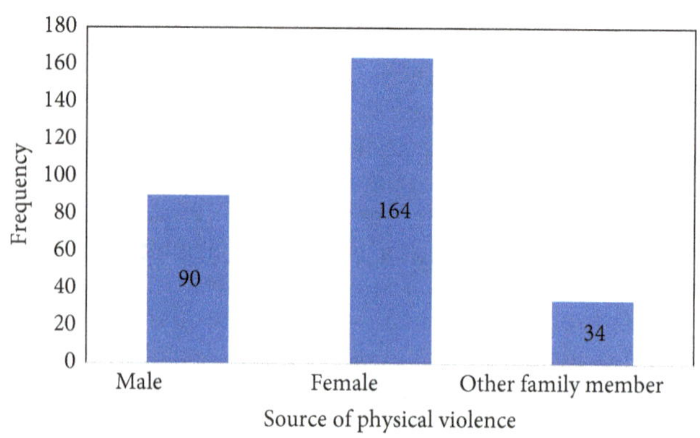

Figure 1: Housemaid physical violence with perpetrators at Debre Tabor town, Ethiopia 2018.

4. Discussion

In this study, it is tried to estimate the prevalence of physical violence and identify associated factors among housemaids at the Debre Tabor town, northwest Ethiopia. The prevalence of physical violence during their lifetime, while they became housemaid, was (37.1%) (95% CI: 33.1, 41.0). The finding was consistant with a finding in Bangladesh [12]. However, it is slightly higher compared to a study conducted in the Gondar zuria district, northwest Ethiopia [13], and Germany [14], and significantly higher than a study conducted in the Mekele town, northern Ethiopia [6]. This could partly be due to the

TABLE 3: Logistic regression analysis to identify factors associated with lifetime physical violence among housemaid, Debre Tabor town, Ethiopia 2018.

Variables		Housemaid violence		*COR* (95% CI)	*AOR* (95% CI)
		Yes	No		
Previous residence	Urban	21	94	1.00	1.00
	Rural	214	305	3.14 (1.89, 5.20)	2.82 (1.61, 4.94)
Work experience	[0.5–2) years	51	161	1.00	1.00
	[2–4) years	99	170	1.84 (1.23, 2.75)	1.35 (0.86, 2.13)
	4+ years	85	68	3.95 (2.52, 6.18)	2.17 (1.27, 3.71)
Age of housemaid in years	15–19	132	254	1.00	
	20–24	71	93	1.47 (1.01, 2.14)	
	25+	32	52	1.18 (0.73, 1.93)	
Salary housemaid	100–300	86	196	1.00	
	301–500	132	174	1.73 (1.23, 2.42)	
	501+	17	29	1.34 (0.69, 2.56)	
Family living situation	Both alive	59	192	1.00	1.00
	Only father alive	53	59	2.92 (1.82, 4.69)	2.02 (1.18, 3.46)
	Only mother alive	60	70	2.79 (1.78, 4.38)	1.97 (1.18, 3.28)
	Both dead	63	78	2.63 (1.69, 4.09)	1.95 (1.20, 3.18)
Family size of employer	1–3	59	90	1.00	
	4–6	161	264	0.93 (0.64, 1.36)	
	7+	15	45	0.51 (0.26, 0.99)	
Marital status of employer	Married	190	348	1.00	1.00
	Single	11	17	1.19 (0.54, 2.58)	1.62 (0.67, 3.91)
	Divorced + widowed	34	34	1.83 (1.10, 3.04)	2.34 (1.31, 4.20)
Extended family	No	164	341	1.00	1.00
	Yes	71	58	2.54 (1.72, 3.77)	2.26 (1.42, 3.59)
Employer alcohol consumption	No	164	378	1.00	1.00
	Yes	71	21	7.79 (4.63, 13.11)	4.97 (2.81, 8.79)

COR: crude odds ratio, AOR: adjusted odds ratio.

difference in the population of interest; the current study included housemaids. Housemaids might not get sufficient information about violence, and they cannot easily protect themselves. Larger prevalence, (43.7%) of physical violence was also reported in the Gozamin district northwest Ethiopia [15].

The odds of physical violence were almost three folds among housemaids who previously lived in rural areas. This finding was consistent with a study conducted in Gondar town northwest Ethiopia [13]. Similar findings have been reported in different areas [16, 17]. The possible reason could be most of the time, housemaids who came from the rural areas might relatively make many mistakes in household activities, and their employers might not be satisfied with their work. Additionally, housemaids who came from rural areas are not empowered to deal effectively with their employers, and they do not know when they could change their employers when their employers attempt to act violently.

In our study, the odds of having physical violence were 2.17 times higher among women with four and above years of working experience as a housemaid. This might be because this study measures a lifetime physical violence, an individual with longer working experience as a housemaid might have a higher chance of experiencing physical violence.

The housemaid who had no or less family support could increase the risk of housemaid violence. In this finding, housemaids who had neither father nor mother or both were about two times more likely to have lifetime physical violence compared to those who had both father and mother. This finding was consistent with another study in northern Ethiopia [6]. The possible reason might be parents' support could increase the confidence in housemaid, and this helps to protect them from any violence. This might also make employers understand that conflict may happen with the parents of the housemaids. Hence, employers may refrain from causing violence.

Divorced or widowed employers increased the odds of housemaid physical violence by a factor of 2.34 compared to married employers. This finding is supported by other studies [12, 18, 19]. This is because divorced or widowed employers might have different problems like psychosocial problems that may lead to envy and depression. A study in 53 countries conducted by the WHO showed that divorced or widowed individuals increased the likelihood of depression [20]. These groups of individuals most likely to be aggressive due to their incompetence in their marriage may be an additional reason.

The odds of physical violence were five times higher among either male or female alcoholic employers. The finding was similar to that of studies conducted in Slovenia, Ghana, Uganda, eastern Sudan, Shimelba refugee camp northern

Tigray, Mekele, and Gondar town which revealed that alcohol consumption of employers increased the likelihood of physical violence [5, 6, 13, 19, 21–23]. Many victims of housemaids reported that when the employers took excess alcohol than usual, they assaulted the housemaids. A qualitative study in Debre Tabor town also supported this finding [24]. This is because alcohol has a depressive mental impairment and thus, human beings are encouraged to undertake violence.

An employer having extended family was 2.56 times more likely to increase the probability of housemaids' physical violence. This is because when there are a number of families in the household, the possible sources of violence increased as well, and this increases the likelihood of housemaid violence. Besides, employers with extended family may not have sufficient material assets and income for their expenditure and became more aggressive on their employees.

Though the study did its best to determine the magnitude of physical violence and associated factors in the study setting, it is not free from some limitations. The study was quantitative, and it was better if the qualitative approach was also employed to investigate attitudes of study subjects towards gender-based violence. It may also be exposed to recall bias due to the nature of the cross-sectional design.

5. Conclusion

The magnitude of physical violence among housemaids was high. Housemaids coming from rural areas, having more than four years working experience, not having either a mother or a father or both, and employers' alcohol use, having extended family, and being divorced or widowed are the independent factors for housemaid physical violence.

The labor and social affair office and women and children's office have to give special attention and develop strategies to prevent violence of housemaids. It is also important to interrupt the contract of housemaids and employers, and change the behavior of employers so that they do not use alcohol. Further research is needed to address the psychological, sexual, and economic violence of housemaids.

Abbreviations

AOR: Adjusted odds ratio
CI: Confidence interval
COR: Crude odds ratio
GBV: Gender based violence
SPSS: Statistical package for social science
WHO: World health organization.

Authors' Contributions

Kefyalew Amogne Azanaw designed the study, developed the proposal, participated in data collection, performed analysis, and interpretation of data and drafted the paper. Abebaw Addis Gelagay, Ayenew Molla Lakew, and Destaw Fetene Teshome assisted in the design of the study, proposal writing, data analysis, and interpretation of the study. Ayenew Molla Lakew carried out the manuscript preparation. All authors reviewed and approved the final manuscript.

Acknowledgments

We are highly grateful to the study participants, data collectors, and supervisors.

References

[1] Z. Iliyasu, I. S. Abubakar, M. H. Aliyu, H. S. Galadanci, and H. M. Salihu, "Prevalence and correlates of gender-based violence among female university students in Northern Nigeria," *African Journal of Reproductive Health*, vol. 15, no. 3, pp. 123–133, 2011.

[2] L. Heise and E. Fulu, *What Works to Prevent Violence Against Women and Girls? State of the Field of Violence Against Women and Girls: What Do We Know and What Are the Knowledge Gaps*, Medical Research Council, Pretoria, South Africa, 2014.

[3] Y. Berhane, "Ending domestic violence against women in Ethiopia," *The Ethiopian Journal of Health Development (EJHD)*, vol. 18, no. 3, 2017.

[4] S. G. Abeya, M. F. Afework, and A. W. Yalew, "Intimate partner violence against women in western Ethiopia: prevalence, patterns, and associated factors," *BMC Public Health*, vol. 11, no. 1, p. 913, 2011.

[5] F. Girmatsion and G. Mulusew, "Intimate partner physical violence among women in Shimelba refugee camp, Northern Ethiopia," *BMC Public Health*, vol. 12, no. 1, p. 125, 2012.

[6] M. Zenebe, A. Gebresilassie, and H. Assefa, "Magnitude and factors associated to physical violence among house maids of Mekelle town, Tigray, Northern, Ethiopia: a cross sectional study," *American Journal of Nursing*, vol. 3, no. 6, pp. 105–109, 2014.

[7] E. G. Krug, J. A. Mercy, L. L. Dahlberg, and A. B. Zwi, "The world report on violence and health," *The Lancet*, vol. 360, no. 9339, pp. 1083–1088, 2002.

[8] R. Borwankar, R. Diallo, and A. E. Sommerfelt, *Gender-Based Violence in Sub-Saharan Africa: A Review of Demographic and Health Survey Findings and Their Use in National Planning*, Wilson Center, Washington, DC, USA, 2008.

[9] C. R. Mikton, A. Butchart, L. L. Dahlberg, and E. G. Krug, "Global status report on violence prevention 2014," *American Journal of Preventive Medicine*, vol. 50, no. 5, pp. 652–659, 2016.

[10] A. Blackett, "Exploited, undervalued–and essential: domestic workers and the realisation of their rights. Edited by Darcy du Toit. Pretoria: Pretoria University Law Press, 2013. 380 pp. ZAR225. 00, $22 paperback, available online," *Law & Society Review*, vol. 49, no. 3, pp. 801–804, 2015.

[11] World Health Organization, *WHO Multi-Country Study on Women's Health and Domestic Violence Against Women: Summary Report of Initial Results on Prevalence, Health Outcomes and Women's Responses*, World Health Organization, Geneva, 2005.

[12] K. VanderEnde, S. Amin, and R. T. Naved, "Community-level correlates of physical violence against unmarried female adolescents in Bangladesh," *BMC Public Health*, vol. 14, no. 1, p. 1027, 2014.

[13] T. Yigzaw, A. Yibric, and Y. Kebede, "Domestic violence around Gondar in northwest Ethiopia," *Ethiopian Journal of Health Development*, vol. 18, no. 3, pp. 133–139, 2004.

[14] R. Schlack, J. Rüdel, A. Karger, and H. Hölling, "Physical and psychological violence perpetration and violent victimisation in the German adult population," *Federal Health Gazette, Health Research, Health Protection*, vol. 56, no. 5-6, pp. 755–764, 2013.

[15] M. Andualem, G. Tiruneh, A. Gizachew, and D. Jara, "The prevalence of intimate partner physical violence against women and associated factors in Gozaman Woreda, Northwest Ethiopia 2013," *Global Journal of Sex Education*, vol. 2, no. 3, pp. 26–35, 2014.

[16] B. V. Babu and S. K. Kar, "Domestic violence against women in eastern India: a population-based study on prevalence and related issues," *BMC Public Health*, vol. 9, no. 1, p. 129, 2009.

[17] C. Rada, "Violence against women by male partners and against children within the family: prevalence, associated factors, and intergenerational transmission in Romania, a cross-sectional study," *BMC Public Health*, vol. 14, no. 1, p. 129, 2014.

[18] T. Abramsky, C. Watts, H. Garcia-Moreno et al., "What factors are associated with recent intimate partner violence? Findings from the WHO multi-country study on women's health and domestic violence," *BMC Public Health*, vol. 11, no. 1, p. 109, 2011.

[19] P. Selic, K. Pesjak, and J. Kersnik, "The prevalence of exposure to domestic violence and the factors associated with co-occurrence of psychological and physical violence exposure: a sample from primary care patients," *BMC Public Health*, vol. 11, no. 1, p. 621, 2011.

[20] D. Rai, P. Zitko, K. Jones, J. Lynch, and R. Araya, "Country-and individual-level socioeconomic determinants of depression: multilevel cross-national comparison," *The British Journal of Psychiatry*, vol. 202, no. 3, pp. 195–203, 2013.

[21] E. S. O. Adjah and I. Agbemafle, "Determinants of domestic violence against women in Ghana," *BMC Public Health*, vol. 16, no. 1, p. 368, 2016.

[22] B. Kwagala, S. Wandera, O. P. Ndugga, and A. Kabagenyi, "Empowerment, partner's behaviours and intimate partner physical violence among married women in Uganda," *BMC Public Health*, vol. 13, no. 1, p. 1112, 2013.

[23] A. A. Ali, K. Yassin, and R. Omer, "Domestic violence against women in Eastern Sudan," *BMC Public Health*, vol. 14, no. 1, p. 1136, 2014.

[24] A. A. Muche, A. O. Adekunle, and A. O. Arowojolu, "Gender-based violence among married women in Debre Tabor Town, Northwest Ethiopia: a qualitative study," *African Journal of Reproductive Health*, vol. 21, no. 4, pp. 102–109, 2017.

20

Responsiveness of Health Professionals to Postabortion Care at a Regional Level Hospital in Ghana: A Qualitative Study of Patients' Self-Reports

Kenneth Setorwu Adde,[1] Eugene Kofuor Maafo Darteh,[1] Akwasi Kumi-Kyereme,[1] and Hubert Amu[2]

[1] *Department of Population and Health, College of Humanities and Legal Studies, University of Cape Coast, Cape Coast, Ghana*
[2] *Department of Population and Behavioural Sciences, School of Public Health, University of Health and Allied Sciences, Hohoe, Ghana*

Correspondence should be addressed to Kenneth Setorwu Adde; kensadde@gmail.com

Academic Editor: Hind A. Beydoun

Background. The responsiveness of health professionals to patients in the provision of abortion services is essential to influencing patients' perceptions and expectations regarding the quality of medical care to be received and their general satisfaction. This, in turn, determines if patients will revisit a particular health facility to access abortion services. In this study, we examine the responsiveness of health professionals in providing postabortion care at a regional level health facility in Ghana. *Methods.* Qualitative data collected from 20 female patients who assessed abortion services at a regional level health facility in Ghana were used. The sample was achieved through saturation while a systematic qualitative orientated text analysis was adopted in analysing the data. *Results.* Health professionals were responsive to postabortion care at the facility. Most women who sought postabortion care at the facility were referred from other health facilities which could not handle such cases. Other reasons include satisfaction with services received on previous visits to the hospital. We also realized, however, that postabortion services were not covered by the National Health Insurance Scheme. *Conclusions.* All hospitals across the country should be equipped with the basic equipment and personnel to conduct and manage abortions. This would reduce not only referrals but also possible maternal deaths. Abortion services should also be added to the services covered by the country's National Health Insurance Scheme.

1. Introduction

Globally, about 830 women die from pregnancy and childbirth-related complications every day, and abortion accounts for 8% of these maternal mortality cases [1–3]. Although abortion rates in the developed world have declined significantly since the 1990s, unsafe abortions continue to claim the lives of thousands of women annually in developing countries [4]. In some developing countries, substandard postabortion services have been reported by patients seeking postabortion care (PAC) [5]. They indicate that such substandard services are displeasing and, thus, deter them from seeking subsequent postabortion care in some facilities [6, 7]. PAC refers to emergency treatment services for complications of spontaneous or unsafely induced abortions as well as postabortion family planning counseling and services [7].

In Ghana, abortion is the leading cause of maternal mortality, accounting for about 11% of maternal deaths [8, 9]. Abortion in Ghana is relatively liberal, compared to other Sub-Saharan countries [9, 10]. The abortion law of 1985 (PNDC Law 102), for instance, prohibits the act but states three main conditions under which an abortion can be done [8]. Abortion is allowed when pregnancy results from rape or defilement of a female idiot (who is an imbecile, mad, or under 18 years of age and cannot take decisions for herself) or from incest [8]. It is, also, allowed when the continuance of a pregnancy would involve substantive risk to the life of the pregnant woman or injury to her physical or mental health. Abortion is finally acceptable under Ghana's abortion law when there is a substantial risk that the child, if born, may suffer from or later develop a serious physical abnormality or disease [11, 12].

From a policy perspective, Ghana did not integrate safe abortion into national reproductive health policy until 2003 [8]. In 2006, the Ghana Health Service introduced the new standards and protocols for safe abortion services that include a direction for interpreting Ghana's abortion law. However, to a large extent, the law still tends to be interpreted as prohibiting abortion and, hence, the limited access to abortion services in the public sector [11].

To curb the negative effects of unsafe abortions (which include rupture of the uterus, sepsis, anaemia, and death) in Ghana, the government introduced a comprehensive reproductive health strategy that focuses on maternal morbidity and mortality connected with unsafe abortion [13]. Manual Vacuum Aspiration was, for instance, introduced in the curriculum for midwifery education in the country. However, social, religious, policy, and legal restrictions on abortion continue to serve as barriers to having access to comprehensive abortion care, thereby, forcing women to opt for unsafe abortion [14].

Even though, as a country, Ghana has been increasing efforts to improve access to postabortion care, especially when such abortions are conducted clandestinely, the services have remained underfunded with low visibility and poor quality. As such, they remain inaccessible to most women [15]. Meanwhile, a hospital, be it large or small, can demonstrate successful performance only when it satisfies the factors of quality and satisfaction that a patient expects. The perceptions and expectations of patients regarding the quality of medical care and their general satisfaction are, thus, important in determining if patients will revisit a particular health facility to access abortion services [16]. The responsiveness of the health system and professionals to the provision of services to patients, therefore, becomes very imperative. The World Health Organisation describes responsiveness as "the ability of the health system to meet the population's legitimate expectations regarding their interaction with the health system, apart from expectations for improvements in health or wealth" [17].

Despite the fact that much work has been done by the government to curtail maternal morbidity and mortality as a result of unsafe abortion and postabortion complications, there is a paucity of empirical literature in Ghana with a focus on the responsiveness of health care facilities and professionals to abortion and postabortion care. This study, therefore, examined the responsiveness of health professionals at a regional level health facility to postabortion care from the patients' perspective. An understanding of this issue is an important step towards the implementation of interventions to improve access to PAC in Ghana and other low-resource settings across the globe.

2. Conceptual Framework

The study is underpinned by the health system responsiveness model. This model was developed by the WHO with the goal of developing technical tools to assess, monitor, and raise awareness of how patients are cared for and the environment in which they receive such care when seeking health services. The underlining assumption of the framework is that as a social system the health system is expected to meet a core goal as well as a common social goal expected from all social systems [18].

The health system performance measurement is important because it helps identify the gaps in health systems [19]. It, also, provides indicators for examining a health system over a period. Responsiveness under this framework has been defined to encompass the non-health enhancing and the nonfinancial aspects of the health system. According to Smith [19], words that are commonly used in the discussion of responsiveness are satisfaction and quality of care. Patient satisfaction, in this context, includes perceived need, expectations, and experience of care. The quality of care covers a wide dimension; this includes structural quality, process quality, service quality, and interpersonal quality [20, 21]. This model has been adopted because the WHO proposed it as a desirable measure by which health systems can be judged in the context of performance assessment from patients' views on the quality of care provided and satisfaction with such care, which is what the present study sought to investigate [22].

3. Materials and Methods

This qualitative study was conducted cross-sectionally. The study was cross-sectional because data were collected from participants only once without the intention of conducting future follow-ups. The data collection was conducted at a regional level health facility in Ghana (Ghana is divided into ten administrative regions for the purposes of governance and development). The selected hospital is a state-owned ultramodern regional referral hospital. Obstetrics and Gynecology is one of the several services provided at the hospital. According to the Ghana Maternal Health Survey of 2007, the highest incidence of induced abortion was recorded in the region [23]. For instance, it was noted that 12.3% of women in the reproductive age group in the region had ever had an abortion [23]. Meanwhile, about 94.6% of abortion seekers in the region reported not being provided with abortion services when they visited public health facilities as they were met with negative attitudes from service providers [24].

With the help of health providers, patients with abortion experiences were purposively selected for the study. The PAC patients who were willing to take part in the study were adequately informed about the study and provided with informed consent forms to sign/thumbprint. The patients who agreed to participate in the study were then allowed to select their own time and place for the interview. The interviews were recorded and transcribed. On the average, an interview spanned about 45 minutes. A sample size of 20 women, achieved through saturation, was used for the study.

A self-developed in-depth interview (IDI) guide was used to collect data from women who received postabortion care at the hospital. The IDI was used to acquire in-depth information from participants within the milieu of personal experiences with postabortion care. The instrument was divided into two sections: A and B. While Section A focused on the background information of participants, Section B dealt with issues related to the responsiveness of health professionals at the hospital. In all, the instrument was made up of 10 items which contained further probes. The validity and trustworthiness of the instrument were achieved by giving the instrument to two experts who perused it and made valuable inputs. Based on their review, two questions which did not appropriately address the objectives of the study were expunged while three more questions were introduced to ensure that all issues that the study sought to address were appropriately covered. This review, also, led to the reconstruction of three questions.

Ethical clearance for the study was obtained from the Ghana Health Service Ethical Review Committee (GHS-ERC: 14/10/15) and the University of Cape Coast Ethical Review Board (UCCIRB/CHLS/2015/07). A permission to conduct the study was, also, obtained from the management of the hospital of concern. The data were analysed manually using a qualitative content analysis technique. A systematic qualitative orientated text analysis was, thus, adopted. The data were coded and themes developed based on both a priori and emergent issues. Finally, quotes from the participants were used to substantiate issues discussed.

4. Results

4.1. Sociodemographic Characteristics of Participants. Table 1 presents the sociodemographic characteristics of the participants. Eighty percent were in their 20s while 15% were aged 30–39 years. Those who had attained basic education constituted 35% whereas 30% had tertiary education. Ninety-five percent of the participants were Christians while 5% were Muslims. Fifty-five percent of the participants were never married while 45% were married at the time of the study. The main occupations of the participants were dressmaking (25%), civil service (25%), and trading (20%).

Table 1: Socio-demographic characteristics of participants.

Variable	Frequency	Percentage (%)
Age (In completed years)		
<20	1	5.0
20–29	16	80.0
30–39	3	15.0
Level of education		
No education	2	10.0
Primary	3	15.0
JHS	7	35.0
SHS	2	10.0
Tertiary	6	30.0
Religion		
Christian	19	95.0
Muslim	1	5.0
Marital status		
Never married	11	55.0
Married	9	45.0
Occupation		
Dressmaking	5	25.0
Trading	4	20.0
Farming	2	10.0
Civil service	5	25.0
Schooling	2	10.0
Hairdressing	2	10.0
*Total**	*20*	*100.0*

Source. Fieldwork, 2016 *Total represents the 20 participants which were recruited for the study.

4.2. Responsiveness to Postabortion Care. The major considerations of participants on the responsiveness of health professionals to postabortion care include prompt attention, the attitude of health professionals, patients' satisfaction, and choice of health professionals. Aside from these, the participants noted the challenges they experienced with PAC, their satisfaction with services, and the attitude of providers and the factors which influenced their decision to seek care at the facility.

4.2.1. Prompt Attention. We realized that the hospital placed priority on giving early care to its patients. There were instances where patients were offered treatment upon arrival and prior to the required initial procedure of registering a patient (documenting necessary information such as name, date of birth, and place of residence) for the service. There were also occasions where health professionals took it upon themselves to process the documents on behalf of the patients while they were treated. For instance, a 25-year-old trader who was treated while a hospital staff was processing her card said the following:

> *. . . Oh, they were quick in attending to me. As soon as I got here, I was sent to the ward for treatment to begin but I can't really tell like how many minutes it took them to attend to me because I was in pain and I was really not thinking about that. I was actually in pain from the house so when I got here the door was not opened by then so I approached a young male nurse and as soon as I told him what was happening to me, he took a wheelchair and wheeled me to the ward and they started treatment on me while he went on ahead to process my card . . ..* (Trader, 25 years)

Another participant who received prompt attention indicated the following:

> *Yes when I got here, they didn't even make me stay at the OPD (outpatient department), I was moved to the gynecological ward and my husband processed the folder at the OPD while I was being treated.* (Civil servant, 23 years)

4.2.2. Attitude of Health Professionals. The attitude of health professionals towards patients is an integral part of postabortion care [6]. This study revealed that the participants were generally happy about the attitude of health professionals at the hospital. The professionals were generally praised for being caring and polite. A 33-year-old farmer who expressed satisfaction with the attitude of the professionals said the following:

> *Oh, they are good, caring and are free with us. For some other hospitals, the nurses are not friendly at all and will fight and argue with you at the least thing. But at this hospital, they are very kind and free. Ever since I came all those who came to speak with me talk with some kind of respect for me and if they say something or do something and realized you are not happy, they are quick to apologize.* (Farmer, 33 years)

Another participant indicated the following:

> *Their attitude, in general, is fine. They know how to talk to us and are not abusive in their choice of words and they take very good care of us like coming to check up on us regularly to see if everything is going on well.* (Seamstress, 23 years)

About one-fourth of the participants, however, felt the health professionals exhibited negative attitudes. The negative attitudes they complained about include insulting and provocative behaviour of the health professionals. A 28-year-old hairdresser said the following:

> *I will not say everyone is having a good character. When I was here the other time, they really worried me. Is it insult they did not insult me? But I was in pain so I couldn't talk but those who treated me yesterday were very nice.* (Hairdresser, 28 years)

Corroborating the negative attitude of the health professionals, another participant noted the following:

> *Is this a good hospital? This is just a place for insulting. Hmmm the people are wicked and they don't take care of me. I have not been to a hospital that they have treated me like that before. The people are wicked, they are very wicked papa. Even if you are dying they won't mind you.* (Student, 28 years)

4.2.3. Challenges. Most of the women reported to the hospital with little or no money with the intention of using their health insurance cards. Ghana operates a National Health Insurance Scheme (NHIS) which provides services to residents free of any charges at the point of service delivery after payment of annual premiums [25]. Exemptions are, however, made with regard to such payments for children under 18 years, social security and national insurance trust contributors and pensioners, pregnant women, and the indigent [26]. However, the women only got to know at the facility that the insurance did not cover their treatments. A participant who was disappointed said the following:

> *The only thing that is bothering me is that I had only GH₵30 when I was coming knowing very well the health insurance will also cover some costs but they are telling me I have to pay GH₵130 and that the insurance card does not cover everything. She added that if not for the card, I would have paid about GH₵400.* (Hairdresser, 28 years)

Another disappointed participant noted the following:

> *Well, the government told us that health insurance will help us when we come to the hospital but when you come, then they expect you to pay for the medicine again and when you are done and about to leave they give you bill again and I don't understand why it should be like that. For example, when they wanted to clean my stomach (evacuation of the womb) for me, I was asked to pay for it as well as other things like water and medicines, which I think should be covered by the NHIS.* (Seamstress, 23 years)

4.3. Patients Satisfaction with Postabortion Care. More than three-quarters of the women expressed satisfaction with the postabortion care services at the facility. Overall, the women expressed satisfaction mainly because of the attitude of the health professionals towards them and how they were catered for even when they had no money to pay for the service. The participants said the following about the attitudes of the health professionals towards them:

> *The reason I am very satisfied is that I have been to different hospitals and I have come here too and I have seen the difference. Surprisingly, this happens to be the hospital that I was rather afraid of coming to, but I am really glad I did come here. The health workers here are very nice and caring towards us.* (Trader, 29 years)

Another participant said

> *... they are quick to attend to patients. Unlike other places that when you go and you are in pain, they will just stand and be watching you and how to even attend to patients or give them treatment becomes a problem. But for the three days I spent at the regional hospital, I was amazed at the way everyone who comes is dedicated to their work. Everyone was serious about their work and did it to satisfaction at the same time smiling at us.* (Farmer, 33 years)

Others also expressed satisfaction with the treatment they received mainly because after the treatment they did not suffer any complications again. For instance, a satisfied participant indicated the following:

> *Yes because the day they cleaned my stomach, the following day and I was okay and I did not feel*

> *any pain again but some other sister came and she really suffered after the process. I think she even got a swollen thigh.* (Student, 19 years)

4.3.1. Factors Influencing Patients' Choice of Facility. The major factors which influenced participants' choice of the facility were referrals from other facilities and past experiences. Regarding referrals, the women noted that, to a large extent, they did not decide on the facility to receive their postabortion care by themselves. Most of them were referred from other health facilities where they first sought PAC services. For instance, a participant who was referred from another health facility said the following:

> *. . . I was then sent to a hospital in Togo. When we got there, they pressed my stomach for long before it came out and I was in severe pain. But they said they were not having the machine that they will use to clean my stomach so they referred me to the VRH.* (Hairdresser, 28 years)

To corroborate this statement, another participant indicated the following:

> *I was sent to the hospital in Sokode. They managed to stabilise my condition there and then transferred me to the regional hospital. It was at the regional hospital that they carried out some tests on me and detected that I was pregnant but the pregnancy got spoilt (had spontaneous abortion) so went ahead to clean my stomach for me (evacuation of the uterus).* (Farmer, 33 years)

Some of the women, however, indicated that their choice of the facility was influenced by their past experiences at the hospital. Such experiences include the treatment and the care they received while at the hospital. A participant with a past experience from the Volta Regional Hospital indicated the following:

> *Well! this is the hospital that I had my first child and I liked how I was treated here so I don't see any reason to go anywhere else. Even my first child, I decided to come here because they treat people well. Even if you come alone and have no one to aid you, they themselves will take up that responsibility and take care of you for you to be comfortable. For example, when you come to this hospital and you need to purchase some things, but you don't have money, they will give it to you and you pay for it later.* (Hairdresser, 23 years)

Another participant said the following:

> *Because I don't have anyone who will take care of me at the hospital so I decided to come to the regional hospital. Unlike other hospitals that you need a relative or someone to be coming to wash for you, take care of you among other things, this place, the nurses do all that for you and make sure you are always comfortable.* (Farmer, 37 years)

5. Discussion

An essential factor to consider when assessing the quality of care of a health facility is the viewpoint of the patient. Since patients' needs often vary, their personal satisfaction rests on individual views and expectations [27]. Our findings show that waiting time for treatment at the hospital was relatively short: the women were satisfied with the prompt attention they received at the facility. This according to the conceptual framework is part of patient orientation which offers prompt attention to the patient [28]. This is, however, contradictory to findings made by Tesfaye and Oljira [29] who observed that the waiting time from arrival to treatment is usually very long. Nonetheless, other studies revealed that there is a bias in the delivery of early treatment to patients, with adolescents often not given early attention [30].

In line with postulations of the health system responsiveness, patients are expected to be treated with respect in terms of dignity, autonomy, and confidentiality [28]. We realized in our study that patients were generally satisfied with postabortion care at the hospital mainly because of positive attitudes exhibited towards them by the health professionals. These findings are consistent with that of Melkamu et al. [5] who reported that health professionals are usually caring and polite to patients who sought PAC services. However, some expressed dissatisfaction with PAC services at the hospital due to the provocative nature of some health professionals. This, also, affirms the findings of Arambepola et al. [31] in Sri Lanka, arguing that postabortion patients were displeased with services received from health facilities owing to the verbal harassment meted out to them by some health care providers due to their abortion condition.

The findings, however, show that treating patients with care and respect at a health facility gives them the needed satisfaction with health care services. The health professionals at the hospital were, therefore, applauded by the participants for their attitude towards them. Melkamu et al. [6] opined that most women perceive postabortion services in health facilities to be satisfactory and are, therefore, motivated to access postabortion services in hospitals. The specific factors that prompted this positive perception include the value of care, good conduct of health professionals, and the proximity of the health facilities [5, 6]. This corroborates the current findings as well as the health system responsiveness model which requires health systems to provide structural quality, service quality, and interpersonal quality to attain patient satisfaction [21].

The inability of some hospitals to perform postabortion care services resulted in the referral of some participants to the hospital. Others, however, noted that they chose the facility for the services mainly based on their past experiences at the hospital which they considered satisfactory. This affirms the health systems' responsiveness model's proposal that the ability to exercise preferences could be as a result of treatment by persons of a particular sex, age group, and emotional bonding to a particular facility [18]. This, also, agrees with the findings of Wariki [32] who argued that patients seek postabortion care at particular hospitals as a result of their satisfaction with the services at the facility and, hence, their enthusiasm to return for a follow-up and recommend the services to others.

Even though participants had subscribed to the NHIS, they realized at the facility that the scheme did not cover their treatments. This points to the challenges and concerns that have been raised by subscribers concerning the inadequacies of the health insurance over the years. The exclusion of abortion and postabortion services from the scheme may result in needless deaths [33]. Meanwhile, abortion services are considered basic services due to the high possibility of maternal deaths if they are not handled early and appropriately [34].

Despite the important findings made from this study, there are possible limitations inherent in the study that are worth mentioning. For instance, the fact that the study was conducted in only one facility and used a relatively small sample size greatly limits its generalizability to the general Ghanaian society. This limitation, however, does not limit the reliability and trustworthiness of the study in any way as the necessary steps needed to make the instrument valid and trustworthy were adhered to. Also, the study was conducted cross-sectionally. Trends in the responsiveness of the facility may, however, change in future as such trends may differ from current findings made in our study.

6. Conclusion

We established that health professionals were responsive to postabortion care at the facility. Patients were offered early treatment at the hospital. PAC patients were also found to be generally satisfied with postabortion care services at the facility. Women sought postabortion care at the facility generally as a result of referrals from other health facilities that could not handle such cases and also based on satisfaction with services received on previous visits to the hospital.

The referral of postabortion cases by some facilities could result in complications with serious maternal health implications for the patients. Pragmatic steps should be taken by the Ministry of Health and Ghana Health Service to equip all health facilities across the country with the needed facilities and personnel with the requisite skills to provide complete postabortion care. Also, efforts should be made by the NHIA to add postabortion care to the range of services covered by the NHIS.

Disclosure

The paper does not represent the views of the Volta Regional Hospital.

Authors' Contributions

Kenneth Setorwu Adde conceived the study. Kenneth Setorwu Adde, Eugene Kofour Marfo Darteh, and Akwasi Kumi-Kyereme designed and performed the analysis. Kenneth Setorwu Adde and Hubert Amu drafted the manuscript. Akwasi Kumi-Kyereme and Eugene Kofour Marfo Darteh reviewed the manuscript and provided substantial contributions to the interpretation of data and discussion of findings which greatly improved the intellectual content. All authors read the final manuscript and approved it.

Acknowledgments

The authors acknowledge the immense assistance from the Volta Regional Hospital, Ho.

References

[1] C. R. Kim, Ö. Tunçalp, B. Ganatra, and A. M. Gülmezoglu, "WHO Multi-Country Survey on Abortion-related Morbidity and Mortality in Health Facilities: study protocol," *BMJ Global Health*, vol. 1, no. 3, p. e000113, 2016.

[2] World Health Organisation, "Fact sheet: Maternal mortality," 2016, http://www.who.int/mediacentre/factsheets/fs348/en/.

[3] H. Amu and S. H. Nyarko, "Preparedness of health care professionals in preventing maternal mortality at a public health facility in Ghana: a qualitative study," *BMC Health Services Research*, vol. 16, article 252, 2016.

[4] G. Sedgh, J. Bearak, S. Singh et al., "Abortion incidence between 1990 and 2014: global, regional, and subregional levels and trends," *The Lancet*, vol. 388, no. 10041, pp. 258–267, 2016.

[5] Y. Melkamu, F. Enquselassie, A. Ali, H. Gebresilassie, and L. Yusuf, "Assessment of quality of post abortion care in government hospitals in Addis Ababa, Ethiopia," *Ethiopian Medical Journal*, vol. 43, no. 3, pp. 137–149, 2005.

[6] Y. Melkamu, M. Betre, and S. Tesfaye, "Utilization of post-abortion care services in three regional states of Ethiopia," *Ethiopian Journal of Health Development*, vol. 24, no. 1, pp. 123–129, 2010.

[7] S. Kumbi, Y. Melkamu, and H. Yeneneh, "Quality of post-abortion care in public health facilities in Ethiopia," *Ethiopian Journal of Health Development*, vol. 22, no. 1, 2008.

[8] K. Esia-Donkoh, E. K. M. Darteh, H. Blemano, and H. Asare, "Who cares? Pre and post abortion experiences among young females in Cape Coast metropolis, Ghana," *African Journal of Reproductive Health*, vol. 19, no. 2, pp. 43–51, 2015.

[9] B. O. Asamoah, K. M. Moussa, M. Stafström, and G. Musinguzi, "Distribution of causes of maternal mortality among different socio-demographic groups in Ghana: a descriptive study," *BMC Public Health*, vol. 11, article 159, 2011.

[10] A. Sundaram, F. Juarez, A. Bankole, and S. Singh, "Factors Associated with Abortion-Seeking and Obtaining a Safe Abortion in Ghana," *Studies in Family Planning*, vol. 43, no. 4, pp. 273–286, 2012.

[11] "GSS and GHS and Calverton, Macro International," in *Proceedings of the GSS and GHS and Calverton, Macro International*, Accra, Ghana, 2007.

[12] F. Baiden, K. Amponsa-Achiano, A. R. Oduro, T. A. Mensah, R. Baiden, and A. Hodgson, "Unmet need for essential obstetric services in a rural district in northern Ghana: Complications of unsafe abortions remain a major cause of mortality," *Public Health*, vol. 120, no. 5, pp. 421–426, 2006.

[13] J. Taylor, A. Diop, J. Blum, O. Dolo, and B. Winikoff, "Oral misoprostol as an alternative to surgical management for incomplete

abortion in Ghana," *International Journal of Gynecology and Obstetrics*, vol. 112, no. 1, pp. 40–44, 2011.

[14] M. R. Corbett and K. L. Turner, "Essential elements of postabortion care: Origins, evolution and future directions," *International Family Planning Perspectives*, vol. 29, no. 3, pp. 106–111, 2003.

[15] L. Hessini, E. Brookman-Amissah, and B. B. Crane, "Global policy change and women's access to safe abortion: the impact of the World Health Organization's guidance in Africa.," *African Journal of Reproductive Health*, vol. 10, no. 3, pp. 14–27, 2006.

[16] R. Gopal and SS. Bedi, "Impact of hospital services on outpatient satisfaction," vol. 2, pp. 37–44, 2014.

[17] World Health Organisation, "Health system responsiveness," 2017, http://www.who.int/responsiveness/hcover/en/.

[18] World Health Organisation, "Health system responsiveness," 2015, http://www.who.int/responsiveness/en/.

[19] C. Smith, "Validation of a patient satisfaction system in the united kingdom," *International Journal for Quality in Health Care*, vol. 4, no. 3, pp. 171–177, 1992.

[20] J. P. Logerfo, "Explorations in Quality Assessment and Monitoring. Volume I: The Definitions of Quality and Approaches to its Assessment," *Medical Care*, vol. 19, no. 10, pp. 1066-1067, 1981.

[21] J. W. Kenagy, D. M. Berwick, and M. F. Shore, "Service quality in health care," *Journal of the American Medical Association*, vol. 281, no. 7, pp. 661–665, 1999.

[22] N. Valentine, A. Prasad, N. Rice, S. Robone, and S. Chatterji, "Health systems responsiveness: A measure of the acceptability of health-care processes and systems from the user's perspective," *Performance Measurement for Health System Improvement: Experiences, Challenges and Prospects*, pp. 138–186, 2010.

[23] Ghana Statistical Service, "2010 Population and housing census: National analytical report," in *World population policies 2013*, Ghana Statistical Service, Accra, Ghana, 2013.

[24] B. M. Domhnaill, G. Hutchinson, A. Milev, and Y. Milev, "The social context of schoolgirl pregnancy in Ghana," *Vulnerable Children and Youth Studies*, vol. 6, no. 3, pp. 201–207, 2011.

[25] A. Kumi-Kyereme, H. Amu, and E. K. M. Darteh, "Barriers and motivations for health insurance subscription in Cape Coast, Ghana: A qualitative study," *Archives of Public Health*, vol. 75, no. 1, article no. 24, 2017.

[26] H. Amu and K. S. Dickson, "Health insurance subscription among women in reproductive age in Ghana: do socio-demographics matter?" *Health Economics Review (HER)*, vol. 6, article 24, 2016.

[27] M. Brawley, *The client perspective: What is quality health care service? A literature review*, 2000.

[28] C. J. Murray and J. Frenk, *A WHO framework for health system performance assessment*, Evidence and Information for Policy, World Health Organization, 1999.

[29] G. Tesfaye and L. Oljira, "Post abortion care quality status in health facilities of Guraghe zone, Ethiopia," *Reproductive Health*, vol. 10, no. 1, article no. 35, 2013.

[30] A. A. Fawole and A. P. Aboyeji, "Complications from unsafe abortion: presentations at Ilorin, Nigeria," *journal of the National Association of Resident Doctors of Nigeria*, vol. 11, no. 2, pp. 77–80, 2002.

[31] C. Arambepola, L. C. Rajapaksa, and C. Galwaduge, "Usual hospital care versus post-abortion care for women with unsafe abortion: A case control study from Sri Lanka," *BMC Health Services Research*, vol. 14, no. 1, article no. 470, 2014.

[32] W. M Wariki, *Post-abortion care in North Sulawesi, Indonesia: Patients determinants in selection of health facility , Quality in Primary Care*, Patients determinants in selection of health facility, Indonesia, 2014.

[33] A. Bankole, I. F. Adewole, R. Hussain, O. Awolude, S. Singh, and J. O. Akinyemi, "The incidence of abortion in Nigeria," *International Perspectives on Sexual & Reproductive Health*, vol. 41, no. 4, pp. 170–181, 2015.

[34] L. B. Haddad and N. M. Nour, "Unsafe abortion: unnecessary maternal mortality," *Reviews in Obstetrics and Gynecology*, vol. 2, no. 2, p. 122, 2009.

21

Hookworm Infection among Pregnant Women at First Antenatal Visit in Lira, Uganda

Felister Apili ,[1,2] Stephen Ochaya,[3,4] Charles Peter Osingada,[1] Scovia Nalugo Mbalinda ,[1] David Mukunya,[5] Grace Ndeezi,[6] and James K. Tumwine[6]

[1]*Department of Nursing, College of Health Sciences, Makerere University, Kampala, Uganda*
[2]*Faculty of Health Sciences, Lira University, Lira, Uganda*
[3]*Department of Clinical Pathology, Academic Hospital, Uppsala, Sweden*
[4]*Department of Immunology and Microbiology, Gulu University, Gulu, Uganda*
[5]*Center for Intervention Science in Maternal and Child Health, University of Bergen, Bergen, Norway*
[6]*Department of Paediatrics and Child Health, College of Health Sciences, Makerere University, Kampala, Uganda*

Correspondence should be addressed to Felister Apili; fapili@lirauni.ac.ug

Academic Editor: Samir Hamamah

Background. Hookworm infection in expectant mothers has adverse health effects on both the mothers and their unborn babies. Foetal effects are known to include intrauterine growth retardation and physical and mental growth retardation, while the mothers may develop anemia which could potentially result in death. Unfortunately, little is known about factors that may predispose a pregnant woman to infection by hookworm. In this study, we strived to determine not only the prevalence of hookworm infection among pregnant women attending their first antenatal visit during the current pregnancy in a local health center in northern Uganda but also factors that might predispose them to hookworm infection. *Method.* This cross-sectional study was conducted among 346 pregnant women from Ogur Health Center IV located in Lira district, northern Uganda. Stool samples were collected from each study participant and analyzed for hookworms. The independent variables listed in this study (participant's sociodemographic characteristics, preconception care, and sanitation factors) were obtained using a structured questionnaire. Data analysis, including calculation of adjusted ratios, was performed using STATA software (version 14). *Results.* Prevalence of hookworm infection among pregnant women who attended their first antenatal visit at Ogur Health Center IV was 11% ($n = 38$). After controlling for confounders, factors found to be significantly associated with this infection among pregnant women here were gardening barefooted (adjusted odds ratio (AOR), 3.4; 95% confidence interval (CI), 1.6 to 7.5; $P < 0.001$) and fetching unsafe water shared with animals for domestic uses (AOR, 2.8; 95% CI, 1.3 to 6.2; P value of 0.002). *Conclusion.* Hookworm infection among pregnant women at Ogur Health Center IV in Lira district, at 11%, is a public health concern and significantly associated with barefoot gardening and fetching water from unsafe sources shared with animals. We, therefore, recommend that special emphasis during routine prenatal health education be placed on the use of protective footwear during farming and fetching water for domestic use from protected safe sources. *Author Summary.* Hookworm infection is a parasitic condition that more often goes unnoticed, yet it presents immense detrimental effects, especially to pregnant women and their unborn children. It is a chronic disease with accruing effects of blood depletion resulting in anemia. Anemia is, by far, one of the major causes of maternal morbidity and mortality in Uganda. Pregnant women are more prone to hookworm infection by virtue of their compromised immunity, secondary to the physiological process of pregnancy. We demonstrated here that hookworm infection still exists among pregnant women in Uganda. We also showed that gardening barefooted and fetching water for domestic uses from unsafe sources shared with animals were major factors associated with this helminthic infection. This study provides evidence necessary to influence decision making on prevention of hookworm infection in the study area.

1. Background

Hookworm infection is a major public health concern. The two known species of concern are *Ancylostoma duodenale* (*A. duodenale*, causes ancyltomiasis) and *Necator americanus* (*N. americanus*, causes necatoriasis) [1]. These species have similar lifecycles and are difficult to differentiate by the traditional light microscopy. The larval stages require unique but sometimes overlapping environments, mostly soil, water, and temperature for sustenance. *A. duodenale* was found mostly in the Middle East, North Africa, India, and Southern Europe before it was eradicated. In contrast, *N. americanus* is found in America (tropical and semitropical regions), Sub-Sahara Africa, Southeast Asia, China, and Indonesia. Both species of hookworm infect primarily by way of the mature infective third-stage larva penetrating human skin [2] and through oral ingestion in case of *A. duodenale* [3]. Children and pregnant women are particularly vulnerable to hookworm infection [4]. Hookworm infection during pregnancy is associated with adverse health effects in expectant women and the unborn children [5]. Hookworm, a blood-feeding parasite that lives in the small intestine, is common in tropical countries largely due to a favourable climate in those countries [6], and in poor countries due to socioeconomic factors such as low quality of water for domestic use fetched from sources shared with animals, lack of, or poor utilisation of pitlatrine and poor personal hygiene in general [7]. This infection is characterized by ground itch at the point of entry, fever, nagging cough, fluctuating appetite, weight loss, and diarrhoea [8].

Hookworm infection has been reported to predispose victims to anemia [9], and in Uganda, hookworm infection is one of the few common factors that cause anemia; a disease that is among the top 10 causes of maternal morbidity and mortality [3]. Anemia is also one of the top five causes of hospital-based mortality in women and children [3] and is generally associated with poor birth outcomes like preterm labor, low birthweight [10], intrauterine growth retardation, extrauterine growth retardation, delayed sexual development, and early infant death [11, 12]. The prevalence of anemia among pregnant women in Uganda is estimated to be 32% [13]; 20.2% of which is attributable to hookworm infection [14]. Because of this, the Uganda ministry of health adopted the WHO recommendation of routine biannual deworming for girls and women of reproductive age and twice in pregnancy during the second and third trimesters [15].

Factors that may predispose an individual to hookworm infections are demographics, social, economic, and biological status. Socioeconomic status of families greatly influences the quality of life [16]. Poor communities often fail to access basic sanitation facilities, walk barefooted, and use farm tools with bare hands, all of which escalate the risk of hookworm infection [17]. Farming, the main economic activity in rural areas, keeps the rural population in constant contact with infected soil [12].

In Uganda, the prevalence of hookworm infection as reported from previous studies was relatively similar across different geographical locations. For instance, 45% of Entebbe population are infected [18], 40.5% in Mayuge, and 51% in Tororo. In Ethiopia, it is reported to be 36.1% [19]. Unfortunately, very few published studies have been done specifically among pregnant women in these and other geographical areas. We believe this to be an oversight because preventing hookworm infection improves pregnancy outcomes since the unborn is always the most affected in this scenario. It was, therefore, imperative to study the prevalence of hookworm infection among pregnant women and identify the factors involved. In this study, we have taken a first step in that direction in northern Uganda with pregnant women attending their first antenatal visit at Ogur Health Center IV in Lira district. The goal was to assess the prevalence of hookworm infection and identify preliminarily factors that predispose a pregnant woman in this area of Uganda to this parasitic infection.

2. Methods

2.1. Study Design. This was a cross-sectional study conducted between December 2017 and February 2018 among pregnant women attending their first antenatal visit (for that particular pregnancy regardless of the gestational age at the time of contact). Only pregnant women who consented to participate in the study and had not received routine mebendazole treatment during the current pregnancy were enrolled. Also, excluded were severely ill pregnant women who could not disclose personal information or bring stool samples. Similarly, those who met the criteria, consented to participate but failed to provide stool samples were excluded as well. Each participant provided approximately 10 g of valid stool sample uncontaminated with water or urine. No visual evidence of water or urine in a stool sample assured validity.

2.2. Study Area. The study was done at Ogur Health Center IV, a rural site located approximately 30 km from Lira town (Lira district, northern Uganda) along Kitgum road. The health center is a mid-level health facility that offers basic and emergency obstetric services and operates an antenatal clinic every weekday except public holidays. Pregnant women attending their first antenatal care (ANC) are booked on all those days. Although it has only 24 beds, the health center offers general health care services for a catchment area of 106 villages with about 40,269 people according to Lira district population statistics of 2018. On average, the monthly outpatient attendance is about 12,000 patients of which 2,600 are pregnant women seeking antenatal care. We chose to study this rural site because of the suitable environment and practices that favor hookworm proliferation. For example, land cultivation which is the major economic activity among the rural population [20] provides a favourable climate alongside contact with infected soil on bare hands and feet during cultivation for hookworm infection [21]. Additionally, Lira district, the location of Ogur Health Center IV, is currently recovering from a 20-year civil war and is extremely poor. Former war refugees have since relocated to villages at the end of the war where they live in semipermanent houses made of mud blocks without concrete floors. They often share water from unprotected wells with animals, more so, during the dry seasons when water is scarce. The latter scenario further exposes the rural population to hookworm infection [22].

2.3. Sample Size Determination. The sample size for this cross-sectional study was calculated using the Kish Leslie formula [23]: $n = z^2pq/d^2$, where n is the minimum sample size, z is the standard score corresponding to 5% level of significance (i.e., 0.05 and $z = 1.96$), p is 1% (the prevalence of hookworm infection among pregnant women), q is 99%, and d is 5% confidence limit (the proportion of sampling error). We assumed that the prevalence of hookworm infection among pregnant women in Ogur was similar to the 45% obtained from a randomized controlled trial done in Entebbe, Uganda [18]. With an alpha value of 5% and a precision value of 5%, this study needed 380 participants.

2.4. Sampling Method. To attain the required sample size within the study timeframe, consecutive sampling was used to recruit participants as follows. A team was stationed at the antenatal clinic who interviewed women as they arrived before the antenatal services commenced. Their arrival usually began at around 10 to11 am local time (the late start time is to give the same staff shared between the delivery ward and antenatal clinic at the health facility ample time to complete the latter). Interviewing was continued daily (except on public holidays and weekends) until the targeted sample size was achieved. A comprehensive interviewer-administered questionnaire was developed in English language and translated into Lango, the native language spoken in the study area. For applicability and accuracy and to find out how clearly respondents understood and responded to questions as intended, the questionnaire was pretested one week prior to data collection. Broadly, the questionnaire was used to gather data on social demographic factors, obstetric characteristics, and environmental-related factors. Six items in the questionnaire (presented in Table 1) measured sociodemographic characteristics and ten items measured preconception factors. Prevalence was derived from microscopic stool analysis where the number of all positive slides for ova, larva, or adult hookworm were summed up and divided by the respondent sample size. The results are expressed as percentages in this study.

2.5. Study Variables

2.5.1. Dependent Variables. The dependent variable in this study was hookworm infection among pregnant women at their first ANC visit in Ogur Health Center IV. Stool samples were examined for hookworms using direct and formol-ether-based light microscopic methods. The presence of ova, larva, or adult hookworms indicated hookworm infection; the absence meant no hookworm infection.

2.5.2. Independent Variables. The independent variables were sociodemographic characteristics of the pregnant women, preconception care, and sanitation factors. Age was categorized in years as ≤20, 21-30, and>30; a participant's religion was considered to be either Christian or Moslem; marital status was taken to be married or single; education status as either no formal education, primary, or secondary or higher; a person was considered a resident if she lived in this community or visited for a month or more. Occupation was civil servant and/or businesswoman (paying employment), housewife, and/or peasant farmer (nonpaying employment). Proper pit latrine utilisation was considered if one reported disposing all faecal materials of both children and adults into the pit latrine. Boreholes, protected spring wells, and taps were taken as safe sources of domestic water supply while unprotected spring wells were considered unsafe water sources. These variables were measured using a pretested twenty-one-item tool developed in-house.

Table 1: Sociodemographic characteristics of pregnant women attending their first ANC at Ogur Health Center IV ($n = 346$).

Characteristic	Frequency	Percentage (%)
Age (years)		
≤20	171	49.4
21 to 30	138	39.9
>30	37	10.7
Religion		
Christian	333	96.2
Moslem	13	3.8
Marital status		
Married	302	87.3
Single	44	12.7
Education level		
None	299	86.4
Primary	34	9.8
Secondary or higher	13	3.8
Resident		
Yes	328	94.8
No	18	5.2
Occupation		
Unpaying employment	279	80.6
Paying employment	67	19.4

2.6. Participant Recruitment and Data Collection Procedure. Each participant was required to provide a stool sample before she could respond to the questionnaire. All 380 stool sample containers used in this study were paired up and precoded similarly with corresponding questionnaires to avoid mixing up of samples. Participants were educated about avoiding sample contamination with urine or water during collection; they provided freshly voided stool samples. The samples were collected from a cleaned toilet provided with toilet paper and hand washing facility at the health center. Even then, 34 participants failed to empty their bowel hence could not proceed to answer the questionnaires. Stool analysis was done within 30 min of collection. The interviewer-administered questionnaires were used to gather information about sociodemographic and potential factors associated with hookworm infection (see Sampling Method). The interviewer checked all questions immediately after questionnaire completion for completeness before disengaging with a participant and, where necessary, sought clarifications. Laboratory results were disclosed to participants on the same day of testing and before they left the health center. A brief health talk was conducted pertaining to hookworm infection in pregnancy and measures of preventing exposure including proper use of pit latrine for both children and adults, building protected water sources, and wearing hand and foot protective gears during farming to avoid contact with hookworm-infected soil.

2.7. Specimen Processing and Analysis. Stool analysis was done at the Ogur Health Center IV laboratory by two qualified and experienced laboratory technicians. Semisolid samples were examined within 30 minutes of collection, while the rest were examined within an hour of collection without refrigeration to prevent destruction of the morphology of ova and adult warms.

Two methods of stool analysis were used simultaneously. Fresh warm stool was analyzed by direct microscopy at two different magnifying powers (10x and 40x) to observe eggs, larva, and adult hookworms. Some portions of the samples were examined by light microscopy after performing formol-ether concentration. Although direct microscopy is cheap and easy to perform under our field conditions, it is only sensitive to heavy infections. Formol-ether concentration method for intestinal parasites, on the other hand, is more sensitive at low hookworm infection and therefore was used to minimize false negatives. As such, all samples which qualified as negative for hookworms by direct microscopy were also subjected to the formol-ether concentration method.

2.8. Statistical Analysis. A statistical software package STATA 14.0 (Stata Corp, College Station, TX, USA) was used to summarize the data we collected in tables. Continuous descriptive variables were presented as means and standard deviations. Categorical variables were presented as proportions. We performed bivariable and multivariable logistic regressions to determine the association between independent factors and hookworm infection. Factors known from the literature to be predictors of hookworm infection and those with a bivariable P value < 0.25 (as long as they were not in the casual pathway and they were not strongly collinear with other independent variables) were considered for the initial multivariable model [1]. To assess for collinearity, factors were considered strongly collinear if their variance inflation factor was greater than 10. In case of collinearity, the factor with a stronger measure of association with the outcome variable was retained and the other dropped. We generated the final model using the method of purposeful selection of variables as described by Hosmer and Lemeshow [24]. A variable was called a confounder if it changed the unadjusted measure of association by 10% or more. The final model included all confounders and was tested for goodness-of-fit using the Hosmer and Lemeshow goodness-of-fit test [24].

2.9. Ethics. The Research and Ethics Committee of Makerere University School of Health Sciences approved this study (reference number #SHSREC REF: 2017-060). Prior to enrolment, written informed consent was obtained from each participant, clearly explaining the study processes, benefits, discomforts, and their rights to refuse or withdraw from the study at any time without consequences. Confidentiality and privacy were maintained throughout the study, and no direct identifier was captured on questionnaires. Pregnant women under the age of 18 years were regarded as emancipated minors who could consent [25]. Declining to provide stool samples or to respond to questions asked did not in any way obscure access to routine ANC. Results were provided to the participants. All individuals with positive results were helped to access treatment. Education about preventing hookworm infection was provided to every participant.

Table 2: Results of stool sample analysis of pregnant women attending their first ANC at Ogur Health Center IV, Lira district, northern Uganda.

Method	Stool sample (n = 346) Positive	Negative
Direct microscopy	(18)	328
Light infection (<1,000 ova/larva/adult hookworms)	11	—
Heavy infection (>1,000 ova/larva/adult hookworms)	7	—
Formol-ether concentration	(20)	308
Light infection (<1,000 ova/larva/adult hookworms),	19	—
Heavy infection (>1,000 ova/larva/adult hookworms)	1	—

3. Results

3.1. Sociodemographic Characteristics of Participants. We interviewed 346 participants ranging in age from 15 to 42 years (mean 23 ± 6 SD). Most participants were Christians, married, had less than 7 years of formal schooling, and were mainly peasant farmers and/or housewives. The overall social demographic characteristics of the participants are summarized in Table 1.

3.2. Prevalence of Hookworm Infection. This was obtained from the summation of the number of positive results by both direct microscopy and formol-ether methods then expressed as a percentage of the response sample size (346) as is shown in Table 2. Eighteen out the 346 tested samples were found positive for hookworm infection using direct microscopy. Eleven of which were quantified as light infection whereas seven were heavy hookworm infection.

3.3. Distribution of Hookworm Infection. Hookworm infection was more common among resident, young, married, Christian pregnant women, with less than seven years of formal education, and peasant farmers. This helminthic infection was also predominant among women who reported to have given birth before and currently in their first trimester of pregnancy and fetched domestic water from unsafe sources shared with animals. The infection was similarly higher among participants who practiced open defecation. The results are presented in Table 3.

3.4. Factors Associated with Hookworm Infection. Results of both bivariable and multivariable analyses of the data are presented in Table 4. During bivariable analysis, all factors apart from marital status were significant (P values < 0.05). The multivariable analysis, however, revealed only two statistically significant factors: gardening barefooted and fetching domestic water from sources shared with animals. These results are presented in Table 4.

4. Discussion

This study finds that hookworm infection is prevalent among pregnant women at their first ANC visit during the current pregnancy in Ogur Health Center IV. Women who reported to have given birth before were found to have a higher prevalence (71.1%, $n = 38$) than those pregnant for the first time. Several potential factors known to be associated with hookworm infection were confirmed as confounders. Gardening barefooted and fetching unsafe water from sources shared with animals were strongly associated with hookworm infection in this population of pregnant women.

This finding that hookworm infection is prevalent in a rural community of Uganda confirms the notion that this helminthic parasite is predominate in tropical areas [6] owing to conducive environmental conditions for sustenance. It also confirms that the proximity to hookworm-infected soil is a major health concern for pregnant women. The 11% prevalence of hookworm infection among pregnant women as at their first ANC visit found here was lower than those obtained from other studies in Uganda. This is not surprising since this study was conducted during the dry season in northern Uganda (December 2017 and February 2018) when no land cultivation was being done, open wells were mostly dry and temperature was probably too high for hookworms to survive in the soil. We believe this thesis fits here because studies elsewhere have demonstrated seasonal discrepancy. In Bangladesh, for example, a low prevalence of hookworm infection was found during the winter season (19.4%) when compared to the rainy season (29.3%) [26]. In India, a higher prevalence of hookworm infection (80.5%) was reported in autumn than the 43.9% in spring [27].

The prevalence of hookworm infection as determined in this study is similar to those observed in Kenya (3.9%) [28] and Ghana (13.9%) [29]. This could probably be attributed to the routine deworming practice within this vulnerable group. Locally, the prevalence observed here is much lower than the 45% obtained in a double-blinded randomized controlled trial among a similar study group in Entebbe, Uganda [18]. The discrepancy could have resulted from the fact that Ndibazza et al. [18] had a big sample size of 2,507 participants and conducted their study all year round for nearly two years and among a fishing community living around the shores of Lake Victoria where majority of the people do not have proper sanitation facilities and the area has a weather conducive to hookworm proliferation [30]. In

Table 3: Distribution of hookworm infection among pregnant women attending first antenatal visit at Ogur Health Center IV, Lira district, northern Uganda.

Variable	Hookworm positive ($n = 38$)	Hookworm negative ($n = 308$)
Age (years)	n (%)	n (%)
≤20	17 (44.7)	154 (50)
21-30	14 (36.8)	124 (40.3)
>30	7 (18.4)	30 (9.7)
Religion	n (%)	n (%)
Christian	36 (94.7)	297 (96.4)
Moslem	2 (5.3)	11 (3.6)
Marital status	n (%)	n (%)
Single	9 (23.7)	35 (11.4)
Married	29 (76.3)	273 (88.6)
Education	n (%)	n (%)
None	11 (29.0)	46 (14.9)
Primary	26 (68.4)	218 (70.8)
Secondary or higher	1 (2.6)	44 (14.3)
Occupation	n (%)	n (%)
Peasant farmer/HW[a]	33 (86.8)	248 (80.5)
Civil servant/BW[b]	5 (13.2)	60 (19.5)
Resident	n (%)	n (%)
Yes	38 (100)	291 (94.5)
No	0 (0)	17 (5.5)
Gestational age	n (%)	n (%)
1st trimester	20 (52.6)	154 (50.0)
2nd-3rd trimester	18 (47.4)	154 (50.0)
Gravidity	n (%)	n (%)
Primegravida	11 (28.9)	70 (22.7)
Multigravida	27 (71.1)	238 (77.3)
Water source	n (%)	n (%)
Unsafe	14 (36.8)	47 (15.3)
Safe	24 (63.2)	261 (84.7)
Boiling drinking water	n (%)	n (%)
Yes	2 (5.3)	58 (18.8)
No	36 (94.7)	250 (81.2)
Pit latrine utilisation	n (%)	n (%)
Yes	6 (15.8)	14 (4.6)
No	32 (84.2)	294 (95.5)
Gardening shoes	n (%)	n (%)
Yes	10 (26.3)	121 (39.3)
Never	28 (73.7)	187 (60.7)
Floor type	n (%)	n (%)
Concrete	3 (7.9)	58 (18.8)
Earth	35(92.1)	250 (81.2)

[a]Housewife. [b]Businesswoman.

TABLE 4: Factors associated with hookworm infection among pregnant women attending their first ANC visit at Ogur Health Center, Lira district, northern Uganda.

Variable	Crude OR[a] (95% CI)	P value	Adjusted OR[a] (95% CI)
Mother's age			
≤20	1		—
21-30	1.0	0.953	
>30	2.1	0.128	
Religion			
Moslem	1		—
Christian	0.67	0.607	
Marital status			
Single	1	1	—
Married	0.41 (0.18-0.94)	0.036	
Mother's education			
None	1		1
Primary	0.50 (0.23-1.08)	0.078	0.70 (0.30-1.6)
Secondary or higher	0.10 (0.01-0.77)	0.027	0.17 (0.02-1.4)
Gestational age			
1st trimester	1		
2nd-3rd trimester	0.90 (0.46-1.77)	0.760	—
Water source			
Safe	1		1
Unsafe	3.2 (1.6-6.7)	0.002	2.8 (1.3-6.2)
Boiling drinking water			
Yes	1		—
No	4.2 (0.98-17.8)	0.054	
Pit latrine utilization			
Yes	1		1
No	3.9 (1.4-11.0)	0.009	3.2 (1.1-9.8)
Gardening shoes			
Yes	1		1
No	4.3 (2.0-9.2)	<0.001	3.4 (1.6-7.5)
Floor type			
Concrete	1		—
Earth	2.7 (0.80-9.1)	0.108	

[a]OR: odds ratio.

other studies, the prevalence of hookworm infection in two communities in Uganda was 40.5% in Mayuge [14] and 51.6% in Tororo located in eastern Uganda [1]. These studies were, however, conducted among the general population and not pregnant women; which explains the difference in results in relation to this study findings. Additional studies from two other Sub-Saharan countries involving large sample sizes found that the prevalence of hookworm infection in Ethiopia was 36.1% [19] and among pregnant women in Ghana was 13.9% [29]. The latter is similar to the prevalence of hookworm infection among pregnant women at their first ANC visit in Ogur.

4.1. Factors Associated with Hookworm Infection. This study has shown that gardening barefooted (AOR, 3.4; 95% CI, 1.6 to 7.5; $P < 0.001$) and fetching water for domestic uses from unsafe sources shared with animals (AOR, 2.8; 95% CI, 1.3 to 6.2; $P = 0.002$) were strongly associated with hookworm infection among pregnant women attending first antenatal visit in Ogur Health Center IV as is seen in Table 4. The association between gardening barefoot and infection with hookworm emanates from the fact that rural women do many fieldwork including harvesting and weeding crops without protective footwear, hence exposing them to infective hookworm larva thereby increasing risk of getting infected. In addition, most women in rural northern Uganda, from personal observation, are often barefooted. Barefooting was reported to result from the social norms of not wearing them while in the garden or when at home generally and from the inability to afford shoes. Again, from personal observation and experience, shoes in the study area are spared for special occasions like church and marriage functions.

Association between gardening barefooted, fetching water for domestic uses from unsafe sources shared with animals, and hookworm infection demonstrated in this study is consistent with the life cycle of the more prevalent *N. Americanus* [3]. Preventative measures should therefore target curbing these factors to break the cycle of hookworm infection. A cohort study conducted in Thailand among the rural population reported associations between barefooting or raising buffalos near the house and hookworm infection [31], a result very similar to our finding. Similar findings were also obtained in a study from Ethiopia in which hookworm infection was demonstrated to be significantly associated with walking barefooted as well [19]

In 2014, Strunz and colleagues conducted a meta-analysis and systematic review of 94 studies to determine the association of improved water, sanitation, hygiene (WASH) and soil-transmitted infections including hookworm. Five of those studies were randomized controlled trials and the rest cross-sectional studies. Their review demonstrated a significant association between wearing shoes and decreased odds of hookworm infection [22]. However, a recent cross-sectional study in Ethiopia among 283 elementary and secondary school students failed to demonstrate any significant associations between hookworm infection and sources of domestic water or shoe wearing [7] contrary to our study findings.

Open-ground defecation and poor utilisation of the pit latrine were some of the factors independently found to be associated with hookworm infection in this study. This was probably because the study site is rural which increases risk of hookworm infection when the occupants choose to go to the bush to help themselves, without putting on shoes. Secondly, barefooting and improper use of latrines by defecating on the floors can contribute to hookworm infection. However, these variables were ruled out as confounding factors during the multivariable data analysis process of this study.

5. Conclusion

We have shown in this study that hookworm infection during pregnancy in Ogur, at a prevalence of 11%, is still a public health concern that is associated with gardening barefooted and fetching water for domestic uses from unsafe sources shared with animals. This is notwithstanding our main limitation of low predictive power here to study factors associated with hookworm infection. In the interim, we encourage income-generating activities as part of the routine prenatal care education so that pregnant women can afford protective footwear and access to safe water in order to prevent hookworm infection.

Consent

The patients gave written informed consent to the publication of their case details.

Authors' Contributions

Felister Apili helped in the conceptualization, methodology, software, formal analysis, investigation, data curation, writing of original draft, and review and editing of the manuscript. Stephen Ochaya helped in the critical reviewing of the study, manuscript writing, and critical editing. Osingada Charles Peter helped in the supervision, data analysis, and review and editing of the draft manuscript. Scovia Mbalinda Nalugo helped in supervision, data analysis, and review and editing of the draft manuscript. David Mukunya helped in drafting the manuscript and analysis and reviewing. Grace Ndeezi helped in the supervision and reviewing. James K Tumwine helped in the conceptualization, supervision, and reviewing.

Acknowledgments

The first author acknowledges the Makerere University and Swedish International Corporation Development Agency collaboration under project 344 for funding this study as part of a strategy to accelerate reduction in maternal and child morbidity and mortality. The authors acknowledge the management, staff, and participants from Ogur Health Center IV for making this study possible and Professor Okot Nyormoi (retired) of North Carolina Central University Durham, NC, USA and Dr. Ochan Otim of the University of California, Los Angeles for the critical reviews of the draft manuscript.

References

[1] R. L. Pullan, N. B. Kabatereine, H. Bukirwa, S. G. Staedke, and S. Brooker, "Heterogeneities and consequences of Plasmodium species and hookworm coinfection: a population based study in Uganda," *Journal of Infectious Diseases*, vol. 203, no. 3, pp. 406–417, 2011.

[2] A. Echazú, D. Bonanno, M. Juarez et al., "Effect of poor access to water and sanitation as risk factors for soil-transmitted helminth infection: selectiveness by the infective route," *PLoS Neglected Tropical Diseases*, vol. 9, no. 9, 2015.

[3] CDC and US Centers for Disease Control and Prevention, *Life cycle of hookworms*, 2013, https://www.cdc.gov/parasites/hookworm/biology.html.

[4] A. Loukas, P. J. Hotez, D. Diemert et al., "Hookworm infection," *Nature Reviews Disease Primers*, vol. 2, no. 1, 2016.

[5] H. Mpairwe, J. Ndibazza, E. L. Webb et al., "Maternal hookworm modifies risk factors for childhood eczema: results from a birth cohort in Uganda," *Pediatric Allergy and Immunology*, vol. 25, no. 5, pp. 481–488, 2014.

[6] S. M. Bartsch, P. J. Hotez, L. Asti et al., "The global economic and health burden of human hookworm infection," *PLoS Neglected Tropical Diseases*, vol. 10, no. 9, 2016.

[7] I. Ali, G. Mekete, and N. Wodajo, "Intestinal parasitism and related risk factors among students of Asendabo Elementary and Junior Secondary school, South Western Ethiopia," *Ethiopian Journal of Health Development*, vol. 13, no. 2, 1999.

[8] H. Cedron-Cheng and O. Carlos, "Hookworm infestation diagnosis by capsule endoscopy," *Journal of Gastrointestinal & Digestive System*, vol. 1, 2011.

[9] G. Kumera, K. Haile, N. Abebe, T. Marie, and T. Eshete, "Anemia and its association with coffee consumption and hookworm infection among pregnant women attending antenatal care at Debre Markos Referral Hospital, Northwest Ethiopia," *PloS One*, vol. 13, no. 11, p. e0206880, 2018.

[10] G. Obai, P. Odongo, and R. Wanyama, "Prevalence of anaemia and associated risk factors among pregnant women attending antenatal care in Gulu and Hoima Regional Hospitals in Uganda: a cross sectional study," *BMC Pregnancy and Childbirth*, vol. 16, no. 1, 2016.

[11] T. W. Gyorkos and N. L. Gilbert, "Blood drain: soil-transmitted helminths and anemia in Pregnant women," *PLoS neglected tropical diseases*, vol. 8, no. 7, p. e2912, 2014.

[12] A. F. Gabrielli, A. Montresor, and L. Savioli, "Soil-transmitted helminthiasis.," in *Helminth Infections and their Impact on Global Public Health*, F. Bruschi, Ed., pp. 275–297, Springer Vienna, Vienna, 2014.

[13] UDHS, *Uganda demographic and health survey*, 2016.

[14] G. F. Chami, A. A. Kontoleon, E. Bulte et al., "Profiling nonrecipients of mass drug administration for schistosomiasis and hookworm infections: a comprehensive analysis of praziquantel and albendazole coverage in community-directed treatment in Uganda," *Clinical Infectious Diseases*, vol. 62, no. 2, pp. 200–207, 2015.

[15] WHO, *WHO recommendations on antenatal care for a positive pregnancy experience*, 2016, https://www.who.int/reproductivehealth/publications/maternal_perinatal_health/anc-positive-pregnancy-experience/en/.

[16] D. Kattula, R. Sarkar, S. S. Rao Ajjampur et al., "Prevalence & risk factors for soil transmitted helminth infection among school children in South India," *Indian Journal of Medical Research*, vol. 139, no. 1, pp. 76–82, 2014.

[17] R. L. Pullan and S. J. Brooker, "The global limits and population at risk of soil-transmitted helminth infections in 2010," *Parasites & Vectors*, vol. 5, no. 1, 2012.

[18] J. Ndibazza, L. Muhangi, D. Akishule et al., "Effects of deworming during pregnancy on maternal and perinatal outcomes in Entebbe, Uganda: a randomized controlled trial," *Clinical Infectious Diseases*, vol. 50, no. 4, pp. 531–540, 2010.

[19] Y. Belyhun, G. Medhin, A. Amberbir et al., "Prevalence and risk factors for soil-transmitted helminth infection in mothers and their infants in Butajira, Ethiopia: a population based study," *BMC Public Health*, vol. 10, no. 1, 2010.

[20] D. Humphries, W. A. Twum, K. Bosompem et al., "Epidemiology of hookworm infection in Kintampo north municipality, Ghana: patterns of malaria coinfection, anemia, and albendazole treatment failure," *The American Journal of Tropical Medicine and Hygiene*, vol. 84, no. 5, pp. 792–800, 2011.

[21] A. Alemu, A. Atnafu, Z. Addis et al., "Soil transmitted helminths and Schistosoma mansoni infections among school children in Zarima town, Northwest Ethiopia," *BMC Infectious Diseases*, vol. 11, no. 1, 2011.

[22] E. C. Strunz, D. G. Addiss, M. E. Stocks, S. Ogden, J. Utzinger, and M. C. Freeman, "Water, sanitation, hygiene, and soil-transmitted helminth infection: a systematic review and Meta-Analysis," *PLoS Medicine*, vol. 11, no. 3, 2014.

[23] L. Kish, *Survey Sampling*, John Wiley and Sons, Inc., New York, NY, 1965.

[24] D. W. Hosmer Jr., S. Lemeshow, and R. X. Sturdivant, *Applied Logistic Regression*, John Wiley and Sons, Inc., Hoboken, New Jersey, Third edition, 2013.

[25] UNCST, *National Guidelines for Research Involving Human Subjects as Research Participants*, 2007, https://www.uncst.go.ug/download/national-guidelines-for-research-involving-humans/.

[26] H. Khanum, M. R. Islam, and S. Parvin, "Occurrences of eggs and larvae of gastrointestinal nematodes in nails of street inhabitants in Dhaka City," *Journal of Life and Earth Science*, vol. 5, pp. 75–79, 2010.

[27] H. Kumar, K. Jain, and R. Jain, "A study of prevalence of intestinal worm infestation and efficacy of anthelminthic drugs," *Medical Journal Armed Forces India*, vol. 70, no. 2, pp. 144–148, 2014.

[28] A. Wekesa, C. Mulambalah, C. Muleke, and R. Odhiambo, "Intestinal helminth infections in pregnant women attending antenatal clinic at Kitale district hospital, Kenya," *Journal of Parasitology Research*, vol. 2014, 5 pages, 2014.

[29] S. Baidoo, S. Tay, and H. Abruquah, "Intestinal helminth infection and anaemia during pregnancy: a community based study in Ghana," *African Journal of Microbiology Research*, vol. 4, no. 16, pp. 1713–1718, 2010.

[30] G. Bwire, A. Munier, I. Ouedraogo et al., "Epidemiology of cholera outbreaks and socio-economic characteristics of the communities in the fishing villages of Uganda: 2011-2015," *PLoS Neglected Tropical Diseases*, vol. 11, no. 3, 2017.

[31] V. Jiraanankul, W. Aphijirawat, P. Piyaraj et al., "Incidence and risk factors of hookworm infection in a rural community of Central Thailand," *The American Journal of Tropical Medicine and Hygiene*, vol. 84, no. 4, pp. 594–598, 2011.

22

Flow Cytometry Detection of Sperm DNA Fragmentation and Apoptotic Markers in the Semen of Infertile Males

Huda Mossa Omran,[1,2] **Moiz Bakhiet**,[1] **and Volker Ehemann**[3]

[1]*Department of Molecular Medicine, College of Medicine and Medical Sciences, Princess Al-Jawhara Center for Genetics and Inherited Diseases, Arabian Gulf University, Manama, Bahrain*
[2]*Pulse Health Training Center, Manama, Bahrain*
[3]*Institute of Pathology, University Hospital Heidelberg, Heidelberg, Germany*

Correspondence should be addressed to Huda Mossa Omran; hudamossa.omran@gmail.com

Academic Editor: Julio Rosa e Silva

The effect of sperm molecular defects on fertilization and pregnancy outcome after assisted reproductive therapy (ART) is widely documented by both research and clinical societies. Sperm DNA fragmentation and abnormal chromatin condensation represent critical causes of male infertility. Advanced androgenic techniques for accurately identifying molecular defects help in selecting an appropriate treatment strategy. Additionally, specific markers of apoptosis are increasingly important in predicting male infertility. The ability of flow cytometry to estimate the quantity of sperm with DNA fragmentation or damage and multifactor measurements in immotile sperm have made this developed technique essential in fertility centers. The study is aimed at assessing the level of DNA fragmentation and apoptosis by measuring flow cytometry using new techniques. Flow cytometry analysis revealed a varying degree of DNA damage. It was able to quantify the degree of impairment even in samples with minimal DNA fragmentation. DNA damage was observed even in samples that were considered normal with a routine semen analysis. Flow cytometry was sensitive to changes in sperm apoptosis. Elevated p53 activity levels were associated with high DNA fragmentation. Meanwhile, B-cell lymphoma 2 (Bcl-2) activities showed a different pattern. In conclusion, flow cytometry for sperm DNA fragmentation and markers of apoptosis can be a valuable tool in assisted reproductive centers.

1. Introduction

Exploring the impact of sperm DNA and apoptotic changes on male subfertility is being important along with the standard semen analysis [1–3]. Zini et al. [4] reported that sperm DNA damage comprises a predictive factor for pregnancy loss after ART. The need for a precise approach to accurately measure this factor is increased. Several techniques in the andrology lab have been used to evaluate these markers [5]. The sperm chromatin dispersion (SCD) test is a method based on the shape of the characteristic halo that is created when sperm nuclear proteins are removed by acid denaturation [6, 7]. It is a direct method but with interlaboratory variability. The comet is another technique that qualitatively measures sperm DNA damage by visualising single- and double-strand breaks using electrophoresis [5]. A double-strand DNA appears at the head of a comet. The full head and tail emerge, while damaged double- and single-strand DNA fragments move towards the tail part. Therefore, this essay is an immensely useful tool to measure the DNA fragmentation index (DFI, %), which indicates the number of cells with DNA damage [8], and high DNA stainable (HDS) (%), which indicates the proportion of the histone-to-protamine transition in the immature sperm [9]. The disadvantages of this test are that the testing requires expensive equipment and a high concentration of sperm and that the reference range for the sample needs to be calibrated [5].

Flow cytometry is a potent molecular technique that has the ability in measuring several markers accurately and in a short time. In an andrology laboratory, it can be used to differentiate between several types of DNA abnormalities, apoptosis markers, the detection of antisperm antibodies, and others [10, 11].

FCM principles depend on calculating the ratio of single- and double-stranded DNA staining of sperm nuclei with DNA fluorescent stain. During FCM, exposure to acid usually results in denaturing of double-stranded DNA in spermatozoa whose chromatin structure is altered [12, 13].

Apoptosis or programmed cell death (PCD) in male germ cells normally occurs in the prospermatogonia (gonocytes) layer in the differentiating testis during fetal life [14]. Apoptosis usually occurs during normal spermatogenesis and accounts to the loss of up to 75% of potential sperm number, where only 25% of the expected number of primary spermatocytes is produced from the spermatogonia A [15]. Impairment of apoptosis at this stage generates a male infertility phenotype, while apoptosis in the mature spermatozoa appears to be significantly involved in the production of a subfertile state [16].

Apoptotic features that detected in the PCD of germ line include the following: condensation of the chromatin, membrane leakage, endoplasmic reticulum Ca^{2+} pool depletion, release of cytochrome c from mitochondria, downstream caspase activation, generating substrate cleavage, endonuclease activation, and DNA fragmentation [17–20]. Apoptotic markers that may be detected in ejaculated spermatozoa include Bcl-xl, p53, B-cell lymphoma-2 Bcl-2, caspase-3, caspase-8, caspase-9, Fas receptors, and DNA strand breaks. However, DNA strand breaks and apoptotic markers do not always exist together [14].

The guardian of the genome or p53 is an important apoptotic marker. It is called so because of its molecular weight. It is a sequence-specific transcriptional factor that plays an important role in controlling the quality of sperm production. It is usually present in very small amounts in normal sperm [14, 20]. Genital tract infection, varicocele, and testicular cancers are commonly linked with abnormal spermatogenesis and high level of fragmented DNA and p53 [21, 22]. Omran et al. [23] also revealed that smoking could induce DNA fragmentation of human spermatozoa [23].

2. Materials and Methods

2.1. Ethics. The study was approved by the Ethics Committee of Arabian Gulf University and Bahrain Ministry of Health. All participants gave written informed consent.

2.2. Sample Collection. Semen samples were obtained by masturbation after at least 3 days of abstinence. The samples were subjected to analysis according to the World Health Organization criteria (2010) [24]. The samples were ejaculated into sterile containers and allowed to liquefy for at least 30 min before being processed, and all experiments were performed at least in two replicates. The study inclusion criteria were applied scheduled for a routine semen analysis as a patient at Princess Al-Jawhara fertility hospital, age 20 years and more, infertility of 1 year or more whether primary or secondary, and not currently receiving hormonal treatment. Exclusion criteria were incomplete sample and incomplete questionnaire.

TABLE 1: Values of standard parameters of normal and abnormal samples by WHO* analysis.

Parameter	Normal (mean ± 2SD)	Abnormal (mean ± 2SD)
Concentration ($\times 10^6$/ml)	83.18 ± 9.93	23.73 ± 5.34
Motility (% grade a)	6 0.18 ± 1.96	33.70 ± 3.96
Vitality (% alive)	68.37.84 ± 2.42	47.73 ± 4.56
Morphology (% normal form)	9.83 ± 0.68	3.46 ± 0.70
Leukocyte count ($\times 10^6$/ml)	0.85 ± 0.15	1.23 ± 0.27

WHO: World Health Organization.

2.3. Assessment of Semen according to the WHO Guidelines (2010). After liquefaction, the freshly collected semen samples were assessed according to WHO criteria [24]. Seminal physical characteristics (appearance, odor, viscosity, volume, and semen pH) were evaluated. Sperm motility was assessed on the wet preparation. Sperm concentration was determined, and the presence of leukocytes and spontaneous agglutinates was noted. For sperm morphology evaluation, the slides were stained with freshly prepared Giemsa stain. Teratozoospermia index (TZI) was used to categorize the sperm morphology [25].

2.4. Flow Cytometry (FCM) Analysis. Cytometry analysis for sperm DNA and apoptotic markers required cell fixation with citric acid and staining with fluorescent stains (DAPI–phosphate) prior to analysis. Aliquots (100 μl) of the liquefied sample were fixed with 5 ml of a citric acid solution and stored at 4°C.

For sperm DNA analysis, a 0.5 ml of the citric acid fixed cells was stained with a 3.5 ml of DAP–phosphate staining solution, mixed gently, and analyzed by FCM (8).

For apoptotic marker p53 and Bcl-2 analysis, the methods were done according to Gogolin et al. [26] and Berger et al. [27], respectively. The freshly collected samples were fixed with 80% ethanol for 24 hours prior to being analyzed by flow. 200 μl of the fixed cells was filled up with 2 ml of PBS, centrifuged at 1500 rpm for 10 minutes.

The supernatant was discarded, and the rest (about 100 μl) was labeled by p53-PE antibody/FITC for p53 or Mouse Anti-Human Bcl-2 for Bcl-2 analysis. Then, it was reserved in the dark for 30 minutes at room temperature. The labeled cells were counter stained with 3.5 ml of DAPI–phosphate staining solution. Finally, the stained cells were kept at room temperature in the dark for 30 minutes to be analyzed by flow cytometry. Calibrations were performed by p53 or Bcl-2 isotypes, and then, analysis was done.

SPSS 16.0 software (SPSS Inc., Chicago IL, USA) was used for statistical evaluation.

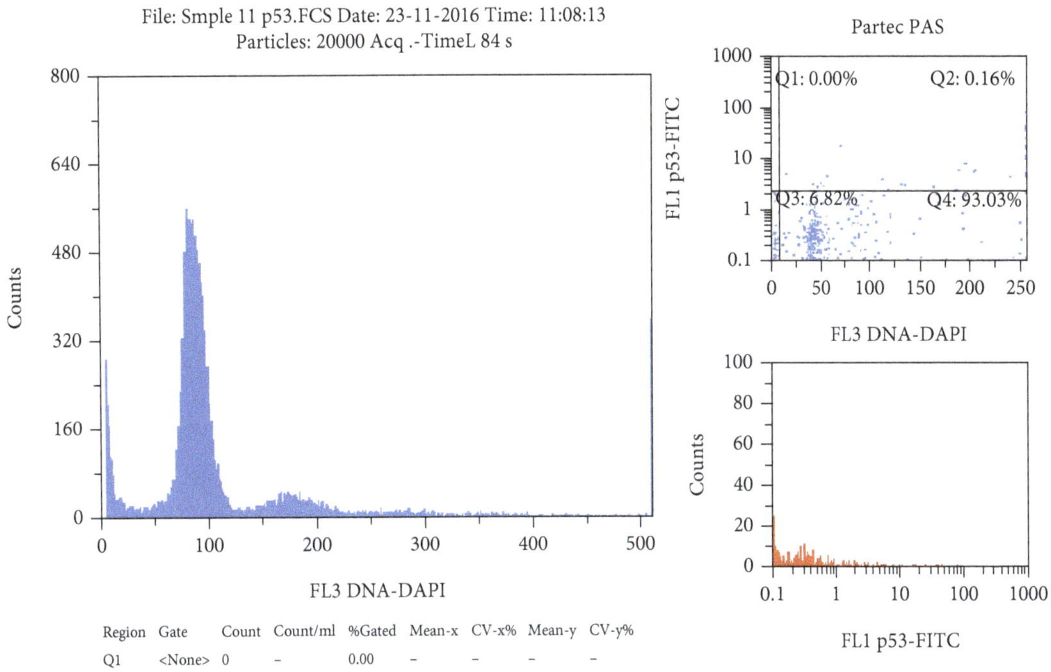

Region	Gate	Count	Count/ml	%Gated	Mean-x	CV-x%	Mean-y	CV-y%
Q1	<None>	0	-	0.00	-	-	-	-
Q2	<None>	31	-	0.16	178.85	47.44	12.72	136.90
Q3	<None>	1363	-	6.82	4.25	42.13	0.11	86.31
Q4	<None>	18606	-	93.03	60.48	71.76	0.11	67.36

(a)

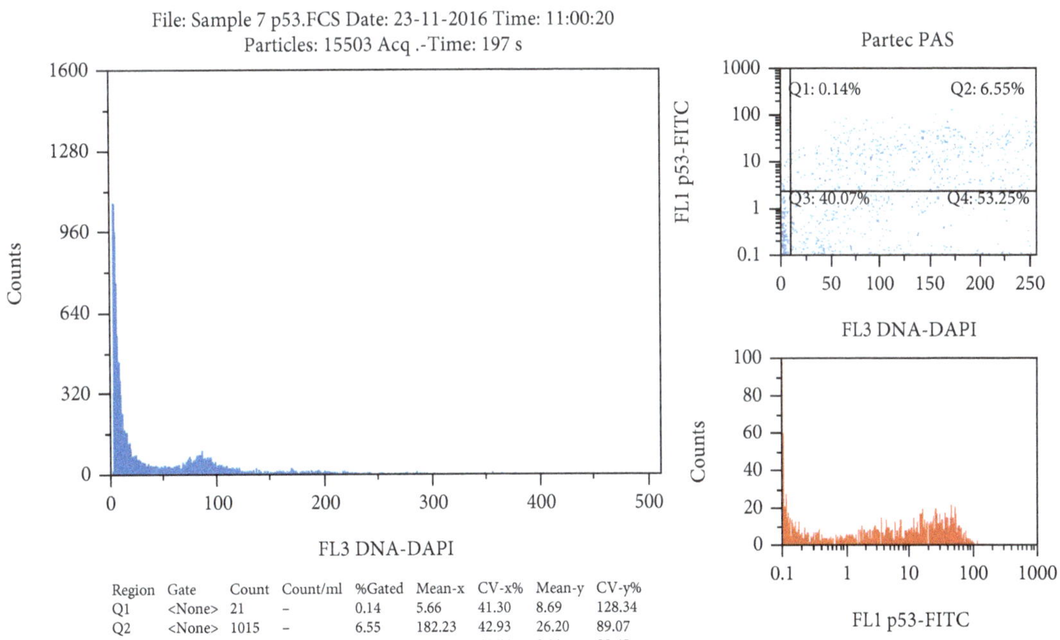

Region	Gate	Count	Count/ml	%Gated	Mean-x	CV-x%	Mean-y	CV-y%
Q1	<None>	21	-	0.14	5.66	41.30	8.69	128.34
Q2	<None>	1015	-	6.55	182.23	42.93	26.20	89.07
Q3	<None>	6212	-	40.07	4.35	41.64	0.11	80.45
Q4	<None>	8555	-	53.25	83.15	93.06	0.13	151.21

(b)

FIGURE 1: Cytometry result of p53 labeled samples: (a) normal sample with 0.16% of positively labeled cells; (b) abnormal sample with 6.55% of positively labeled cells.

3. Results

Male partners of 139 infertile couples agreed to participate in the study; only eighty-four of them fulfilled the criteria for inclusion. More than half of the patients (63.1%) were in the age group of 26-35 years. Around 64.3% of patients had normal semen samples. The normozoospermic semen samples had better seminal parameters than the abnormal as shown in Table 1.

Cytometry DNA analysis had shown the different statuses of chromatin maturity and DNA integrity. The samples were classified according to Hacker-Klom et al. classification

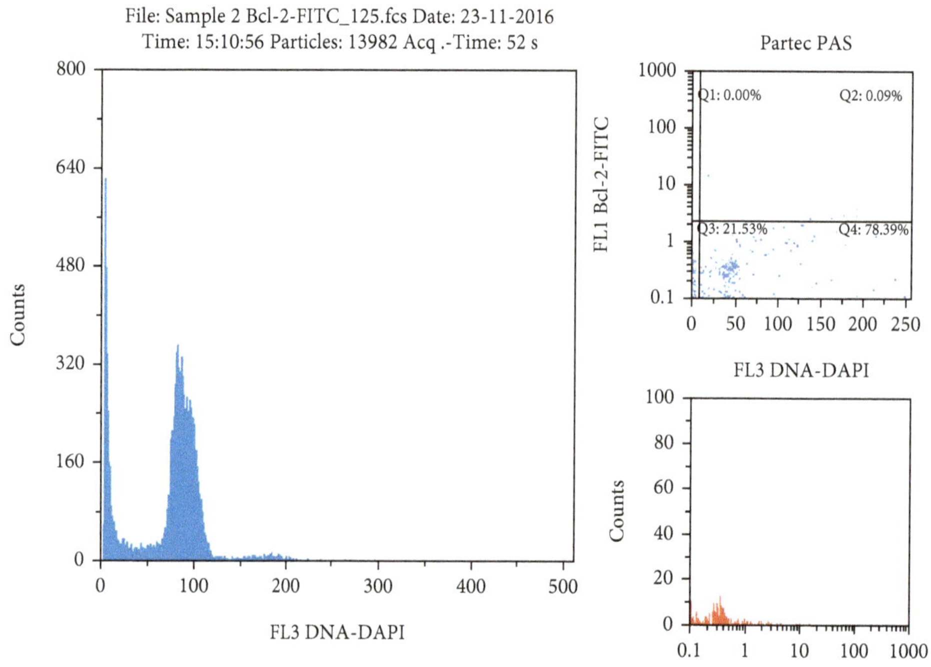

Region	Gate	Count	Count/ml	%Gated	Mean-x	CV-x%	Mean-y	CV-y%
Q1	<None>	0	-	0.00	-	-	-	-
Q2	<None>	12	-	0.09	181.91	48.11	5.34	74.02
Q3	<None>	3010	-	21.53	3.98	43.38	0.10	26.60
Q4	<None>	10960	-	78.39	46.98	47.17	0.11	66.01

(a)

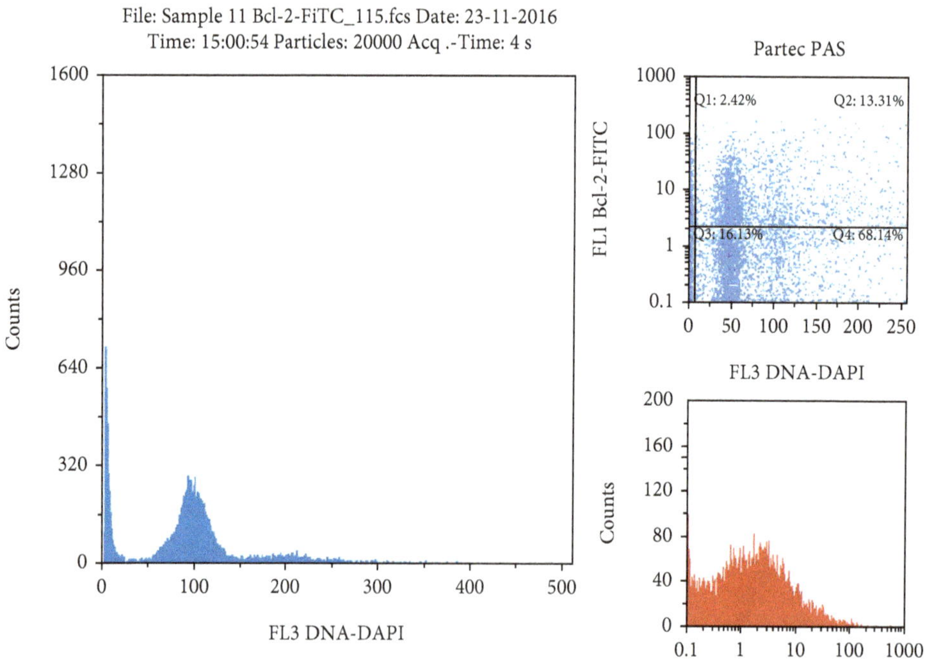

Region	Gate	Count	Count/ml	%Gated	Mean-x	CV-x%	Mean-y	CV-y%
Q1	<None>	484	-	2.42	3.80	42.09	9.38	114.25
Q2	<None>	2662	-	13.31	92.65	75.56	14.69	204.67
Q3	<None>	3225	-	16.13	3.80	42.00	0.28	150.21
Q4	<None>	13629	-	68.14	76.32	73.74	0.28	156.84

(b)

Figure 2: Cytometry result of Bcl-2-FITC labeled samples: (a) normal sample with 0.9% of positively labeled cells; (b) abnormal sample with 13.3% of positively labeled cells.

[28] into eight classes that considered only class one and two as normal. Class 4 was characterized by an increase in the percentage of diploid spermatozoa samples > 5%, whereas Class 5 contained samples' histograms with skewing of the 1 CC peak to the left.

DNA analysis was not normal in all normozoospermic samples. About 54.8% of the semen samples demonstrated abnormal chromatin status. Samples with normal class one chromatin condensation were represented only 32.1% of the study population. Aneuploidy cells were detected in three samples with an abnormal semen analysis. Sample with abnormal p53 activity had a high level of positively labeled cells with anti-p53 antibodies (≥5%) (Figure 1). Also, samples with abnormal Bcl-2 activity had ≥5% of positively labeled cells (Figure 2).

Apoptotic markers' analysis reveals that contrary to expectation, normal chromatin condensation did not reflect standard cell cycle analysis. About 65.5% of the semen samples had an abnormally high level of positively labeled cells with FITC Mouse Anti-Human Bcl-2; some of them had normal chromatin condensation (Figure 3), while 51.2% of the semen samples had an abnormally high level of positively labeled cells with a p53-PE antibody.

The Bcl-2 protein activity was higher in Classes 4 and 5 than in other classes; however, no Bcl-2 activity was detected in Classes 7 and 8 (Figure 3). Comparably, Classes 7 and 8 had elevated measures of p53 activity (Figure 4). Moreover, Bcl-2 activity was even high in samples with normal chromatin condensation and normal p53 activity (Figure 5).

4. Discussion

Despite the widespread decline in human fertility, science has not established perfect methods for diagnosis. To date, all the IVF techniques rely in their final sperm selection on its gross morphology, not the nuclear content or DNA normality. Besides, most of the urological procedures rely principally on traditional semen analysis to assess treatment success.

The study demonstrated considerable differences in the results of the traditional analysis in comparison to those of the molecular procedures. Research showed normality of 64.3% of the study group by the routine semen analysis, whereas this figure dropped to only 34.5% after the application of the molecular methods.

The cytometry analysis of DNA integrity revealed considerable damage in sperm DNA even within the grossly normal samples. These findings indicate that selection of sperm for IVF and ICSE on the bases of gross morphology and routine analysis is not sensitive.

Because of their role in sperm maturity, analysis of apoptotic markers was performed. The p53 family of genes has an established task in the regulation of male and female germ-line production of gametes, especially in stress response. The p53 family protects against developmental defects in the progeny. Also, there is abundant evidence that p53 protein plays a critical role in female reproduction and embryonic implantation [29]. The proper response to stress signals through the adequate control of these metabolic pathways is a central element of development. Ordinarily, p53 is present in low quantity in spermatozoa; therefore, its presence in large amounts may reflect stress conditions such as cancer, oxidative stress, or testicular disease [30, 31].

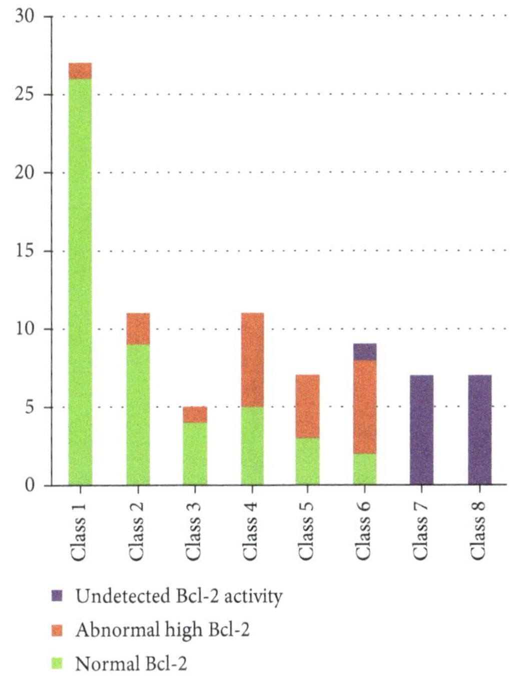

FIGURE 3: Distributions of patients according to cytometry classes vs. Bcl-2 activity.

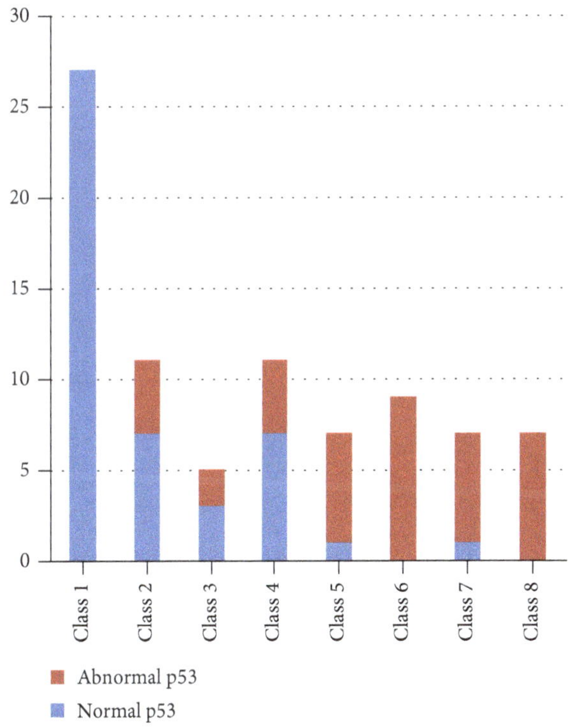

FIGURE 4: Distributions of patients according to cytometry classes vs. p53 activity.

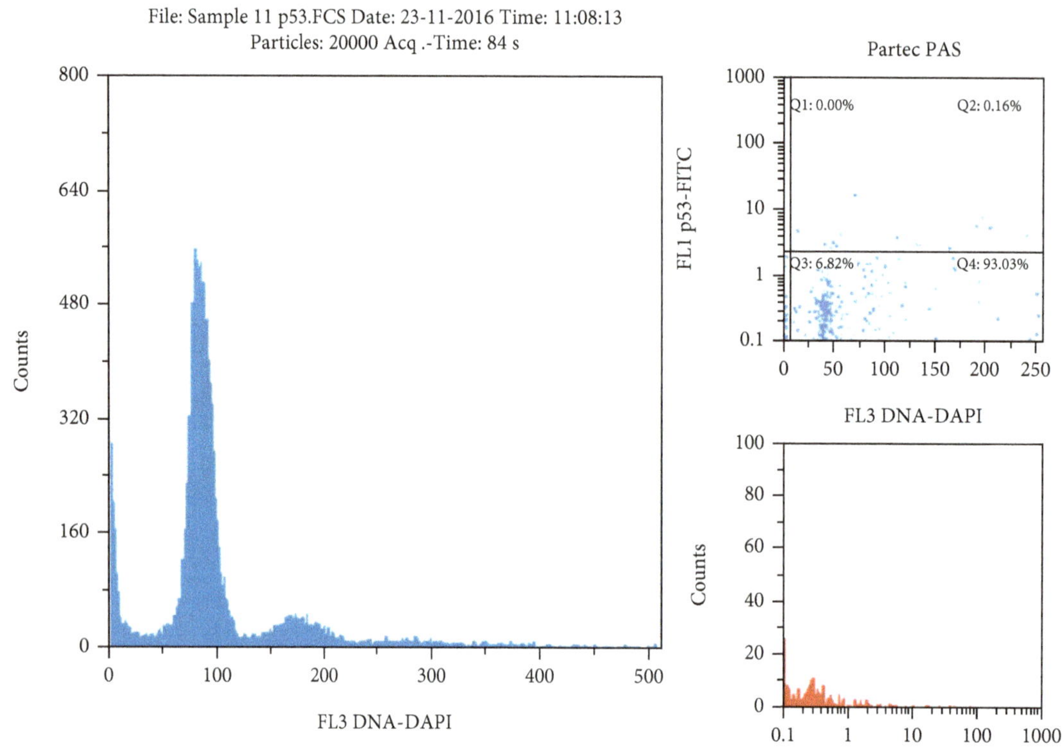

Region	Gate	Count	Count/ml	%Gated	Mean-x	CV-x%	Mean-y	CV-y%
Q1	<None>	0	-	0.00	-	-	-	-
Q2	<None>	31	-	0.16	178.85	47.44	12.72	136.90
Q3	<None>	1363	-	6.82	4.25	42.13	0.11	86.31
Q4	<None>	18606	-	93.03	60.48	71.76	0.11	67.36

(a)

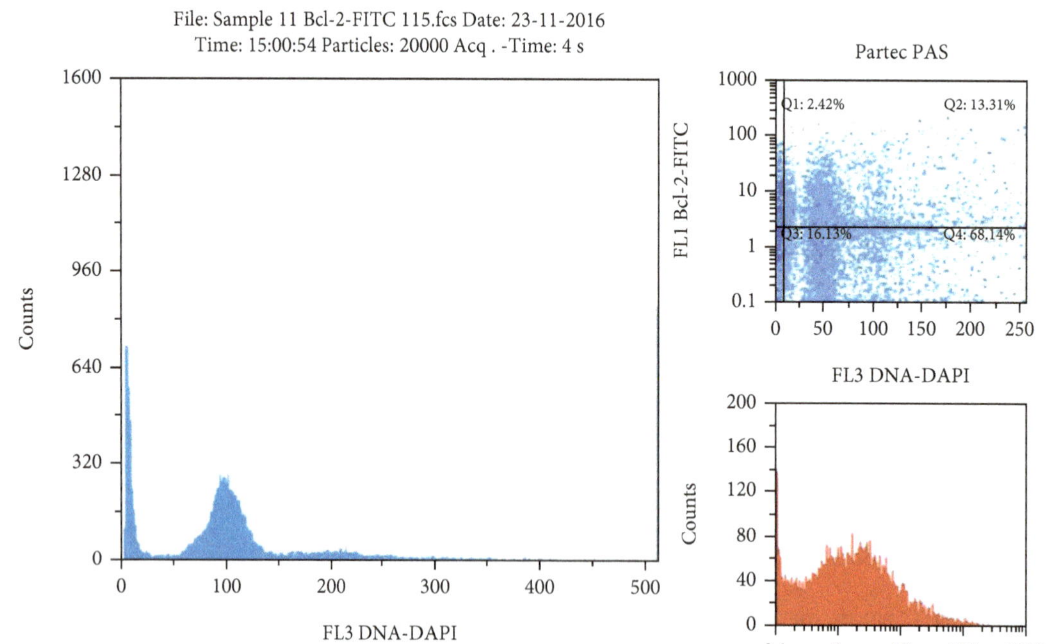

Region	Gate	Count	Count/ml	%Gated	Mean-x	CV-x%	Mean-y	CV-y%
Q1	<None>	484	-	2.42	3.80	42.09	9.38	114.25
Q2	<None>	2662	-	13.31	92.65	75.56	14.69	204.67
Q3	<None>	3225	-	16.13	3.80	42.00	0.28	150.21
Q4	<None>	13629	-	68.14	76.32	73.74	0.28	156.84

(b)

FIGURE 5: Cytometry result of sample 11: (a) normal chromatin condensation sample with normal p53 activity (0.16% of positively labeled cells); (b) abnormal Bcl-2 activity of the same sample with 13.3% of positively labeled cells.

The present study had the importance in measuring p53 level in human sperm population by using flow cytometry. It revealed that around 51.2% of the study population had abnormal measures of p53 protein with a significant correlation between the degree of DNA damage and p53 level (Figure 3). These findings agreed with that of Raimondo et al. [31] who found a positive correlation between the corrected p53 values measured by ELISA and the degree of DNA damage in sperm cells.

Bcl-2 was another apoptotic marker assessed in this study. Bcl-2 is expressed predominantly during sperm development. It works as an apoptotic regulator (a protooncogene) that is inserted into the outer mitochondrial, nuclear, and endoplasmic reticulum membranes with the bulk of the protein facing the cytosol [32].

Stress stimulates cytoplasmic proapoptotic proteins that move to the mitochondrial level, where antiapoptotic proteins also exist ([33], 30). The communication between proapoptotic and antiapoptotic proteins interrupts the antiapoptotic Bcl-2 function leading to the formation of mitochondrial pores and proapoptotic molecule release from the intermembrane space [33] (31). By binding to Apaf-1, these elements activate caspase-9 and through targeting caspase effectors lead eventually to cell death [34]. The Bcl-2 family enhances the cell viability, and low level of Bcl-2 harms cell survival and differentiation [35].

Around 65.5% of the study population had abnormal levels of Bcl-2. These levels were detected even in samples with normal chromatin condensation (Figure 5). The Bcl-2 protein activity was considerably high in Classes 4 and 5. However, no Bcl-2 activity was detected in Classes 7 and 8 (Figure 3). Classes 4 and 5 are considered an intermediate stage of chromatin condensation defects [28]. The increase in the Bcl-2 activity in those types of DNA defects may reflect their vital role in protection against apoptosis by interference with the mitochondrial apoptotic pathway [36], while its activity in the sample with normal chromatin condensation may indicate that sperm mitochondrial defect can exist without the existence of nuclear DNA damage and could be the cause of male infertility [37]. The absence of this activity in more severe types of chromatin defect may reflect the failure of the defense mechanism and the failure of sperm production.

The technique used in this study had many advantages including accuracy and the speed of measurements, and it can simultaneously measure the sperm chromatin condensation and aneuploidy rate. Still, a significant limitation of this technique is the expensive instrumentation and the requirement of skilled people to analyze the samples [11].

5. Conclusion

We have many gaps in our knowledge regarding male infertility, partly because of the restricted number of researches in our area in this crucial field and partly because of the limited value of traditional semen analysis in the assessment of infertile males. The study emphasized that future studies should apply the molecular markers in male infertility diagnosis, primarily for those involved in ART cycles. This could have a positive impact on ART results, especially if we correlate the outcome of these procedures with the findings of these assays.

Consent

Informed written consent was obtained from participants.

Authors' Contributions

H. Omran developed the idea, and M. Bakhiet assisted and supported the corresponding author throughout the research work and manuscript writing. V. Ehemann made a substantial contribution to the development, editing, and writing of this article.

Acknowledgments

We would like to thank the Arabian Gulf University, College of Medicine and Medical Sciences, Department of Molecular Medicine for providing us with support to conduct this study all around.

References

[1] E. Evgeni, G. Lymberopoulos, M. Gazouli, and B. Asimakopoulos, "Conventional semen parameters and DNA fragmentation in relation to fertility status in a Greek population," *European Journal of Obstetrics, Gynecology, and Reproductive Biology*, vol. 188, pp. 17–23, 2015.

[2] M. Z. Pipan, J. Mrkun, B. J. Strajn et al., "The influence of macro- and microelements in seminal plasma on diluted boar sperm quality," *Acta Veterinaria Scandinavica*, vol. 59, no. 1, p. 11, 2017.

[3] F. Matter, *A Clinician's Guide to Sperm DNA and Chromatin Damage*, Springer International Publishing, 2018.

[4] A. Zini, J. M. Boman, E. Belzile, and A. Ciampi, "Sperm DNA damage is associated with an increased risk of pregnancy loss after IVF and ICSI: systematic review and meta-analysis," *Human Reproduction*, vol. 23, no. 12, pp. 2663–2668, 2008.

[5] G. Y. Kim, "What should be done for men with sperm DNA fragmentation?," *Clinical and Experimental Reproductive Medicine*, vol. 45, no. 3, pp. 101–109, 2018.

[6] M. T. Le, T. A. T. Nguyen, H. T. T. Nguyen et al., "Does sperm DNA fragmentation correlate with semen parameters?," *Reproductive Medicine and Biology*, vol. 18, no. 4, pp. 390–396, 2019.

[7] J. L. Fernández, L. Muriel, M. T. Rivero, V. Goyanes, R. Vazquez, and J. G. Alvarez, "The sperm chromatin dispersion test: a simple method for the determination of sperm DNA fragmentation," *Journal of Andrology*, vol. 24, no. 1, pp. 59–66, 2003.

[8] D. P. Evenson, K. L. Larson, and L. K. Jost, "Sperm chromatin structure assay: its clinical use for detecting sperm DNA fragmentation in male infertility and comparisons with other techniques," *Journal of Andrology*, vol. 23, no. 1, pp. 25–43, 2002.

[9] N. Tarozzi, D. Bizzaro, C. Flamigni, and A. Borini, "Clinical relevance of sperm DNA damage in assisted reproduction," *Reproductive Biomedicine Online*, vol. 14, no. 6, pp. 746–757, 2007.

[10] H. M. Omran, M. Bakhiet, and M. G. Dashti, "DNA integrity is a critical molecular indicator for the assessment of male infertility," *Molecular Medicine Reports*, vol. 7, no. 5, pp. 1631-1635, 2013.

[11] P. Ahlering and P. Sutovsky, "Biomarker-based flow cytometric semen analysis for male infertility diagnostics and clinical decision making in ART," in *Screening the Single Euploid Embryo: Molecular Genetics in Reproductive Medicine*, pp. 33–51, Springer International Publishing, 2015.

[12] V. Ehemann, B. Hashemi, A. Lange, and H. F. Otto, "Flow cytometric DNA analysis and chromosomal aberrations in malignant glioblastomas," *Cancer Letters*, vol. 138, no. 1-2, pp. 101–106, 1999.

[13] V. Ehemann, J. Sykora, J. Vera-Delgado, A. Lange, and H. F. Otto, "Flow cytometric detection of spontaneous apoptosis in human breast cancer using the TUNEL-technique," *Cancer Letters*, vol. 194, no. 1, pp. 125–131, 2003.

[14] J. Marie Hardwick and L. Soane, "Multiple functions of BCL-2 family proteins," *Cold Spring Harbor Perspectives in Biology*, vol. 5, no. 2, 2013.

[15] A. C. Varghese, F. M. Bragais, D. Mukhopadhyay et al., "Human sperm DNA integrity in normal and abnormal semen samples and its correlation with sperm characteristics," *Andrologia*, vol. 41, no. 4, pp. 207–215, 2009.

[16] T. Mostafa, L. Rashed, N. Nabil, and R. Amin, "Seminal BAX and BCL2 gene and protein expressions in infertile men with varicocele," *Urology*, vol. 84, no. 3, pp. 590–595, 2014.

[17] B. Uttara, A. Singh, P. Zamboni, and R. Mahajan, "Oxidative stress and neurodegenerative diseases: a review of upstream and downstream antioxidant therapeutic options," *Current Neuropharmacology*, vol. 7, no. 1, pp. 65–74, 2009.

[18] T. Finkel, "Signal transduction by reactive oxygen species," *The Journal of Cell Biology*, vol. 194, no. 1, pp. 7–15, 2011.

[19] S. Salim, "Oxidative stress and psychological disorders," *Current Neuropharmacology*, vol. 12, no. 2, pp. 140–147, 2014.

[20] T. Rahman, I. Hosen, M. M. T. Islam, and H. U. Shekhar, "Oxidative stress and human health," *Advances in Bioscience and Biotechnology*, vol. 3, no. 7, pp. 997–1019, 2012.

[21] M. J. Ruiz-Lopez, D. P. Evenson, G. Espeso, M. Gomendio, and E. R. S. Roldan, "High levels of DNA fragmentation in spermatozoa are associated with inbreeding and poor sperm quality in endangered ungulates 1," *Biology of Reproduction*, vol. 83, no. 3, pp. 332–338, 2010.

[22] Y. Shi, R. Buffenstein, D. A. Pulliam, and H. Van Remmen, "Comparative studies of oxidative stress and mitochondrial function in aging," *Integrative and Comparative Biology*, vol. 50, no. 5, pp. 869–879, 2010.

[23] H. M. Omran, M. G. Dashti, and M. Bakhiet, "Significant effects of smoking habit on male fertility," *Bahrain Medical Bulletin*, vol. 35, no. 2, pp. 74–77, 2013.

[24] World Health Organization, *WHO|WHO Laboratory Manual for the Examination and Processing of Human Semen*, WHO, 2018.

[25] D. Ickowicz, M. Finkelstein, and H. Breitbart, "Mechanism of sperm capacitation and the acrosome reaction: role of protein kinases," *Asian Journal of Andrology*, vol. 14, no. 6, pp. 816-821, 2012.

[26] S. Gogolin, R. Batra, N. Harder et al., "MYCN-mediated overexpression of mitotic spindle regulatory genes and loss of p53-p21 function jointly support the survival of tetraploid neuroblastoma cells," *Cancer Letters*, vol. 331, no. 1, pp. 35–45, 2013.

[27] I. Berger, H. H. Paessler, H. Weckauf, V. Ehemann, and B. Helmchen, "Strong expression of Bcl-2 in pigmented villonodular synovitis of the knee with aggressive clinical behaviour," *Scandinavian Journal of Rheumatology*, vol. 34, no. 1, pp. 68–70, 2005.

[28] U. B. Hacker-Klom, W. Göhde, E. Nieschlag, and H. M. Behre, "DNA flow cytometry of human semen," *Human Reproduction*, vol. 14, no. 10, pp. 2506–2512, 1999.

[29] V. A. Belyi, P. Ak, E. Markert et al., "The origins and evolution of the p 53 family of genes," *Cold Spring Harbor Perspectives in Biology*, vol. 2, no. 6, 2010.

[30] C. Shaha, R. Tripathi, and D. Prasad Mishra, "Male germ cell apoptosis: regulation and biology," *Philosophical Transactions of the Royal Society B: Biological Sciences*, vol. 365, no. 1546, pp. 1501–1515, 2010.

[31] S. Raimondo, T. Gentile, F. Cuomo, S. De Filippo, G. E. Aprea, and J. Guida, "Quantitative evaluation of p 53 as a new indicator of DNA damage in human spermatozoa," *Journal of Human Reproductive Sciences*, vol. 7, no. 3, pp. 212–217, 2014.

[32] C. M. Sorenson, "Bcl-2 family members and disease," *Biochimica et Biophysica Acta (BBA) - Molecular Cell Research*, vol. 1644, no. 2-3, pp. 169–177, 2004.

[33] H. Taheri, M. Salehi, T. Eslami Arshaghi, and M. Mosahebi, "Studying of the expression of BAX and BCL-2 genes in men with sperm DNA fragmentation based on DFI and comet," *ASJ*, vol. 12, no. 1, pp. 29–36, 2015.

[34] C. Wang and R. J. Youle, "The role of mitochondria in apoptosis," *Annual Review of Genetics*, vol. 43, no. 1, pp. 95–118, 2009.

[35] J. C. Martinou and R. J. Youle, "Mitochondria in apoptosis: Bcl-2 family members and mitochondrial dynamics," *Developmental Cell*, vol. 21, no. 1, pp. 92–101, 2011.

[36] J. Dalal, A. Kumar, M. Honparkhe, D. Deka, and N. Singh, "Minimization of apoptosis-like changes in cryopreserved buffalo bull sperm by supplementing extender with Bcl-2 protein," *Veterinary World*, vol. 9, no. 5, pp. 432–436, 2016.

[37] D. P. Kumar and N. Sangeetha, "Mitochondrial DNA mutations and male infertility," *Indian Journal of Human Genetics*, vol. 15, no. 3, pp. 93–97, 2009.

23

Proportion of Maternal Near-Miss and Its Determinants among Northwest Ethiopian Women

Mengstu Melkamu Asaye

Women and Family Health Department, School of Midwifery, College of Medicine and Health Sciences, University of Gondar, P.O. Box 196, Ethiopia

Correspondence should be addressed to Mengstu Melkamu Asaye; mengstum@gmail.com

Academic Editor: Samir Hamamah

Background. Life-threatening situations might arise unexpectedly during pregnancy. Maternal near-miss can be a proxy for maternal death and explained as women who nearly died due to obstetric-related complications. It is recognized as the predictor of level of care and maternal death. Maternal near-miss evaluates life-threatening pregnancy-related complications, and it directs the assessment of the quality of obstetric care. *Objective.* To determine the proportion and factors associated with maternal near-miss at maternity wards at the University of Gondar Referral Hospital, Northwest Ethiopia, 2019. *Methods.* A cross-sectional study design was carried out from March 1 to June 20, 2019, using WHO criteria for maternal near-miss at the University of Gondar Referral Hospital. The data are from the interviews and review of 303 systematically selected participants' medical files at maternity wards. Bivariate and multivariable logistic regression analyses were performed to analyze factors associated with maternal near-miss, including estimation of crude and adjusted odds ratios and their respective 95% confidence intervals and p value less than 0.05 through SPSS version 20. *Result.* The study revealed that the proportion of maternal near-miss was found to be 15.8% (95%CI = 11.9%-20.1%). In the adjusted analyses, maternal near-miss was significantly associated with low (≤1000 ETB) monthly income (AOR = 399; 95%CI = 1.65, 9.65), seven or more days of hospital stay (AOR = 5.43; 95% CI = 2.49, 11.83), vaginal bleeding (AOR = 2.75, 95%CI = 1.17, 6.47), and pregnancy-induced hypertension (AOR = 5.13; 95% CI = 2.08, 12.6). *Conclusion and Recommendation.* The near-miss proportion was comparable to that in the region. Associated factors were low monthly income, seven or more days of hospital stay, vaginal bleeding, and pregnancy-induced hypertension. Thus, giving attention on early identification and treatment of these potential factors can be the opportunity in the reduction of maternal morbidity and mortality.

1. Introduction

Maternal near-miss (MNM) refers to a situation where a women who nearly died but survived from a comprehensive range of life-threatening obstetric complication [1] that occurred during pregnancy, child birth, or within 42 days of termination of pregnancy [2].

According to WHO criteria, maternal near-miss is a sign of organ dysfunction that follow life-threatening conditions and it enables the assessment of the quality of care provided to pregnant women [3]. The inclusion criteria for maternal near-miss are categorized in three areas: clinical, laboratory, and management-based criteria. The reason is that these identification criteria may be used in a comparable way across the settings and over time. It is important to understand the process of care that the patient has undergone in order to improve the quality of care, and its applicability depends on the local context [4].

Developing countries account for approximately 99% (302,000) of global maternal deaths, and Sub-Saharan Africa alone accounts for roughly 66% (201 000) to this death [5]. The magnitude also varies among different countries and regions depending on the health care quality and availability [6]. The number of maternal death is high worldwide. This death might be associated with inadequate and poor quality of health care services. Thus, identifying the potential factors that leads to severe maternal life-threatening complications is necessary [7].

We can prevent maternal death through utilization of the near-miss data. Thus, the mother that survives a near-miss can provide more comprehensive information when reviewing maternal death cases. So it is a better predicate for preventive planning [8], and it is a useful means to improve the quality of obstetric care especially in low-income countries.

In developing countries, about 75% of the women were in a critical condition upon arrival. Availability, accessibility, cost of health care, and behavioral factors play an important role in the utilization of maternal health services [2]. Maternal near-miss events were associated with postpartum hemorrhage, sever preeclampsia, eclampsia, sepsis or severe systematic infection, ruptured uterus, and septic abortion [9, 10]. But in the current study, the main approaches to the reduction of maternal near-miss and maternal deaths are emergency obstetric care, skilled care by skilled birth attendants, and unmet obstetric need [2]. Studying maternal near-miss allows the assessment of quality interventions, identifies the health system failures, and provides alternative strategies to reduce maternal mortality [11]. Delays in initiating timely and adequate treatment for obstetric complications were a major factor to develop maternal near-miss [12, 13].

The pregnancy-related mortality ratio, in Ethiopia, is estimated to be approximately 412 death/100,000 live birth according to 2016 EDH [14]. One target of SDG is to achieve a reduction of global maternal mortality ratio to less than 70 per 100,000 live births by 2030 [15]. To achieve this goal and solve the problem, respectively, we have to review both maternal mortality and maternal near-miss cases. The present study is aimed at assessing the proportion of maternal near-miss and factors associated with it at Gondar Tertiary Hospital.

2. Methods

2.1. Study Design and Period. An institution-based cross-sectional study design was employed at the University of Gondar Referral Hospital from March 1 to June 20, 2019.

2.2. Setting. The study was conducted at the University of Gondar Referral Hospital, maternity wards. It is located in the North Gondar administrative zone, in Amhara region, 727 km Northwest of Addis Ababa and 175 km far from Bahirdar. Currently, Gondar town has one tertiary hospital and five health centers. The hospital provides service for 5-7 million people of the north Gondar neighboring zones. The average annual birth rate at the University of Gondar Referral Hospital is 9600 deliveries with 800 births each month.

2.3. Source Population. All pregnant women who were in labor, delivered or aborted, or within 42 days of postpartum period and admitted in maternity wards at Gondar Referral Hospital.

2.4. Inclusion Criteria. All pregnant women who came to the hospital due to early complication of pregnancy including abortion, ectopic pregnancy, and molar pregnancy and patients presenting care in labor, delivery, or postnatal units within 42 days of delivery were included.

2.5. Exclusion Criteria. Women with obstetric near-miss complications due to incidental or accidental causes and those who were revisiting (within data collection time) and unable to respond or seriously ill at interview time were excluded.

2.6. Sample Size Determination. The sample size was calculated by using the following assumptions.

$Z\alpha/2 = \text{confidence level at } 95\% = 1.96$, margin of error $(d) = 5\%$, and prevalence of maternal near − miss = 23.3% [11]

$n = (Z\alpha/2)^2(1-p)/d^2 = (1.96)(1.96)(0.233)(0.767)/(0.05)(0.05) = 275$ and 10% nonresponse rate; the final sample size was 303 women

2.7. Sampling Procedure. The calculated sample size was proportionally allocated to each four maternity wards based on the previous consecutive five-month average monthly client flow of the units which were obtained by referring client registration log books. The average monthly client flow for maternity 1, 2, and 3 and gynecology ward were 800, 500, 310, and 400, respectively. A total of 2010 women were booked. The study participants were selected by using a systematic random sampling technique among women who visited Gondar Tertiary Hospital during the data collection period. The first study participant was selected by a lottery method. I compute K^{th} for each ward, and it ranges from 1.2 to 2.6; then, every 3rd women were selected during the study period.

2.8. Operational Definitions. Maternal near-miss: a woman who nearly died but survived a complication that occurred during pregnancy, childbirth, or within 42 days of termination of pregnancy according to WHO criteria (if the woman full fill one criteria) [3].

Maternal mortality: death of a woman while pregnant or within 42 days of termination of pregnancy, irrespective of the duration and the site of the pregnancy, from any cause related to or aggravated by the pregnancy or its management, but not from accidental or incidental causes [16].

Delay of the decision to seek care: The time taken greater than one hour in deciding to seek care after the onset of labor.

Delay of reaching health facility: a woman is unable to arrive within one hour of travelling to reach the health facility by foot.

Delay of receiving appropriate care: a woman did not get an emergency obstetric care within the first five minutes of arrival to health facility.

Delays to intuitional delivery: at least one or more delay from the three delay model [17].

Income: refers to total household income.

TABLE 1: Sociodemographic characteristics of study participants at the University of Gondar Referral Hospital, Northwest Ethiopia, June, 2019 ($N = 303$).

Variables		Frequency (n)	Percent (%)
Age	≤20	44	14.5
	21-34	228	75.2
	≥35	31	10.2
Religion	Orthodox	269	88.8
	Muslim	32	10.6
	Protestant	2	0.7
Residence	Urban	190	62.7
	Rural	113	37.3
Marital status	Married	297	98
	Unmarried	6	2
Maternal education	Not formal education	146	48.2
	Grades 1-8	53	17.5
	High school and more	104	34.3
Maternal occupation	Housewives	225	74.3
	Government employee	48	15.8
	Merchant	22	7.3
	Farmer	1	0.3
	Daily laborer	5	2.3
Husband occupation	Farmer	114	38.4
	Government employee	90	30.3
	Merchant	85	28.6
	Daily laborer	8	2.7
Monthly income	≤1000	100	33
	1001-2000	30	9.9
	2001-3000	33	10.9
	≥3001	140	46.2

2.9. Data Collection Tools and Procedures. The data was collected by using semistructured interviewer-administrated questionnaires and patient charts. Questionnaires were developed in English. For interview purpose, questionnaires were translated first into Amharic and then back to English for its consistency. Four midwifery students in each ward were allocated for data collection purpose. Participants were interviewed by the data collectors after completion of examination.

2.10. Data Quality Control. The quality of data was assured by proper designing of the questionnaires. Half day training was given for data collectors. Every day after data collection, questionnaires were reviewed and checked for completeness by the data collector and principal investigator.

2.11. Data Processing and Analysis. All the questionnaires were checked, entered to Epi-info 7, and coded into SPSS version 20 software package for analysis. The degree of association between independent and dependent variables was assessed using odds ratio with 95% confidence interval. The results were presented in the form of tables, figures, and text using frequencies, and summary statistics such as percentage and logistic regression was used.

3. Results

A total of 303 women have responded to the questionnaires making a response rate of 100%. The age of the study participants was between 15 and 50 years with mean age of 26.41 ± 5.27 years. The majority of the participants (88.8%) were orthodox Christians, 98% of them were married, and nearly half of the study participants (48.2%) had never attended formal education.

Among the participants, 225 (74.3%) were house wives, 114 (38.4%) of their husbands were farmers in occupation, and 33% of the study participants' monthly incomes were less than or equal to 1000 EBR birr (Table 1).

3.1. Past Obstetric-Related Characteristics of Study Participants. Among the 303 study participants, 6.6% had previous history of caesarean section and 3.0%, 2%, and 3.3% had previous history of APH, PPH, and PIH, respectively. Nearly three-fourth of the study participants, 65.7%,

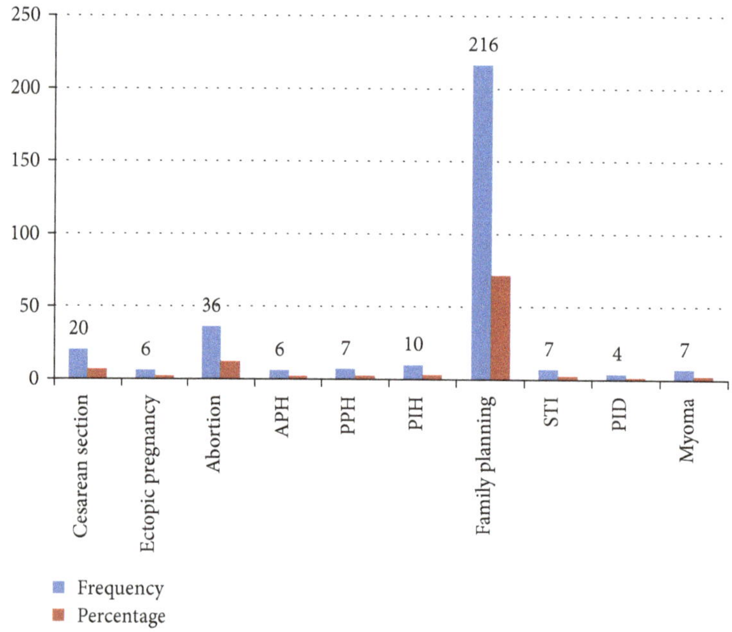

Figure 1: Past obstetric-related characteristics respondents at the University of Gondar Referral Hospital, Northwest Ethiopia, June 2019.

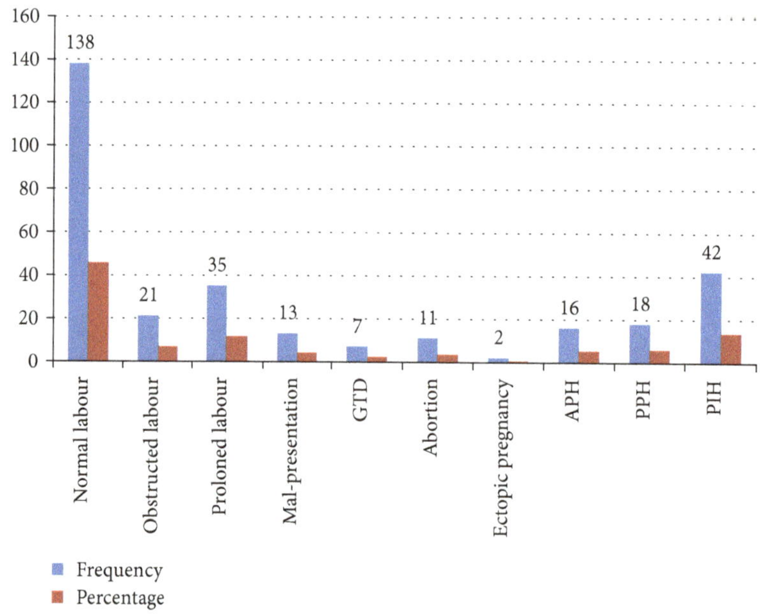

Figure 2: Initial admission diagnosis characteristics of respondents at the University of Gondar Referral Hospital, Northwest Ethiopia, June, 2019 ($n = 303$).

had family planning utilization history, and 11.9% of them had abortion history (Figure 1).

3.2. Current Obstetric-Related Characteristics of Study Participants. Nearly half, 149 (49.2%), of the study participants had two to four children while 121 (39.9%) of them had only one child. Among the study participants, 267 (88.1%) of mothers had attended antenatal care and 253 (83.5%) of the gestational age were term.

3.3. Maternal Health Service-Related Characteristics. Nearly half of the women, 50.8%, had been referred. The majority, 96.4%, of the study participants were tested for hematocrit, and 72.79% of them had greater than 33%. The suggested reasons why they seek the services were 36.6% due to labor pain, 13.5% due to prolonged labor, and 61 (20.1%) of the respondents were due to vaginal bleeding. On the other hand, 45.5%, 6.9%, and 13.8% of the respondents were admitted with an initial diagnosed of normal labor, obstructed labor, and pregnancy-induced hypertension, respectively (Figure 2).

One hundred sixty-seven (60%) women had spontaneous vaginal deliveries. On the other hand, 11.5% of study participants delivered by cesarean section. In addition to this,

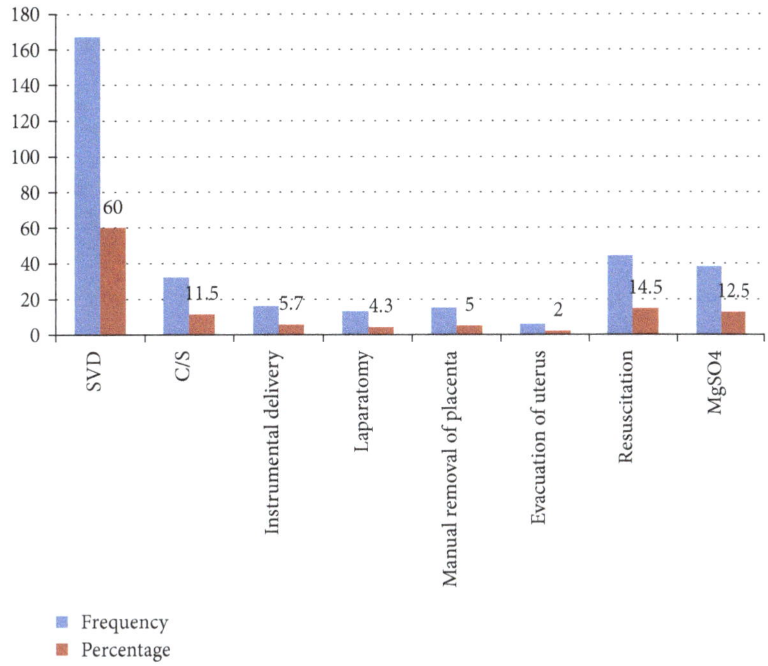

FIGURE 3: Type of intervention that was given to respondents at the University of Gondar Referral Hospital, Northwest Ethiopia, June, 2019 ($n = 303$).

12.5% of study participants were treated with magnesium sulphate (MgSO4) (Figure 3).

3.4. Three Delay Model-Related Variables of Respondents. Two hundred two study participants (80%) came to the hospital by their own decision. Delay in decision to seek care occurred in 48 (15.8%) women. The most common reason why they were delayed to reach the hospital was 16 (61.53%) due to lack of transport. One hundred sixty-seven (55.1%) respondents reported transport greater than or equal to one hour to reach the health facility (Table 2).

3.5. Proportion of Maternal Near-Miss. The present study revealed that the estimated proportion of maternal near-miss was 15.8% (95%CI = 11.9%-20.1%) by WHO criteria.

3.6. Factor Associated with Maternal Near-Miss. In bivariate binary logistic regression, residence, income, parity, duration of hospital stay, admission mode, visual disturbance, severe headache, vaginal bleeding, and pregnancy-induced hypertension (PIH) were directly associated with maternal near-miss. However, in the adjusted analyses, monthly income, duration of hospital stay, vaginal bleeding, and pregnancy-induced hypertension factors were significantly associated with maternal near-miss.

In this study, the odds of developing maternal near-miss among women who had lowest (≤1000 ETB) monthly income were 3.99 times than those who had greater than or equal to 3001 ETB per month (AOR = 3.99, 95%CI = 1.65-9.65).

In the current study, the odds of developing maternal near-miss among women who stayed seven and more days in hospital were 5.43 than those women who stayed less than seven days in the hospital (AOR = 5.43, 95%CI = 2.49-11.83). The study also suggested that women who presented with vaginal bleeding were 2.75 times more likely to develop maternal near-miss as compared to those who did not have vaginal bleeding (AOR = 2.75, 95%CI = 1.17-6.47). Lastly, the analysis showed that the odds of developing maternal near-miss among women with pregnancy-induced hypertension were 5.13 than those who did not have PIH (AOR = 5.13, 95%CI = 2.08-12.6) (Table 3).

4. Discussion

The aim of this study was to determine the proportion and factors associated with maternal near-miss at the University of Gondar Referral Hospital in 2019.

The present study revealed that the proportion of maternal near-miss at the University of Gondar Referral Hospital was 15.8% (95%CI = 11.9%-20.1%). This finding is comparable with a study conducted in Nigeria 17.4% [6] and Morocco 12% [18]. This similarity might be somewhat similar with sociodemographic characteristics of study participants. However, it is higher than a study done in Kerala 9.27% [13]; Harare, Zimbabwe 9.3% [19]; and Brazil 10.2% [20]. The variation might be as a result of the fact that the study institution is a tertiary hospital that receives complicated cases from remote primary hospitals and health centers within the zone and surrounding zones of the region. The second possible reason might be that in this study, 37.3% of the participants were from rural communities. This might be also correlated with delay of life-saving interventions which may impact maternal near-miss. Moreover, the last reason might be that, because of the limited facilities at the private hospitals, women with complicated pregnancies are not usually referred to these health institutions.

Table 2: Three delay model-related characteristics of study participants at the University of Gondar Referral Hospital, Northwest Ethiopia June, 2019 ($n = 303$).

Three delay model variables		Frequency	Percent
Decision maker	Self	239	78.9
	Husband	48	15.8
	Relatives	16	5.3
Delay in making decision	Yes	48	15.8
	No	255	84.2
Did you go straight to the hospital?	Yes	277	91.4%
	No	26	8.58%
Why you were delayed to reach the hospital?	Lack of transport	16	61.53
	Lack of money	4	15.38
	Bad road construction	6	23.07
Time to reach the hospital	<1 hr	136	44.9
	≥1 hr	167	55.1
Time it take to get the care in the hospital	<30	180	59.4
	≥30	123	40.6
Type of problems you faced in the hospital	Delay in making correct diagnosis	7	2.3
	No assessment by senior health care provider	3	1.0
	Lack of supply and equipment	4	1.3
	Poor monitoring of patient	5	1.7

In contrast, this study is lower as compared with the studies conducted in South Sudan 94.1% [21], Northeast Region of Brazil 31.5% [22], Southeast Iran 25.2% [8], Brazilian demographic health survey 21.1% [23], and Debre-Markos hospital, Ethiopia, 29.7% [23]. The primary possible explanation might be due to the small sample size and short study period in the current study. The second reason might be due to the implementation of currently endorsed nonpneumatic antishock garment for postpartum hemorrhage management at the University of Gondar Referral Hospital. Lastly, it could be due to the availability of magnesium sulphate for prevention of eclampsia and broad spectrum antibiotics for the prevention of sepsis at the University of Gondar Referral Hospital.

The current study found that those mothers who had the lowest income (≤1000 ETB) per month were 3.99 times more likely to develop maternal near-misses as compared to their counter parts. This study is consistent with a study conducted in the Kathmandu Medical College of Teaching Hospital [24] and Muzaffarnagar, India [25]. This might be due to financial constraints that women face, leading to delays in access care, even when they have obstetric complications. The lack of economic power may make women dependent on the decision-making of others, even to access health care services.

The study also revealed that those women who stayed 7 or more days at the hospital were 2.49 times more likely to develop maternal near-misses than those who stayed less than 7 days. This finding is consistent with studies conducted in Amhara regional state hospitals [11]. This might be due to participants who had a longer hospital stay that could be at a higher risk of infection development. One contributing factor to this might be surgical site infections which commonly occur from the first few weeks after operation which might be related to the lack of aseptic technique with procedures, equipment, and inadequate postoperative care.

The study suggested that the odds of developing maternal near-miss among women who had vaginal bleeding were 2.75 times more likely to develop life-threatening complication as compared to their counter parts. This report is supported with studies conducted in Nepal [10], southeast Iran [8], and Tigray, Ethiopia [12]. The possible explanation might be that women with excessive blood loss are more susceptible to shock with treatment regimens which often required blood transfusion. Hemorrhage can occur suddenly and unexpectedly. Management of obstetric hemorrhage at facilities where there is no available blood supply and no highly trained health care workers who are skilled with management of obstetric hemorrhage may increase the morbidity of women with bleeding.

This study showed that women who had initially diagnosed with pregnancy-induced hypertension were 5.3 times more likely to develop maternal near-miss than those without pregnancy-induced hypertension. This is consistent with the study done in Kathmandu Hospital [24]; Tigray, Ethiopia [12]; Sudan [21]; and southeast Iran [8].This might be a reflection of poor management of pregnancy-induced hypertension cases in the peripheral health centers as 50.8% of them were referral cases. On the other hand, this might be due to delay in seeking appropriate treatment because of lack of proper referral system and early detection of life-threatening conditions like eclampsia.

TABLE 3: Factors associated with maternal near-miss at the University of Gondar Referral Hospital, Northwest Ethiopia, June 2019 (n = 303).

Variables		Near-miss Yes (%)	Near-miss No (%)	COR (95% CI)	AOR (95% CI)
Residence	Urban	22 (11.6)	168 (88.4)	1	
	Rural	26 (23.0)	87 (77.0)	0.01 (1.22-4.26)	
Monthly income	≤1000	29 (29.0)	71 (71)	3.99 (1.95, 8.16)	3.99 (1.65, 9.65)*
	1001-2000	2 (6.7%)	28 (93.3)	0.69 (0.15, 3.26)	0.89 (0.14, 5.57)
	2001-3000	4 (12.1)	29 (87.9)	1.34 (0.41, 4.43)	1.65 (0.41, 6.67)
	≥3001	13 (9.3)	127 (90.7)	1	1
Parity	1	18 (14.2)	109 (85.8)	1	
	2-4	23 (15.4)	126 (84.6)	1.10 (0.56, 2.15)	
	≥5	7 (25.9)	20 (74.1)	2.11 (0.87, 5.73)	
Duration of hospital stay	<7days	22 (9.3)	215 (90.7)	1	
	≥7days	26 (39.4)	40 (60.6)	6.4 (3.28, 12.30)	5.43 (2.49, 11.83)**
Admission mode	Not referred	16 (10.7)	133 (89.3)	1	
	Referred	32 (20.8)	122 (79.2)	2.18 (1.14, 4.17)	
Reason for seeking care					
Visual disturbance	Yes	17 (50)	17 (50)	7.68 (3.56, 16.56)	
	No	31 (11.5)	238 (88.5)	1	
Severe headache	Yes	16 (42.1)	22 (57.9)	5.29 (2.52, 11.12)	
	No	32 (12.1)	233 (87.9)	1	
Vaginal bleeding	Yes	18 (29.5)	43 (70.5)	2.96 (1.51, 5.78)	2.75 (1.17, 6.47)**
	No	30 (12.4)	212 (87.6)	1	
Initial diagnosis					
PIH	Yes	18 (42.9)	24 (57.1)	5.77 (2.81, 11.86)	5.13 (2.08, 12.63)**
	No	30 (11.5)	231 (88.5)	1	

NB: *p value < 0.005 and **p < 0.05.

5. Conclusion

The proportion of maternal near-miss was found to be high. Variables like low monthly income, seven or more days of hospital stay, vaginal bleeding, and pregnancy-induced hypertension were significantly associated factors with maternal near-miss.

5.1. Recommendation. Early identification and management of vaginal bleeding, pregnancy-induced hypertension, and decrement of long hospital stay are recommended to the hospital. Lastly, income generation activity needs attention by region.

5.2. Limitation of the Study. In this study, no follow-up was done for the women after their discharge from the hospital. This may be underestimating the magnitude of maternal near-miss.

Abbreviations

AOR: Adjusted odds ratio
APH: Antepartum hemorrhage
CI: Confidence interval
CS: Caesarean section
EDHS: Ethiopian demographic health survey
ETB: Ethiopian birr
GTD: Gestational troplastic disease
HCT: Hematocrit
HIV: Human immune-virus
MDG: Millennium development goal
MNM: Maternal near-miss
PID: Pelvic inflammatory disease
PIH: Pregnancy-induced hypertension
PPH: Postpartum hemorrhage
SDG: Sustainable development goal
SPSS: Statistical package for the social science
STI: Sexually transmitted infection
SVD: Spontaneous vaginal delivery
WHO: World Health Organization.

Consent

The reasons why the research was to be done was explained to the study subjects; verbal informed consent was obtained from each study subject after explanation of the purpose of the study, and involvement (to be participant) was after their complete consent.

Authors' Contributions

MMA wrote the proposal, participated in data collection, analyzed the data, and drafted the paper. MMA read, edited, and approved the final manuscript.

Acknowledgments

The author is very grateful to the University of Gondar for the approval of the ethical clearance. My last gratitude goes to the Gondar referral hospital administrator. I would like to extend my appreciation to the study participants and data collectors.

References

[1] J. P. Souza, J. G. Cecatti, S. M. Haddad et al., "The WHO maternal near-miss approach and the maternal severity index model (MSI): tools for assessing the management of severe maternal morbidity," *PLoS One*, vol. 7, no. 8, p. e44129, 2012.

[2] K. Begum, "Maternal near miss: an indicator for maternal health and maternal care," *Journal of Bangladesh College of Physicians and Surgeons*, vol. 36, no. 1, pp. 1–3, 2018.

[3] R. Pattinson, L. Say, J. P. Souza, Broek Nv, C. Rooney, and WHO Working Group on Maternal Mortality and Morbidity Classifications, "WHO maternal death and near-miss classifications," *Bulletin of the World Health Organization*, vol. 10.1186/s12978-016-0232-y, no. 10, p. 734, 2009.

[4] E. Nelissen, E. Mduma, J. Broerse et al., "Applicability of the WHO maternal near miss criteria in a low-resource setting," *PLoS One*, vol. 8, no. 4, article e61248, 2013.

[5] WHO, UNICEF, UNFPA, World Bank Group and the United Nations Population Division, *Trends in maternal mortality: 1990 to 2015*, WHO, 2015, WHO Library Cataloguing-in-Publication Data.

[6] O. P. Aduloju, T. Aduloju, and O. M. Ipinnimo, "Profile of maternal near miss and determinant factors in a teaching hospital, Southwestern Nigeria," *International Journal of Reproduction, Contraception, Obstetrics and Gynecology*, vol. 7, no. 9, pp. 3450–3458, 2018.

[7] F. C. Oliveira Jr., M. L. Costa, J. G. Cecatti, J. L. Pinto e Silva, and F. G. Surita, "Maternal morbidity and near miss associated with maternal age: the innovative approach of the 2006 Brazilian demographic health survey," *Clinics*, vol. 68, no. 7, pp. 922–927, 2013.

[8] T. Naderi, S. Foroodnia, S. Omidi, F. Samadani, and N. Nakhaee, "Incidence and correlates of maternal near miss in Southeast Iran," *International Journal of Reproductive Medicine*, vol. 2015, Article ID 914713, 5 pages, 2015.

[9] A. K. Tura, J. Zwart, J. van Roosmalen, J. Stekelenburg, T. van den Akker, and S. Scherjon, "Severe maternal outcomes in eastern Ethiopia: application of the adapted maternal near miss tool," *PLoS One*, vol. 13, no. 11, article e0207350, 2018.

[10] B. S. Gurung, R. B. Koju, and Y. Dongol, "Near-miss obstetric events in a tertiary care teaching hospital in Nepal: an audit," *Nepal Journal of Obstetrics and Gynaecology*, vol. 19, no. 1, pp. 30–35, 2015.

[11] T. Abate, M. Dile, and T. Syoum, "Proportion of maternal near misses and associated factors in referral hospitals of Amhara regional state, Northwest Ethiopia: institution based cross sectional study," *Gynecology & Obstetrics*, vol. 5, no. 8, pp. 1–8, 2015.

[12] D. E. Mekango, M. Alemayehu, G. B. Gebregergs, A. A. Medhanyie, and G. Goba, "Determinants of maternal near miss among women in public hospital maternity wards in northern Ethiopia: a facility based case-control study," *PLoS One*, vol. 12, no. 9, article e0183886, 2017.

[13] R. P. Reena and K. R. Radha, "Factors associated with maternal near miss: a study from Kerala," *Indian Journal of Public Health*, vol. 62, no. 1, pp. 58–60, 2018.

[14] Government of Ethiopia et al., *Demographic and Health Survey*, Central Statistical Agency, 2016.

[15] A. Langer, A. Meleis, F. M. Knaul et al., "Women and health: the key for sustainable development," *The Lancet*, vol. 386, no. 9999, pp. 1165–1210, 2015.

[16] S. Z. Brown, H. Newby, D. Chou et al., "Understanding global trends in maternal mortality," *International Perspectives on Sexual and Reproductive Health*, vol. 39, no. 1, pp. 32–41, 2013.

[17] T. E. Yarinbab, "Delays in utilization of institutional delivery service and its determinants in Yem Special Woreda, Southwest Ethiopia: health institution based cross-sectional study," *Journal of Gynecology and Womens Health*, vol. 10, no. 4, pp. 1–6, 2018.

[18] B. Assarag, B. Dujardin, A. Delamou, F.-Z. Meski, and V. De Brouwere, "Determinants of maternal near-miss in Morocco: too late, too far, too sloppy?," *PLoS One*, vol. 10, no. 1, article e0116675, 2015.

[19] H. Chikadaya, M. G. Madziyire, and S. P. Munjanja, "Incidence of maternal near miss in the public health sector of Harare, Zimbabwe: a prospective descriptive study," *BMC Pregnancy and Childbirth*, vol. 18, no. 1, p. 458, 2018.

[20] R. M. Domingues, M. A. Dias, A. O. Schilithz, and M. D. Leal, "Factors associated with maternal near miss in childbirth and the postpartum period: findings from the birth in Brazil National Survey, 2011-2012," *Reproductive Health*, vol. 13, no. S3, article 115, 2016.

[21] F. M. Alemu, M. Fuchs, T. Martin Vitale, and M. Abdalla Mohamed Salih, "Severe maternal morbidity (near-miss) and its correlates in the world's newest nation: south sudan," *International Journal of Women's Health*, vol. 2019, pp. 177–190, 2019.

[22] J. G. Cecatti, R. T. Souza, R. C. Pacagnella, M. C. Leal, E. C. Moura, and L. M. P. Santos, "Maternal near miss among women using the public health system in the Amazon and Northeast regions of Brazil," *American Journal of Public Health*, vol. 37, pp. 232–238, 2015.

[23] M. Gedefaw, H. Gebrehana, A. Gizachew, and F. Taddess, "Assessment of maternal near miss at Debre Markos referral hospital, Northwest Ethiopia: five years experience," *Journal of Epidemology*, vol. 4, no. 4, pp. 199–207, 2014.

[24] N. S. Shrestha, R. Saha, and C. Karki, "Near miss maternal morbidity and maternal mortality at Kathmandu Medical College Teaching Hospital," *Kathmandu University Medical Journal*, vol. 8, no. 30, pp. 222–226, 2010.

[25] S. Tyagi, "Near miss maternal mortality, who is responsible? Administration, healthcare system or the people themselves," *International Journal of Reproduction, Contraception, Obstetrics and Gynecology*, vol. 6, no. 10, pp. 4318–4322, 2017.

Emergency Contraceptives: Knowledge and Practice towards Its Use among Ethiopian Female College Graduating Students

Kirubel Minsamo Mishore,[1] **Abebaw Demissie Woldemariam**,[2] **and Solomon Assefa Huluka**[3]

[1]*School of Pharmacy, Haramaya University, Harar, Ethiopia*
[2]*Department of Anesthesia, Harar Health Sciences College, Harar, Ethiopia*
[3]*Department of Pharmacology and Clinical Pharmacy, School of Pharmacy, Addis Ababa University, Addis Ababa, Ethiopia*

Correspondence should be addressed to Solomon Assefa Huluka; solomon.assefa@aau.edu.et

Academic Editor: Stefania A. Nottola

Introduction. Ethiopia has a high incidence of unwanted pregnancies and incomplete and unsafe abortions, particularly among adolescents. This can be avoided by using different contraceptive methods including emergency contraceptives (EC). This study aimed to assess the knowledge and practice of EC among female college graduating students in Harar, Eastern Ethiopia. *Methods.* Institution based cross-sectional study was conducted on 214 female students selected from two randomly selected colleges. Data was collected using a self-administered questionnaire and analyzed using SPSS for Windows version 20.1. Level of significance was taken at $P < 0.05$. *Results.* The mean (±SD) age of the participants was 21.06 (±2.14) years. Of the 200 (93.5%) study participants who had ever heard of ECs, 140 (70.0%) had good knowledge. Among the 214 graduating female students, 66 (33.0%) had ever used EC. Being above the age of 20 years old, father's and mother's literacy were found to be determinants of knowledge of EC. Moreover, knowledge was the only determinant factor of practice of EC. *Conclusion.* Most of the respondents had relatively good knowledge of EC. The study revealed that female students of older age and higher educational status of parents had higher knowledge and practice of EC.

1. Introduction

Unintended pregnancy and unsafe abortion can be prevented by access to contraceptive methods including emergency contraceptives (EC). EC is a method used to avoid pregnancy after unprotected sexual intercourse. It is used before the potential time of implantation, unlike the regular contraceptive methods that are administered before the act [1]. EC can reduce the risk of unintended pregnancy by 75% to 99% if taken within 72 hours of sexual intercourse [2, 3]. ECs are cost-effective, medically safe, and highly effective to be used for the prevention of unplanned pregnancy and subsequently avoid unsafe abortion and other consequences [4].

An estimated 80 million unintended pregnancies occurred in 2012 in the developing world, resulting in 40 million abortions and 10 million miscarriages [5]. About one-third of unintended pregnancies each year result from the incorrect use or failure of contraceptives [6]. World Health Organization (WHO) estimates that every year, nearly 5.5 million African women have unsafe abortions. Moreover, 59% of all unsafe abortions in Africa are among young women aged 15-24 years [7].

Unsafe abortion due to an unplanned pregnancy is one of the main causes of maternal morbidity and mortality in Ethiopian women [8, 9]. Several studies in the country have revealed that women who tend to undergo induced abortions are below the age of 30 and above the secondary educational level [10–12]. Young people today start sex before marriage. Thus, they face a greater risk of unintended pregnancy [13].

Studies conducted in Ethiopia [1, 14–16] indicated that awareness of EC is less than 50% and utilization is below 10%. These limited studies conducted on the issue of EC in the country were mostly focused on university students, who are believed to have better overall knowledge than college students [17]. Studies conducted in college students were not specific to their year of study, which was found to be determinant of knowledge of EC among female college students [18]. Thus, the aim of the present study was to assess determinants of knowledge and practice of ECs among female college graduating students in Harar town, eastern Ethiopia.

2. Methods

2.1. Study Setting. The study was conducted in Harar town, eastern Ethiopia, which is located 525 kilometers east of Addis Ababa. There are eight colleges (private and governmental) in the city. Harar Health Science College (HHSC), Harar Poly Technique College, and Harar Teachers Training College are governmental colleges. Rift Valley University Harar Campus (RVUHC), AferenQallo College, Horn International College, Dakmas College, and Lucy University College are privately owned colleges. Two of the colleges, namely, HHSC and RVUHC, were selected by simple random sampling methods from the list.

2.2. Study Design and Data Collection. An institution based cross-sectional study was conducted in June 2016 among graduating female college students from selected colleges in Harar town. Sample size was determined using the simple proportion formula for cross-sectional study and taking the proportion of 21.9% for good knowledge of EC [18]. The multistage sampling techniques were used to approach the participants. Since the source population was less than 10,000, finite population correction was made, which brought the sample size to 214. Then, the sample size to each selected college and respective departments was then allocated proportionally using total number of female graduating students. Finally, the study participants were selected randomly (Figure 1). The study was conducted by means of a self-administered questionnaire survey. The questionnaire included questions on demographic variables, sexual practice, and knowledge and practice of EC.

2.3. Data Analysis. Following data collection, a unique code was assigned to each questionnaire. Data was then entered, cleaned, and imported to SPSS version 20.1 for analysis. Both bivariate and multivariate analysis techniques were applied to identify the factors associated with knowledge towards EC. The variables that were significant in the bivariate analysis were reexamined using stepwise binary logistic regression, to identify the significant predictors after controlling for other variables. P values less than 0.05 were considered as statistically significant.

The respondent's knowledge scores were aggregated and ranged 0–9. Based on the cumulative score, respondents who scored 5 (mean score) and above were considered to have "good knowledge", while those who scored below the mean score were considered to have "poor knowledge". Practice was determined based on every use of EC after exposure to unprotected sexual intercourse to prevent unintended pregnancy.

2.4. Ethical Consideration. The study was carried out after obtaining ethical clearance from Institutional Ethical Clearance Board of Harar Health Science College and permission from the dean offices of selected colleges. All participants were informed about the objectives and their right to leave the study at any time they wished. A verbal consent was obtained from all participants. Confidentiality of the participants was maintained at all times. To further maintain anonymity, no forms of identifiers were in the questionnaires, as code numbers were used and only data collector and supervisor were involved in the data collection and supervision process.

3. Results

3.1. Sociodemographic Characteristics. A total of 214 female students of the graduating class participated in the study. The mean (±SD) age of the participants was 21.06 years (± 2.14). Ninety (42.1%) of them were midwifery students followed by nursing students (16.4%). As it is shown in Table 1, most of the respondents 164 (76.6%) were urban residents. Nearly three fourths (74.3%) of the respondents were unmarried. The majority (132; 61.7%) of the participants were living with their parents (Table 1).

3.2. Knowledge of Emergency Contraceptives. Majority of the participants (93.5%) reported that they had heard about EC. Only those respondents who had heard of EC (200) were further analyzed for having knowledge and practices. The overall summary index for knowledge disclosed that 140 (70.0%) of the study participants had good knowledge about EC (Figure 2). The main sources of information about EC were college (40.5%) followed by healthcare workers (29%) and mass media (24.5%). Most of the respondents 130 (65.0%) could identify the correct timing for administration of emergency contraceptive pills after unprotected sex. However, only 54 (27.0%) could tell the correct timing of insertion of the intrauterine contraceptive device (IUCD) (Table 2).

3.3. Practice of Emergency Contraception and Sexual Activity. Among female graduating college students who had ever heard of EC, almost one-third (33.0%) of them had ever used EC Pills (Figure 2). However, none of the women had ever used IUCD. Pills missed, failed withdrawal, timing miscalculation, and condom slippage were the commonly stated reasons for using EC each accounted for 15 (22.7%), 9 (14.0%), 9 (13.6%), and 8 (12.1%), respectively. Seventy-one (55.9%) of participants started sex below age of 20 years. Among the sexually active students, 30 (23.6%) had an experience of pregnancy. Unintended pregnancy were observed in 20 (15.7%) of participants (Table 3).

3.4. Determinants on Knowledge and Practice of EC. Sociodemographic factors, age and educational status of the respondents' parents, showed a significant association with good knowledge of EC in multivariate logistic regression analysis. Females who were older (>20 years) were 6.09 times more likely to have good knowledge of EC than their younger

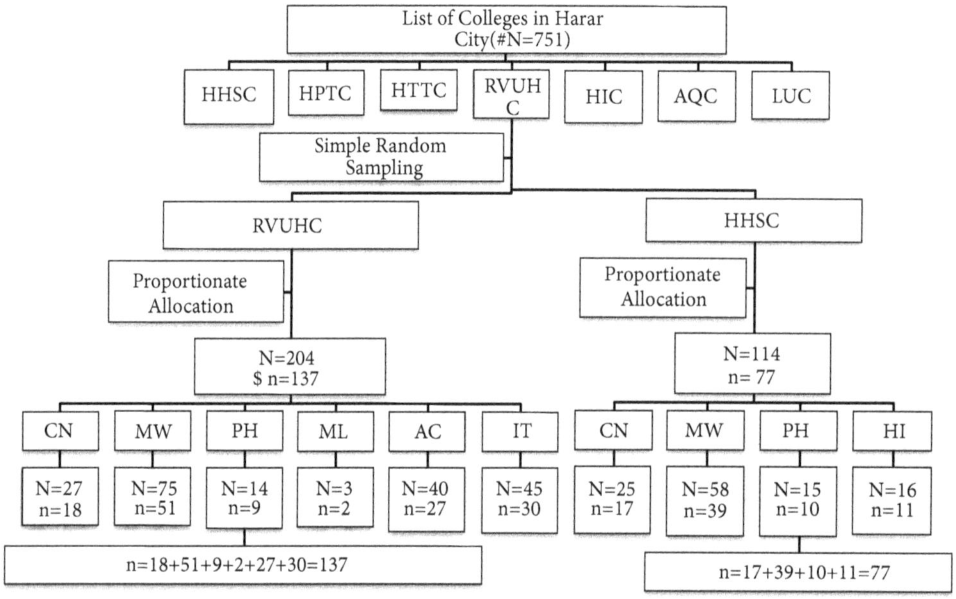

Figure 1: Schematic presentation of sampling procedure. # Total number of graduating class female students in each college and departments. $ Sample size proportionally allocated to each college and departments. Comprehensive Nurse (CN); Midwifery (MW); Pharmacy (PH); Medical Laboratory (ML); Accounting (AC); Information Technology (IT); Health Informatics (HI).

Table 1: Sociodemographic characteristics of female college graduating students in Harar town, eastern Ethiopia, 2016 (N=214).

Variable	Category	Frequency	Percent
Age group (year)	≤20	108	50.5
	21-24	93	43.5
	25^+	13	6.1
Residence	Urban	164	76.6
	Rural	50	23.4
Religion	Christian	133	62.1
	Muslim	81	37.9
Marital status	Single	159	74.3
	Ever married	55	25.7
Field of study	Midwifery	90	42.1
	Comprehensive nurse	35	16.4
	Information technology	30	14
	Accounting	27	12.6
	Pharmacy	19	8.9
	Health informatics	11	5.1
	Medical laboratory	2	0.9
Living with	Parents	132	61.7
	Alone	34	15.9
	Husband	26	12.1
	Friends	22	10.3
Father's Education	Nonliterate	28	13.1
	Completed primary school	44	20.6
	Completed secondary school	59	27.6
	Completed tertiary school	83	38.8
Mother's Education	Nonliterate	34	15.9
	Completed primary school	51	23.8
	Completed secondary school	72	33.6
	Completed tertiary school	58	27.1

TABLE 2: Knowledge of emergency contraceptives among graduating female college students of Harar, eastern Ethiopia, 2016 (N=200).

Characteristics	Category	Frequency	Percent
Ever heard of EC	Yes	200	93.5
	No	14	6.5
Source of information	College	81	40.5
	Healthcare workers	58	29
	Mass media	49	24.5
	Others	12	6
Method reported used as EC	Pills	124	62.0
	IUCD	18	9.0
	Pills and IUCD	29	14.5
	Implants and Injectable	29	14.5
Places where a woman can obtain EC	Hospital /health center	109	54.5
	Pharmacy	59	29.5
	Don't know	10	5.0
	Others	22	11.0
Indication of EC	After unprotected sexual intercourse	114	57.0
	When unwanted pregnancy occurs	62	31.0
	As regular method of contraceptive	24	12.0
Drug strength in EC pills compared to regular pills	The same strength	92	43.0
	Higher dose in the same hormones	35	16.4
	Don't know	73	34.1
Maximum time limit for taking ECPs	Within 72 hours	130	65.0
	Within 48 hours	9	4.5
	Within 24 hours	10	5.0
	Within 12 hours	18	9.0
	Don't know	33	16.5
Maximum time limit for having an IUCD after unprotected sex	Within 5 days	54	27.0
	Within 72 hours	30	15.0
	Within 48 hours	12	6.0
	Don't know	104	52.0
Effectiveness of EC methods in preventing pregnancy when used within the specified time limit	<75%	20	10.0
	≥75% but < 100%	113	56.5
	Not sure	67	33.5
How safe do you think EC are for most women?	Safe	138	69.0
	Unsafe	28	14.0
	No response	34	17.0

counterparts (AOR: 6.09, 95% CI: 2.89-12.86, P≤0.001). On the other hand, respondents with a literate father were 3.5 times more likely to have good knowledge of EC compared to those with a nonliterate father (AOR: 3.50, 95% CI: 1.12-10.94, P=0.031). Similarly, respondents whose mother was literate were 2.84 times more likely to be knowledgeable (AOR: 2.84, 95% CI: 1.02-7.88, P=0.046) compared to their counterparts (Table 4).

Among variables, which showed association with bivariate logistic regression analysis, only having good knowledge of EC showed a significant association with student's ever utilization or practice of EC in multivariate analysis. Accordingly, students who had good knowledge of EC were 2.53 times more likely to practice EC than those who had poor knowledge of EC (AOR: 2.53, 95%CI: 1.29, 4.92) (Table 5).

TABLE 3: Practice of emergency contraception and sexual activity among female college graduating students, Harar, eastern Ethiopia, 2016 (N=200).

Variables	Category	Frequency	Percent
Ever use of EC	Yes	66	33
	No	134	67
Frequency of use	Once	30	45.5
	Twice	14	21.2
	Three times	7	10.6
	Not specified	15	22.7
Recommended by	Friends	20	30.3
	Partner	18	27.3
	Health professional	23	34.8
	Not specified	5	7.6
Reasons for using	Timing miscalculation	9	13.6
	Condom slippage/breakage	8	12.1
	Pills missed	15	22.7
	Forced sex	6	9.1
	Failed withdrawal	9	13.6
	Not specified	19	28.8
History of sexual practice	Yes	127	63.5
	No	73	36.5
Age at first sex	15-19	71	55.9
	≥20	47	37.0
	Not specified	9	7.1
History of pregnancy	Yes	30	23.6
	No	97	76.4
Was the pregnancy planned?	Yes	10	33.3
	No	20	66.7

TABLE 4: Univariate and multivariate analysis of factors associated with knowledge of EC among female college graduating students, Harar, eastern Ethiopia, 2016 (N=200).

Variable	Category	Knowledge		COR (95% CI)	*P* value*	AOR (95% CI)	*P* value*
		Good	Poor				
Age	≤20	52	441.00			1.00	
	>20	88	16	4.65(2.39-9.07)	0.001	6.09(2.89-12.86)	0.001
Marital Status	Unmarried	96	50	1.00		1.00	
	Ever married	44	10	2.29(1.06-4.94)	0.034	1.83(0.64-5.26)	0.261
Field of Study	Health	113	40	2.1(1.06-4.12)	0.034	1.87(0.82-4.3)	0.14
	Not Health	27	20	1.00		1.00	
Fathers' Education	Nonliterate	10	16	1.00		1.00	
	Literate	130	44	4.73(1.99-11.18)	0.001	3.50(1.12-10.94)	0.031
Mothers' Education	Nonliterate	16	19	1.00		1.00	
	Literate	124	41	3.59(1.69-7.63)	0.001	2.84(1.02-7.88)	0.046

COR: crude odds ratio; AOR: adjusted odds ratio; CI: confidence interval.
**P* value <0.05 indicates statistically significant association.

4. Discussion

Unlike other contraceptive medicines, EC is not given regularly. It is given in cases of unprotected sexual relations, which carry the risk of undesired pregnancy [16]. Awareness of the accessibility and being taken within the defined time period are necessary for appropriate and effective use of EC [19, 20].

Majority (94%) of the study participants included in the study were aged 24 or below, which is considered a sexually active age group [21]. This finding is also in line with a similar study done in Nigeria [22]. The overall prevalence of awareness among the study participants was 93.5%. This finding is higher as compared to studies done in different parts of Ethiopia: Haramaya (47.6%)[14], Adama [15] (46.8%),

TABLE 5: Univariate and multivariate analysis of factors associated with practice of EC among female college graduating students, Harar, eastern Ethiopia, 2016 (N=200).

Variable	Category	Practice		COR (95% CI)	*P* value*	AOR (95% CI)	*P* value*
		Ever used	Not used				
Age	≤20	30	66	1.00		1.00	
	>20	36	68	2.14(1.22-3.77)	0.008	1.29(0.66-2.54)	0.449
Marital Status	Single	43	103	1.00		1.00	
	Ever married	23	31	2.36(1.22-4.57)	0.011	1.84(0.87-3.89)	0.113
Knowledge	Good	53	87	2.96(1.57-5.56)	0.001	2.53(1.29-4.92)	0.006
	Poor	13	47	1.00		1.00	

COR: crude odds ratio; AOR: adjusted odds ratio; CI: confidence interval.
**P* value <0.05 indicates statistically significant association.

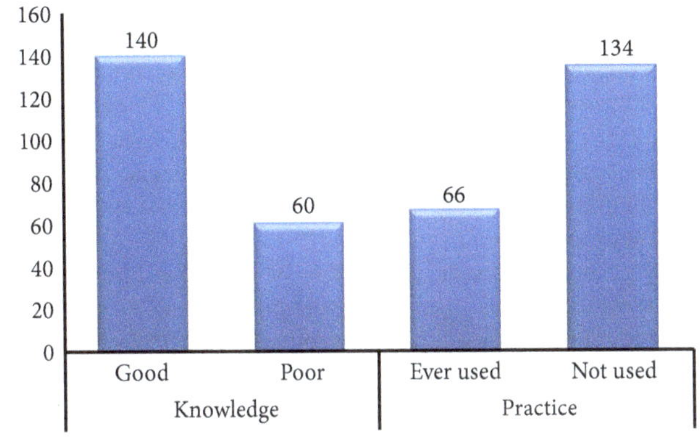

FIGURE 2: Frequency distribution of knowledge and practice of emergency contraceptive among female college graduating students of Harar, eastern Ethiopia, 2016(N=200).

Jimma (41.9%) [16], Ambo (80.7%) [17], Arba-Minch (42.5%) [18], Hosanna (45%) [23], and Debre-Markos (71.1%)[24]. However, this finding is comparable to the result of studies in Mekele (90.7%). Similar levels of awareness prevalence were also recorded in India (92.7%) [25, 26]. In the present study, the major source of information about EC was college, unlike a study done in Addis Ababa [27] whereby participants relied on friends and family for knowledge of EC.

Nearly three quarters (70.0%) of the respondents had good knowledge of EC in this study, which is superior to the result obtained in the studies conducted among Ethiopian colleges and university female students in Haramaya (25.7 %)[14], Arba-Minch (21.9%) [18], and Debre-Markos (62.5%)[24], Mizantepi [28] and elsewhere in India [26] and Nepal [29]. This difference might be attributed to a better free discussion on sex and sexuality among female students in Harar. However, the finding is unexpectedly lower than a study conducted among female preparatory students in Mekelle where 75.7% of the students had good knowledge of EC[25]. Moreover, in this study 130 (65%) of the participants correctly identified the time limit of EC pill use, which is superior to a study done by Abate et al., 18.5% [30]. This could be due to the high health promotion and availability of EC in pharmacies found [31] in Harar.

The finding showed that unintended pregnancies were observed in 20 (15.7%) of the respondents, which is slightly lower than study conducted in northwest Ethiopia (16.5%) [31]. However, it is much lower than the result reported in the national figure EDHS 2011 (24%) [32], and GanjoWoreda (27%)[33]. In the present study, about a third (33.0%) of the respondents had ever used EC. This finding is higher than the study conducted in Dilla (20.9%) [34]. It is also higher than EC use reported in Nigeria and India [26, 35]. This may be explained by wide availability of EC in Ethiopia particularly in major cities [30] and longer college stay.

In this study, age of the student showed a statistically significant association with good knowledge of EC. In agreement with this study, multiple studies [14, 24, 25] have reported a significant association between older age and good knowledge of EC. However, other study done by Melkam et al. [19] reported a contrary finding. This study, furthermore, revealed that EC knowledge was significantly higher for respondents whose parents were literate compared to those with nonliterate parents. This finding is consistent with the conclusion made by different researchers [18, 24], in which literacy improves one's access to information and facilitates discussion of reproductive health issues in the household.

The present study also showed that female students who had adequate knowledge of EC were more likely to use EC than their counterparts, which was in agreement with studies from Ethiopia and other countries [18, 24, 26, 36].

5. Conclusion and Recommendation

In this study, respondents' knowledge of EC is found to be acceptable. This study revealed that age and parents' literacy showed statistically significant association with good knowledge of EC and in turn good knowledge of EC was the only determinant of using EC. To prevent unintended pregnancy among sexually active female college students, sexual education given at high school or counseling provided to college students is highly recommended.

Abbreviations

AOR: Adjusted odds ratio
CI: Confidence interval

COR: Crude odds ratio
EC: Emergency contraception
HHSC: Harar Health Science College
IUCD: Intrauterine Contraceptive Device
RVUHC: Rift Valley University Harar Campus
SD: Standard deviation
WHO: World Health Organization.

Consent

Since none of the respondents are below the age of 16, informed consent to participate in the study was obtained from participants themselves.

Authors' Contributions

Kirubel Minsamo Mishore, Abebaw Demissie Woldemariam, and Solomon Assefa Huluka conceived the study and participated in the design, data analysis, and interpretation of the result. Kirubel Minsamo Mishore was involved in data acquisition and writing of the draft manuscript as well as editing it per the suggestions of the coauthors. Abebaw Demissie Woldemariam and Solomon Assefa Huluka critically reviewed the manuscript. All authors read and approved the manuscript.

Acknowledgments

Authors would like to thank participants of the study. We would like to extend our appreciations to individuals who were involved in data collection. We are also grateful to the colleges that facilitated the study.

References

[1] W. Tamire and F. Enqueselassie, "Knowledge, attitude, and practice on emergency contraceptives among female university students in Addis Ababa, Ethiopia," *Ethiopian Journal of Health Development*, vol. 21, no. 2, pp. 111–116, 2007.

[2] M. E. Hoque and S. Ghuman, "Knowledge, practices, and attitudes of emergency contraception among female university students in KwaZulu-Natal, South Africa," *PLoS ONE*, vol. 7, no. 9, 2012.

[3] J. L. Lenjisa, Z. Gulila, and N. Legese, "Knowledge, attitude and practice of emergency contraceptives among ambo university female students, West Showa, Ethiopia," *Research Journal of Pharmaceutical Sciences*, vol. 2, no. 11, pp. 1-5, 2013.

[4] A. Mir and R. Malik, "Emergency contraceptive pills: Exploring the knowledge and attitudes of community health workers in a developing Muslim country," *North American Journal of Medical Sciences*, vol. 8, pp. 359–364, 2010.

[5] S. Singh and E. J. Darroch, *Adding It Up: The Costs and Benefits of Contraceptive Services; Estimates for 2012*, Guttmacher Institute, New York, NY, USA, 2012.

[6] Population Reference Bureau, *World Population Data Sheet*, 2010.

[7] World Health Organization, *Unsafe Abortion: Global and Regional Estimates of the Incidence of Unsafe Abortion and Associated Mortality in 2003*, WHO, Geneva, Switzerland, 5th edition, 2007.

[8] Y. Berhan and A. Berhan, "Causes of maternal mortality in Ethiopia: a significant decline in abortion related death," *Ethiopian Journal of Health Sciences*, vol. 24, pp. 15–28, 2014.

[9] B. E. Kwast, R. W. Rochat, and W. Kidane-Mariam, "Maternal mortality in Addis Ababa, Ethiopia," *Studies in Family Planning*, vol. 17, no. 6, pp. 288–301, 1986.

[10] F. Hassen, "Analysis of factors for unwanted pregnancy among women in the reproductive age group attending health institutes in Jimma town," *Report*, 2000.

[11] S. Kebede, C. Jirra, and W. D. Mariam, "A survey of illegal abortion in Jimma Hospital; South West Ethiopia," *Ethiopian Medical Journal*, vol. 38, pp. 35–42, 2000.

[12] Y. Melkamu, F. Enquselassie, and A. Ali, "Fertility awareness and future pregnancy intention of postabortion patients in Addis Ababa, Ethiopia," *Ethiopian Journal of Health Development*, vol. 17, no. 3, pp. 167–174, 2003.

[13] H. Rahaman, P. Renjhen, A. Kumar, S. Pattanshetty, A. Sagir, and H. Dubey, "A study on emergency contraceptive practice among nursing staff in Sikkim, India - A cross sectional study," *Australasian Medical Journal*, vol. 3, no. 10, pp. 667–671, 2010.

[14] B. Desta and N. Regassa, "Emergency Contraception among Female Students of Haramaya University, Ethiopia: Surveying the Level of Knowledge and Attitude," *Educational Research*, vol. 2, no. 4, pp. 1106–1117, 2011.

[15] D. Tilahun, T. Assefa, and T. Belachew, "Knowledge, attitude and practice of emergency contraceptive among Adama Universty female student," *Ethiopian Journal of Health Sciences*, vol. 20, no. 3, pp. 195–201, 2010.

[16] N. Tajure, "Knowledge, Attitude and Practice of Emergency Contraception among Graduating Female Students of Jimma University, Southwest Ethiopia," *Ethiopian Journal of Health Sciences*, vol. 20, no. 2, 2011.

[17] J. L. Lenjisa, M. A. Woldu, and D. Ulfina, "Knowledge, Attitude and Practice of Emergency Contraceptives among Ambo TVET College Female Students , Ethiopia," *IJMCH*, vol. 16, no. 1, pp. 1–11, 2014.

[18] A. Worku, "Knowledge, attitude and practice of emergency contraceptives among female college students in Arba Minch town, Southern Ethiopia," *Ethiopian Journal of Health Development*, vol. 25, no. 3, pp. 176–183, 2012.

[19] W. Melkam, G. Teklemariam, S. Abrha, and A. Kahsu, "Knowledge and Practice on Emergency Contraceptives among females who Came for Abortion at Mekelle General Hospital, Mekelle, Ethiopia," *IJMN*, vol. 2, no. 2, pp. 234–239, 2015.

[20] C.-X. Meng, K. Gemzell-Danielsson, O. Stephansson, J.-Z. Kang, Q.-F. Chen, and L.-N. Cheng, "Emergency contraceptive use among 5677 women seeking abortion in Shanghai, China," *Human Reproduction*, vol. 24, no. 7, pp. 1612–1618, 2009.

[21] A. C. Richard, J. D. Ralph, M. W. Gina et al., "Angela: Oral contraceptive use may not preclude condom use: a study of non-pregnant African-American adolescent females," *Sexually Transmitted Infections*, vol. 83, pp. 216–218, 2007.

[22] A. I. Ajayi, E. E. Nwokocha, O. V. Adeniyi, D. Ter Goon, and W. Akpan, "Unplanned pregnancy-risks and use of emergency contraception: a survey of two Nigerian Universities," *BMC Health Services Research*, vol. 17, no. 1, p. 382, 2017.

[23] A. Kassa and M. Wolde-Mariam, "Knowledge, attitude and practice of emergency contraceptive pills among female students of Hosanna College of Health Sciences, Hosanna, South Ethiopia," *Journal of Chemical and Pharmaceutical Sciences*, vol. 7, no. 3, pp. 185–193, 2014.

[24] M. Tessema and H. Bayu, "Knowledge, Attitude and Practice on Emergency Contraception and Associated Factors among Female Students of Debre-Markos University, Debre-Markos Town, East Gojam Zone, North West Ethiopia," *Global Journal of Medical Research: E Gynecology and Obstetrics*, vol. 15, no. 1, pp. 1-7, 2013.

[25] S. Abrha, F. Zeratsion, and F. Molla, "Assessment of Knowledge, Attitude and Practice among Regular Female Preparatory School Students towards Emergency Contraceptives in Mekelle, Northern Ethiopia," *IJPSR*, vol. 5, no. 11, pp. 856–864, 2014.

[26] N. Relwani, A. Saoji, and N. B. Kasturwar, "Emergency Contraception: Exploring the Knowledge, Attitude and Practices of Engineering College Girls in Nagpur District of Central India," *NJCM*, vol. 3, no. 1, pp. 14–19, 2012.

[27] R. Both and F. Samuel, "Keeping silent about emergency contraceptives in Addis Ababa: a qualitative study among young people, service providers, and key stakeholders," *BMC Women's Health*, vol. 14, no. 1, p. 134, 2014.

[28] B. Z. Shiferaw, B. T. Gashaw, and F. Y. Tesso, "Factors associated with utilization of emergency contraception among female students in Mizan-Tepi University, South West Ethiopia," *BMC Research Notes*, vol. 8, no. 817, 2015.

[29] S. Subedi, "Knowledge, attitude and practices of emergency contraception among youths of Parabat District," *JHAS*, vol. 2, no. 1, pp. 50–53, 2012.

[30] M. Abate, N. Assefa, and T. Alemayehu, "Knowledge, attitude, practice, and determinants emergency contraceptive use among women seeking abortion services in Dire Dawa, Ethiopia," *PLoS ONE*, vol. 9, no. 10, 2014.

[31] B. Wasie, Y. Belyhun, B. Moges, and B. Amare, "Effect of emergency oral contraceptive use on condom utilization and sexual risk taking behaviours among university students, Northwest Ethiopia: A cross-sectional study," *BMC Research Notes*, vol. 5, article no. 501, 2012.

[32] D. Habte, S. Teklu, T. Melese, and M. G. M. D. Magafu, "Correlates of unintended pregnancy in Ethiopia: results from a national survey," *PLoS ONE*, vol. 8, no. 12, Article ID e82987, 2013.

[33] F. T. Teshome, A. G. Hailu, and A. N. Teklehaymanot, "Prevalence of unintended pregnancy and associated factors among married pregnant women in Ganji woreda, west Wollega Oromia region, Ethiopia," *Science Journal of Public Health*, vol. 2, no. 2, pp. 92–101, 2014.

[34] M. Soressa, A. Astatkie, Y. Berhane, and S. Mitiku, "Contraceptive Use and Associated Factors among Dilla University Female Students, Southern Ethiopia," *JMCR*, vol. 20, pp. 11–21, 2016.

[35] K. O. Wright, A. O. Fabamwo, and O. I. Akinola, "Emergency contraception: A different perspective on knowledge and use among female undergradutes in a non-residential tertiary institution in Nigeria," *International Journal of Medicine and Medical Sciences*, vol. 6, no. 10, pp. 215–223, 2014.

[36] A. O. Aigbiremolen, C. B. Duru, and S. O. Abah, "Contraception among tertiary students: knowledge, use and behaviour of female undergraduates," *Global Journal of Medical Research*, vol. 14, no. 2, pp. 1–7, 2014.

25

Magnitude of Gender-Based Violence and Its Associated Factors among Female Night Students in Bahir Dar City, Amhara Region, Ethiopia

Habtamu Gebrehana Belay, Tewachew Muche Liyeh, Habtamu Abie Tassew, Abeba Belay Ayalew, Yitayal Ayalew Goshu, and Gedefaye Nibret Mihretie

Department of Midwifery, College of Health Science, Debre Tabor University, Debre Tabor, Ethiopia

Correspondence should be addressed to Habtamu Gebrehana Belay; hgebrehana@yahoo.com

Academic Editor: Maria Grazia Piccioni

Background. Gender-based violence (GBV) is a major public health issue that affects the health and well-being of millions of young people worldwide each year. Gender-based violence was prevalent throughout Sub-Saharan Africa. However, research in Africa is extremely diverse. *Objective.* The purpose of this study is to determine the extent and risk factors of gender-based violence among night female students in Bahir Dar, Ethiopia. *Methods.* This cross-sectional study was conducted among 788 elementary and high school night female students in Bahir Dar from October 15 to November 15, 2019. Data was gathered using self-administered questionnaires. A binary and multiple logistic regression model was used to identify factors associated with gender-based and sexual violence. An adjusted odds ratio (AOR) with a 95 percent confidence interval (CI) was calculated to determine the level of significance. *Results.* The overall lifetime prevalence of gender-based violence (sexual, physical, and emotional violence) was 71.1% with a 95% CI of 67.8%-74.1%. The lifetime prevalence of sexual violence, physical violence, and emotional violence was 49.1%, 57.5%, and 41.6%, respectively. Rural childhood residence (AOR: 3.37, 95% CI: (2.17-5.54)), low school performance (AOR: 3.44, 95% CI: (2.13-5.56)), lack of sexual and reproductive health conversation experience (AOR: 3.68, 95% CI: (2.07-6.54)), poor family control (AOR: 5.62, 95% CI: (3.25-9.71)), and being sexually active (AOR: 3.79, 95% CI: (2.35-6.12)) increased significantly the risk of gender-based violence. The risk factors for sexual violence were young people living with both parents (AOR: 0.28, 95% CI: (0.19-0.41)), peer pressure (AOR: 5.73, 95% CI: (4.11-7.98)), and family support (AOR: 0.31, 95% CI: (0.22-0.43)). *Conclusion.* In the study area, the lifetime prevalence of sexual violence, physical violence, and emotional violence was high. As a result, it is recommended that policymakers, district officials, schools, and other stakeholders pay attention to and act on gender-based values.

1. Background

Gender-based violence is defined as violence directed against an individual based on sex or gender, which results in psychological, physical, or sexual trauma, either directly or indirectly [1]. Gender-based violence (GBV) is one of the most widespread, underreported, and unsolicited human rights violations in the world. It has no social, economic, or national boundaries. Violence against women is a major public health problem affecting the physical, sexual, mental, and social well-being of more than one-third of all women worldwide [2]. Violence against women and girls is one of the most common human rights violations in the world. Providing high-quality care and support services to victims of violence is critical for reducing trauma, assisting victims in healing, and preventing repeat victimization and perpetration [3].

Sexual violence affects people of all genders, sexual orientations, and ages in every community. Anyone can be a victim of sexual violence, but the majority of victims are women [4]. Sexual and gender-based violence is a serious, life-threatening global problem that affects women, girls, boys, and men, and it is widely underreported in all settings.

All forms of violence are strongly linked to social determinants such as poor governance, weak rule of law, cultural, social, and gender norms, unemployment, income, and gender inequality, and limited educational opportunities [5].

Globally, one in every three women has experienced physical and/or sexual intimate partner violence in her lifetime, and one in every three adolescent girls reports having their first sexual experience as a result of coercion [6, 7]. Globally, it is estimated that up to 1 billion children aged 2–17 years have been victims of physical, sexual, or emotional violence [8]. Gender-based violence is common in Sub-Saharan African educational institutions (SSA). Gender-based violence in schools lowers girls' educational attainment and increases absenteeism and dropout rates. More than 40% of women have experienced some form of intimate partner violence at some point in their lives [9]. The consequences of GBV include murder, suicide, HIV/AIDS, shock, infection, chronic pain, alcohol/drug dependence, miscarriage, unwanted pregnancy, unsafe abortion, victim/survivor guilt, anxiety, fear, self-hatred, and self-denial, economic dependence, loss of role or function in society [10].

The systemic review in Ethiopia has shown that the lifetime prevalence of domestic violence against women by husband or intimate partner violence ranges from 20 to 78%. The lifetime prevalence of domestic physical violence by a husband or intimate partner against women ranged from 31 to 76.5%, and the lifetime prevalence of domestic sexual violence against women by husband or intimate partner ranged from 19.2 to 59% [11]. Previous research on gender-based violence in Ethiopia has focused on daytime high school students, but this study is aimed at determining the magnitude and associated factors of gender-based violence among female primary and high school students at night.

2. Methods

2.1. Study Design and Setting. This cross-sectoral institutional study was conducted among 788 elementary and high school night students in Bahir Dar City, Ethiopia, from October 15, 2019, to November 15, 2019. Bahir Dar is the capital of the regional state of Amhara. It is located approximately 565 km away from the capital city of Ethiopia, Addis Ababa.

2.2. Population. All-female night students registered in public institutions in Bahir Dar City for the academic year 2019 were the source population and those identified in the chosen public institution during the data collection period were the study population.

2.3. Inclusion and Exclusion Criteria. All-female night students enrolled in a night program at a public elementary and high school in Bahir Dar were included, while female night students who had lived in the city for less than six months were excluded.

2.4. Sample Size Determination. The single population proportion formula was used to determine the sample size using 58.3% prevalence of lifetime gender-based violence among high school students [12]. Assuming 95% confidence interval (CI), 5% margin of error, design effect 2, and additional 10% for nonresponse rate and the final sample size were 823.

2.5. Sampling Procedure. Based on the percentage of female students in grades 1-8 and 9-10 in each class, the calculated sample size was proportionally allocated to their respective elementary and high school students. Students' rosters or name lists were used as a sampling frame to select study subjects from each grade. The total of students aging 15-24 years in each grade were divided by the proportionally allocated sample size to each grade to get the interval (K). The first respondent was selected by using lottery methods.

2.6. Operational Definition

(i) *Gender-Based Violence.* Results in sexual, psychological, and physical trauma

(ii) *Sexual Violence.* Unwanted or nonconsensual sexual act through force, threat, or intimidation

(iii) *Sexual Harassment.* Unwanted sexual behaviors including jokes, verbal communications, and intentional physical contacts

(iv) *Physical Violence.* In this study, physical violence is defined as a respondent saying "yes" to one of the following items: slapping, kicking, beating with any object, cutting/biting, shaking, shoving, pushing, throwing, and burning/chocking against an individual

2.7. Data Collection Procedure. Data from participants were collected using a pretested interviewer-administered structured questionnaire adapted from literature reviews developed by different authors for similar purposes [13].To ensure the consistency and content of the questionnaire, the questioner was first written in English, then translated into Amharic, and then retranslated back into English. Five Bachelor of Science midwives collected data under the supervision of two Master of Science in clinical midwives.

2.8. Data Quality Assurance. To avoid confusion and to ensure a common understanding of the study, data collectors and supervisors were trained regarding the objectives of the study, data collection methods, and significance of the study. A pretest was conducted for 10% of the total sample at another public institution with similar characteristics to the study population. Throughout the data collection process, interviewers were supervised, and regular meetings were held between the data collectors, the supervisor, and the principal investigator to discuss and address any issues that arose during the interviews. Before entering data, the collected data were reviewed and checked for completeness.

2.9. Data Analysis. The collected data were checked, coded, and entered into Epi-data (version 3.5) software, then exported into SPSS software (version 23) for analysis. Bivariate analysis was performed for all explanatory variables about gender-based violence and sexual violence. Variables having a p value < 0.20 in the bivariate analysis were selected for the multivariate logistic regression modeling, for adjustment of confounding effects between explanatory variables. Adjusted odds ratio (AOR) with 95% CI was computed, and variables having p value < 0.05 in the multivariate logistic regression model were considered as statistically significant. The odds ratio was also used to determine the strength of association between independent variables and the outcome variable.

3. Results

3.1. Sociodemographic Characteristic of Study Participants. A total of 788-night female students were enrolled, with a response rate of 95.75 percent. The mean age of participants in the study was 18.88 years with SD ± 2.73. The majority of respondents 683 (86.7%) were Orthodox religious followers and 718 (91.1%) were Amharic ethnic. More than half of the 463 (58.8%) childhood residences of study participants were urban, and 325 (41.1%) were rural residences. More than two-thirds of participants 514 (65.2%) were grades 1-8, and 274 (34.8%) were from grades 9-10. The current living conditions of the respondents were 118 (15%) alone, 214 (27.2%) with the family, and 245 (31%) with the employer. More than half of 423 (53.7%) were single in marital status. The monthly pocket money of respondents that got less than 2000 Ethiopian birr was 324(41%) and got greater than 4000 Ethiopian birrs was 184(23.4%) (Table 1).

Table 1: Sociodemographic characteristic of female night students in public institution of Bahir Dar City, Amhara Region, Ethiopia, 2019.

Variables	Frequency	Percentage
Age		
15-19	452	57.4
20-24	336	42.6
Religion		
Orthodox	683	86.7
Muslim	64	8.1
Others *	41	5.2
Ethnicity		
Amhara	726	92.1
Others **	62	7.9
Educational level		
Grade 1-8	514	65.2
Grade 9-10	274	34.8
Living condition		
Alone	118	15
With family	214	27.2
With husband/boyfriends	90	11.4
With female friends	121	15.4
With employer	245	31
Marital status		
Married	128	16.2
Had boyfriend	237	30.1
Single	423	53.7
Monthly pocket money		
<2000	324	41
2000-4000	280	35.6
≥4000	184	23.4

*Others include Protestant and Catholic. **Others include Tigray and Oromo.

3.2. Sexual Experience and Sexual Violence. Of the total respondents, 490 (62.2%%) had sexual experience. More than two-thirds of participants 319 (65.1%) started the first sex at the age of between 17-19 years, and 90 (18.4%) started their first sex at age greater than 20 years and above. Three-hundred and ten 310 (63.3%) participants had more than one sexual partner in their lifetime, and 180 (36.7%) had only one sexual partner in their lifetime. The first exposure for the first sexual intercourse was peer pressure 220 (46.7%), forced 59 (12%), and 50 (10.2%) self-interest. Of the total respondents, less than one-third 227(28.8%) were discussed abort sexual and reproductive issues with family and or friends. About four in ten young people (41.2%) had a constant sexual partner. Of the 788 total respondents, 387 (49.1%) had experienced sexual violence in their lifetime. The attempted sexual harassment reported by two-thirds of the respondents was 514 (65.2%), and the lifetime prevalence of rape was 132 (16.7%) (Table 2). There are several consequences of gender-based violence mentioned by the despondences. Those complications were unwanted pregnancy 72 (14.7%), depression 323 (66%), anxiety 303 (62%), self-blame 216 (44), and injury around the genitalia 201 (41%) (Table 3).

3.3. Factors Associated with Gender-Based Violence. Multivariate logistic regression revealed that rural childhood residence, discussing sexual and reproductive health issues with family and/or friends, family control, and being sexually active were all significantly associated with gender-based violence. Living in a rural area during childhood increased the risk of GBV by three times as compared to their counterparts (AOR: 3.37, 95% CI: (2.17-5.54)). Students who had no prior experience discussing sexual and reproductive health matters with family or friends had nearly four times increased the risk of GBV as compared to their counterparts (AOR: 3.68, 95% CI: (2.07-6.54)). Students who performed poorly in school had three times the odds of experiencing GBV as those who performed well in school (AOR: 3.44, 95% CI: (2.13-5.56)). Students who had poor family control were increased almost 4 times the odds of GBV as compared to those who had good family control (AOR: 5.62, 95% CI: (3.25-9.71)) and being sexually active increased almost 4 times the odds of GBV as compared to their counterparts (AOR: 3.79, 95% CI: (2.35-6.12))(Table 4).

Living with a biological partner, peer pressure, and family support was all found to be significantly associated with sexual violence in multivariate logistic regression analyses. Night female students living with their biological partners reduced the risk of gender-based violence by 72% as compared to their counterparts (AOR: 0.28, 95% CI: (0.19-0.41)). Peer pressure increased almost 4 times the odds of GBV (AOR: 5.73, 95% CI: (4.11-7.98)), and family support reduced the

TABLE 2: Sexual characteristic of female night students in public institution of Bahir Dar city, Amhara Region, Ethiopia, 2019.

Variables	Frequency	Percentage
Ever had sexual intercourse		
Yes	490	62.2
No	298	37.8
Age at first sex ($n = 490$)		
10-16	81	16.5
17-19	319	65.1
≥20	90	18.4
Number of sexual partner in life ($n = 490$)		
One	180	36.7
Two and above	310	63.3
How you exposed to first sexual intercourse ($n = 490$)		
With marriage	67	13.7
Self-interest	50	10.2
Peer pressure	220	46.7
Forced	59	12
For money	94	19.2
Discussion SRH issue with family and or friends (788)		
Yes	227	28.8
No	561	71.2
Have constant sexual partner ($n = 490$)		
Yes	202	41.2
No	288	58.8
Lifetime sexual violence ($n = 788$)		
Yes	387	49.1
No	401	50.9
Sexual harassment ($n = 788$)		
Yes	514	65.2
No	274	34.8

TABLE 3: Consequence of gender-based violence among female night students in a public institution of Bahir Dar city, Amhara Region, Ethiopia, 2019.

Variables ($n = 490$)	Frequency	Percentage
Unwanted pregnancy	72	14.7
Abortion	61	12.4
Sexually transmitted infection	132	27
School dropout	152	31
Depression	323	66
Anxiety	303	62
Self-blame	216	44
Rejection from family	44	9
Rejection from friends	29	6
Alcohol dependency	17	3.4
Sexual dependency	33	6.7
Injury around the genitalia	201	41

risk of gender-based violence by 69% as compared to those who did not get monthly pocket money, lack of psychological support, and physical control (AOR: 0.31, 95% CI: (0.22-0.43)) (Table 5).

4. Discussion

The overall lifetime prevalence of gender-based violence was found to be 71.1%. The lifetime prevalence of sexual violence, physical violence, and emotional violence was found to be 49.1%, 57.5%, and 41.6%, respectively. This finding is consistent with studies conducted in Wolaita Sodo town, Debre Markos town, and Aleta Wondo town, which shows that the lifetime prevalence of gender-based violence was 63.2%, 67.7%, and 68.2%, respectively [14–16]. This finding is also supported by studies conducted in different parts of Ethiopia; violence against women was 64.7%; in southwest Ethiopia, the lifetime prevalence of any form of intimates partner violence was 72% in rural Ethiopia, and the prevalence of domestic violence in Fagitalekoma woreda, Awi zone, Amhara regional state was 78% [17–19]. This is might be due to similar sociodemographic characteristics.

This finding is more prevalent than studies conducted in Northern Nigeria, Zimbabwe and Uganda, which revealed that the overall prevalence of gender-based violence was 58.8%, 43.4%, and 47%, respectively [20–22]. Furthermore, this finding is much higher than other different findings; the prevalence of gender-based violence in US women was 25%, 13.9% in South Africa, and 35.6% was among women in Somalia [23–25]. This is might due to differences in culture, sociodemographic, and difference in living status.

The lifetime prevalence of sexual violence among female night students in this study was 49.1%. This finding is similar to studies conducted in Wolaita Sodo University students 45.4% [26]. This could be because young people are unaware of their sexual rights, and the nighttime increases the likelihood of violations. This finding is much higher with different studies in Ethiopia; in Debre Markos town 24.2% [15], Dilla town 13.2% [27], Butajira town 32.8% [28], Aleta Wondo town 26.3% [14], and in Harar town 25% [29].

The factors associated with gender-based violence and sexual violence were investigated in this study. Gender-based violence was associated with rural childhood residence, poor school performance, lack of discussion on sexual and reproductive health issues with family and or friends, poor family control, and sexual activity. Living with a biological partner, family support, and peer pressure were all factors associated with sexual violence.

Students who were rural childhood residence increased three times the odds of GBV as compared to urban childhood residence. This finding is supported by studies from Southeast Nigeria, Nigeria, and Awassa University in Ethiopia [30–32]. This could be due to limited access to information and knowledge about reproductive health issues; the burden of violence against women, girls, and children; and access to health care in rural areas. Students who had poor school performance increased three times the odds of GBV as compared to students who had good school performance. Similar findings were reported in Debre Markos and Mekelle town in

Table 4: Factors associated with gender-based violence among female night students in Bahir Dar city, Amhara region, Ethiopia, 2019.

Variables		Gender-based violence Yes	No	COR (95% CI)	AOR (95% CI)	p value
Childhood residence	Urban	283	180	1	1	
	Rural	277	48	3.67 (2.56-5.26)	3.37 (2.17-5.54)	0.001
School performance	Good	93	92	1	1	
	Poor	467	136	3.40 (2.40-4.80)	3.44 (2.13-5.56)	0.001
Discussion SRH issue with family and/or peers	Yes	90	137	1	1	
	No	470	91	7.86 (5.55-11.14)	3.68 (2.07-6.54)	0.001
Family control	Yes	181	184	1	1	
	No	379	44	8.76 (6.03-12.72)	5.62 (3.25-9.71)	0.001
Being sexually active	Yes	388	132	1.64 (1.19-2.26)	3.79 (2.35-6.12)	0.001
	No	172	96	1	1	

Table 5: Factors associated with sexual violence among night female students in Bahir Dar City, Amhara Region, Ethiopia, 2019.

Variables		Sexual violence Yes	No	COR (95% CI)	AOR (95% CI)	p value
Living with biological partner	Yes	64	168	0.27 (0.19-0.38)	0.28 (0.19-0.41)	0.001
	No	323	233	1	1	
Peer pressure	Yes	229	85	5.40 (3.94-7.37)	5.73 (4.11-7.98)	0.001
	No	158	316	1	1	
Family support	Yes	123	239	0.32 (0.24-0.42)	0.31 (0.22-0.43)	0.001
	No	264	162		1	

Ethiopia, and in the University of Ibadan, Nigeria [15, 33, 34]. Students who were being sexually active increased almost four times the odds of GBV as compared to their counterparts. This finding corresponds with a study from Wolaita Sodo, Aleta Wondo town, and Dilla town, Gedeo zone [14, 16, 27].

Lack of experience of discussion about sexual and reproductive health issues with their family and or friends has increased almost four times the odds of GBV as compared to their counterparts. This finding was a consistent study at Wolaita Sodo University that showed that discussions of sexual issues with her partner reduced 74% of the risks of sexual violence [16]. The fact that discussion of sexual and reproductive health issues between parents and adolescents is one of the strategies that enable adolescents to delay sexual debut or avoid sexual and physical violence. Adolescents should learn the human reproductive system and problems related to the sexual and reproductive issue and appropriate family responsibility.

Living with a biological partner is reducing the risks of sexual violence by 72%. This finding is similar to studies in Harar town, Eastern Ethiopia, Northeastern Nigeria, Uganda, and [29, 35, 36]. Family support significantly reduced sexual violence. This finding is consistent with a study in Butajira town, Ethiopia [28], and studies in Sweden and Australia [37, 38]. This is might be due to the fact that family support in case of income, physical control/supervision, and encouraging concerning on educations leads to avoid exposure for sexual and physical violence. Peer pressure is significantly associated with sexual violence. This finding is consistent with the studies in Harar town, eastern Ethiopia, and World Health Organization (WHO) reports [29, 39]. The supporting study states that adolescence is the time when a person is most susceptible to peer pressure because peers become an important influence on behavior during adolescence, and peers are engaging in similar behavior [40, 41].

5. Conclusion

In the study area, the lifetime prevalence of gender-based violence was high. Gender-based violence has been identified as a prevalent issue among female night students. The lifetime prevalence of sexual violence, physical violence, and emotional violence was 49.1%, 57.5%, and 41.6%, respectively. Factors associated with gender-based violence included rural childhood residence, low school performance, lack of experience in sexual and reproductive health conversations, poor family control, and being sexually active. The risk factors for sexual violence were young people living with their parents, peer pressure, and family support. This finding suggests that the primary prevention of gender-based violence is urgently needed in elementary and high schools. The Ethiopian government and other stakeholders should focus on reducing the risk of gender-based violence at the school level and provide regular health promotion on sexual and reproductive issues through school clubs.

Abbreviations

GBV: Gender-based violence
EDHS: Ethiopia Demographic and Health Survey
WHO: World Health Organization
AOR: Adjusted odds ratio
COR: Crude odds ratio
SV: Sexual violence.

Authors' Contributions

HG, TM, HA, and AB raised the research idea, wrote the proposal, and participated in designing the study, supervising the data collection process, and performed the statistical analyses and writing and the critical reviewing of the manuscript. YA and GN supervised the data collection process, data analysis, and review of the drafting manuscript. All authors read and approved the final manuscript.

Acknowledgments

We would like to thank Debre Tabor University for the approval of the ethical clearance and technical support of this study. This project was financed by the Center for International Reproductive Health Training at the University of Michigan (CIRHT-UM), in partnership with the Ethiopian Federal Ministry of Health (EFMH). All authors declare independence from funding sources. Our grateful appreciation goes to all the study participants, supervisors, and data collectors.

References

[1] World Health Organization, *Violence against women: intimate partner and sexual violence against women: intimate partner and sexual violence have serious short-and long-term physical, mental and sexual, and reproductive health problems for survivors: Fact sheet*, World Health Organization, 2014.

[2] C. Shahpar and T. D. Kirsch, "WhoTs who in humanitarian emergencies," *Health in Humanitarian Emergencies: Principles and Practice for Public Health and Healthcare Practitioners*, vol. 31, p. 25, 2018.

[3] World Health Organization, *Global status report on violence prevention 2014*, World Health Organization, 2014.

[4] Centers for Disease Control and Prevention, *Preventing multiple forms of violence: a strategic vision for connecting the dots*, Division of Violence Prevention, National Center for Injury Prevention and Control, Centers for Disease Control and Prevention, Atlanta, GA, 2016.

[5] T. Palermo, J. Bleck, and A. Peterman, "Tip of the iceberg: reporting and gender-based violence in developing countries," *American journal of epidemiology.*, vol. 179, no. 5, pp. 602–612, 2014.

[6] WHO, *Preventing Intimate Partner and Sexual Violence Against Women*, Taking Action and Generating Evidence, WHO, Geneva, Switzerland, 2010.

[7] United Nations, *Handbook on Effective Police Responses to Violence against Women*, Criminal Justice Handbook series, New York, 2010.

[8] C. Garcia-Moreno and C. Watts, "Violence against women: an urgent public health priority," *Bulletin of the World Health Organization*, vol. 89, no. 1, pp. 2-3, 2011.

[9] D. Durevall and A. Lindskog, "Intimate partner violence and HIV in ten sub-Saharan African countries: what do the Demographic and Health Surveys tell us?," *Lancet Glob Health*, vol. 3, no. 1, pp. e34–e43, 2015.

[10] A. Gevers, N. Jama-Shai, and Y. Sikweyiya, "Gender-based violence and the need for evidence-based primary prevention in South Africa," vol. 11, Tech. Rep. 2, African Safety Promotion: A Journal of Injury and Violence Prevention, 2013.

[11] A. Semahegn and B. Mengistie, "Domestic violence against women and associated factors in Ethiopia; systematic review," *Reproductive Health*, vol. 12, no. 1, p. 78, 2015.

[12] Z. Desalegne, "Gender Based violence and its associated effects on female students: the case Gozamin and Nigus T/Haimanot secondary schools at East Gojjam Administrative Zone," *Arts and Social Sciences Journal*, vol. 9, p. 2, 2018.

[13] A. S. Beyene, C. Chojenta, H. S. Roba, A. S. Melka, and D. Loxton, "Gender-based violence among female youths in educational institutions of sub-Saharan Africa: a systematic review and meta-analysis," *Systematic reviews.*, vol. 8, no. 1, p. 59, 2019.

[14] A. Dogiso, M. Shegaze, A. Alagaw, and B. Wassihun, "Prevalence and associated factors of gender-based violence among high school female students in Aleta Wondo town, Southeast Ethiopia," *Ethiopian Journal of Reproductive Health*, vol. 11, no. 2, p. 10, 2019.

[15] G. Mullu, G. A, D. Amare et al., "Prevalence of gender-based violence and associated factors among female students of Menkorer high school in Debre Markos town, Northwest Ethiopia," *Science*, vol. 3, no. 1, pp. 67–74, 2015.

[16] T. Tantu, S. Wolka, M. Gunta, M. Teshome, H. Mohammed, and B. Duko, "Prevalence and determinants of gender-based violence among high school female students in Wolaita Sodo, Ethiopia: an institutionally based cross-sectional study," *BMC Public Health*, vol. 20, pp. 1–9, 2020.

[17] N. Deyessa, Y. Berhane, A. Alem et al., "Intimate partner violence and depression among women in rural Ethiopia: a cross-sectional study," *Clinical Practice Epidemiology Mental Health*, vol. 5, no. 8, pp. 1–10, 2009.

[18] K. Deribe, K. B. Beyene, A. Tolla, P. Memiah, S. Biadgilign, and A. Amberbir, "Magnitude and correlates of intimate partner violence against women and its outcome in Southwest Ethiopia," *PLoS One*, vol. 7, no. 4, article e36189, 2012.

[19] A. Semahegn, T. Belachew, and M. Abdulahi, "Domestic violence and its predictors among married women in reproductive age in Fagitalekoma Woreda, Awi zone, Amhara regional state, North Western Ethiopia," *Reprod Health*, vol. 10, no. 63, pp. 1–9, 2013.

[20] Z. Iliyasu, I. S. Abubakar, M. H. Aliyu, H. S. Galadanci, and H. M. Salihu, "Prevalence and correlates of gender-based violence among female university students in Northern Nigeria," *African Journal of Reproductive Health*, vol. 15, no. 3, pp. 123–133, 2011.

[21] S. O. Bamiwuye and C. Odimegwu, "Spousal violence in sub-Saharan Africa: does household poverty-wealth matter?," *Reproductive Health*, vol. 11, no. 1, pp. 1 10, 2014.

[22] S. O. Wandera, K. Clarke, L. Knight et al., "Violence against children perpetrated by peers: a cross-sectional school-based survey in Uganda," *Child Abuse & Neglect*, vol. 68, pp. 65–73, 2017.

[23] K. Walsh, K. M. Keyes, K. C. Koenen, and D. Hasin, "Lifetime prevalence of gender-based violence in US women: associations with mood/anxiety and substance use disorders," *Journal of Psychiatric Research*, vol. 62, pp. 7–13, 2015.

[24] M. Schneider, E. Baron, T. Davies, M. Munodawafa, and C. Lund, "Patterns of intimate partner violence among perinatal women with depression symptoms in Khayelitsha, South Africa: a longitudinal analysis," *Global Mental Health.*, vol. 5, 2018.

[25] A. L. Wirtz, N. A. Perrin, A. Desgroppes et al., "Lifetime prevalence, correlates and health consequences of gender-based violence victimisation and perpetration among men and women in Somalia," *BMJ Global Health*, vol. 3, no. 4, article e000773, 2018.

[26] Y. M. Adinew and M. A. Hagos, "Sexual violence against female university students in Ethiopia," *BMC international health and human rights*, vol. 17, no. 1, pp. 1–7, 2017.

[27] D. Tarekegn, B. Berhanu, and Y. Ali, "Prevalence and associated factors of sexual violence among high school female students in Dilla town, Gedeo zone SNNPR, Ethiopia," *Epidemiology (Sunnyvale)*, vol. 7, no. 4, p. 320, 2017.

[28] W. Nimani and B. Hamdela, "Sexual violence and associated factors among high school students in Butajira town, South Ethiopia," *General Medicine*, vol. 3, article 1000196, 2015.

[29] J. M. Markos Cafo, A. S. Demisie, and B. B. Abera, "Assessment of sexual violence and associated factors among high school students in Harari Regional State, Harar town, Eastern Ethiopia," *Science Research*, vol. 2, no. 5, pp. 91–97, 2014.

[30] L. O. Ajah, C. A. Iyoke, P. O. Nkwo, B. Nwakoby, and P. Ezeonu, "Comparison of domestic violence against women in urban versus rural areas of Southeast Nigeria," *International Journal of Women's Health*, vol. 6, p. 865, 2014.

[31] F. O. Benebo, B. Schumann, and M. Vaezghasemi, "Intimate partner violence against women in Nigeria: a multilevel study investigating the effect of women's status and community norms," *BMC Women's Health*, vol. 18, no. 1, p. 136, 2018.

[32] E. G. Sendo and M. Meleku, "Prevalence and factors associated with sexual violence among female students of Hawassa University in Ethiopia," *Science Postprint*, vol. 1, no. 2, article e00047, 2015.

[33] G. Yaynshet, *Prevalence and Factors Related to Gender-Based Violence among Female Students of Higher Learning Institutions in Mekelle Town*, AAU, Tigray, Northern Ethiopia, 2007.

[34] J. E. Umana, O. I. Fawole, and I. A. Adeoye, "Prevalence and correlates of intimate partner violence towards female students of the University of Ibadan, Nigeria," *BMC women's health.*, vol. 14, no. 1, p. 131, 2014.

[35] A. J. Ajuwon, A. Olaleye, B. Faromoju, and O. Ladipo, "Sexual behavior and experience of sexual coercion among secondary school students in three states in North Eastern Nigeria," *BMC Public Health*, vol. 6, no. 1, p. 310, 2006.

[36] M. L. Ybarra, S. S. Bull, J. Kiwanuka, D. R. Bangsberg, and J. Korchmaros, "Prevalence rates of sexual coercion victimization and perpetration among Uganda adolescents," *AIDS Care*, vol. 24, no. 11, pp. 1392–1400, 2012.

[37] S. Lovestad and G. Krantz, "Men's and women's exposure and perpetration of partner violence: an epidemiological study from Sweden," *BMC Public Health*, vol. 12, no. 1, p. 945, 2012.

[38] A. Hunt, K. Webber, J. Montgomery, and A. Duong, *Family, Domestic and Sexual Violence in Australia 2018*, Australian Institute of Health and Welfare, 2018.

[39] World Health Organization, *Preventing intimate partner and sexual violence against women: taking action and generating evidence*, World Health Organization, 2010.

[40] L. Widman, S. Choukas-Bradley, S. W. Helms, and M. J. Prinstein, "Adolescent susceptibility to peer influence in sexual situations," *Journal of Adolescent Health*, vol. 58, no. 3, pp. 323–329, 2016.

[41] V. L. Banyard, A. J. Rizzo, Y. Bencosme, A. C. Cares, and M. M. Moynihan, "How community and peer perceptions promote college students' pro-social bystander actions to prevent sexual violence," *Journal of Interpersonal Violence*, vol. 36, no. 7-8, pp. 3855–3879, 2021.

26

Birth Intervals and Associated Factors among Women Attending Young Child Clinic in Yumbe Hospital, Uganda

M. Aleni,[1] **S. N. Mbalinda**,[2] **and R. Muhindo**[1,2]

[1]*Department of Nursing and Midwifery, Muni University, +256 P.O. BOX, 725 Arua, Uganda*
[2]*Department of Nursing, Makerere University, +256 P.O. BOX, 7062 Kampala, Uganda*

Correspondence should be addressed to M. Aleni; m.aleni@muni.ac.ug

Academic Editor: Robert Gaspar

Introduction. Evidence suggests that both short and long birth intervals are associated with poor maternal and child health outcomes. However, current studies suggest that a number of births still occur at short intervals. The aim of this study was to document birth intervals and associated factors among women of reproductive age in rural Uganda. *Materials and Methods.* This was a cross-sectional study conducted among 296 women aged 15-49 years attending young child clinic at Yumbe Hospital who had at least two successive live births. Data was collected using interviewer-administered questionnaire. Birth interval was categorized according to the WHO-recommended birth interval of ≥24 months and <24 months. *Results.* Of the 296 participants, 86.6% desired a birth interval ≥ 24 months with a desired median birth interval of 36 months. The actual median birth interval was 22 months. Slightly more than half of the women (52.4%) had short birth intervals. Factors which were likely to be associated with short birth intervals included being younger (15-24 years) (AOR = 4.39, 95%CI = 1.49-12.93, $P = 0.007$), not planning to have another pregnancy (AOR = 0.33, 95%CI = 0.18-0.58, $P = 0.001$), not deciding together with husband when to have the next child (AOR = 3.10, 95%CI = 1.53-6.28, $P = 0.002$), not always using contraceptives before the next pregnancy (AOR = 0.28, 95%CI = 0.12-0.64, $P = 0.003$), and lack of influence of husband on when to have the next child (AOR = 2.59, 95% CI = 1.44 – 4.64, $P = 0.001$). *Conclusion.* Prevalence of short birth intervals is still high in rural Uganda (52.4%), although majority (86.6%) of the women desire optimal birth intervals. Factors which were likely to be associated with short birth intervals included young maternal age, not using contraceptives, and lack of male involvement in child spacing activities. Therefore, to optimize birth intervals, focused child spacing strategies targeting young women and men are needed.

1. Introduction

World Health Organization (WHO) defines birth interval as the time period from live birth to a successive pregnancy and the recommended period is at least 24 months (2 years) [1]. Short birth intervals defined as those less than 2 years have implications on maternal and child health [2], and long birth intervals defined as those above 5 years have undesired effects on maternal and child health as well [3, 4]. Adequate birth intervals on the other hand help women recover from macro- and micronutrient depletion which occurs during pregnancy and lactation [5]. This therefore helps to improve subsequent pregnancies and child health. It has been estimated that if all birth to pregnancy intervals were spaced at least 3 years, 1.6 million deaths of under-five would be averted annually [6].

Globally, it was estimated that 25% of births still occur at intervals less than 24 months. Most of the cases of short birth intervals were observed in Central Asia at 33%. Sub-Saharan Africa had short birth intervals at 20% [7]. Study of fertility transition in sub-Saharan Africa shows that the median birth interval at birth order two was 35 months which was longer than in Asia and Latin America of 25 months [8].

Though the sub-Saharan African picture shows optimal median birth intervals, individual countries were observed to be having differences in birth intervals. Demographic and Health Survey (DHS) reports show most of the countries having a significant number of births occurring at short intervals. Most countries in Africa including Uganda do not report about long birth intervals probably because it is not happening frequently. In Nigeria, short birth intervals were

23% [9], and in Zimbabwe, it was estimated at 11% [10]. In East Africa, Kenya and Tanzania had almost similar birth intervals less than 24 months of 18% [11] and 19% [12], respectively. Uganda Demographic and Health Survey (UDHS) 2016 did not report short birth, but [7] analysis of trends in birth intervals from DHS of several countries estimated that Uganda had short birth intervals occurring at a rate of 25.9%.

Studies have shown that short birth intervals contribute to poor maternal and child health [3, 13]. In Uganda, up to 4% of infant mortalities can be attributed to short birth intervals [14]. Some of the poor child health outcomes related to short birth intervals include preterm birth, low birth weight, congenital malformations, and early neonatal deaths [15]. Under-five mortality has also been found to increase with birth intervals below 2 years [16]. Among women, short birth interval is associated with maternal nutritional depletion, placenta previa and abruption, incomplete healing of caesarean section scars, poor lactation, and cross infection among siblings [5]. However, systematic review has shown that birth intervals longer than 5 years are associated with labour dystocia and increases the risk of preeclampsia [4]. Optimal birth intervals could therefore help prevent some of these poor maternal and child health outcomes.

Authors have documented a number of factors associated with birth intervals. Some of these may be direct factors such as being sexually active, use of contraceptives, postpartum infecundability, abortion, and sterility while indirect factors may include sociocultural factors [17]. In their study, Fayehun et al. [18] found that the type of contraceptives used, living in rural or urban settings, wealth index, husbands' occupation, and sex of preceding children determined birth intervals. It was further noted that having more female children and having a female last child significantly reduced birth intervals in quest for a male child. Use of contraceptives for birth spacing was also seen to be affected by son preference where the last child born being a female, a woman would like to use a shorter acting contraceptive in order not to wait too long to get a male child [19].

Uganda like many sub-Saharan African countries still has high fertility, maternal mortality, and neonatal, infant, and under-five mortality rates. Recent estimates show the countries total fertility rate at 5.4, maternal mortality rate at 336/100,000 live births, neonatal mortality rate at 27/1,000 live births, infant mortality rate at 43/1,000 live births, and under-five mortality rate at 64/1,000 live births [20]. However, little is known about the currents trends of birth intervals and its determinants. UDHS 2016 assessed preferred birth intervals for women of reproductive age associating it with only one factor (the number of living children a woman has). The actual birth intervals were not measured. Not many studies in Uganda have comprehensively studied contextual factors associated with birth intervals. Little is known about community awareness regarding dangers associated with short or long birth intervals.

Therefore, understanding birth intervals and its determinants is critical for a country like Uganda so as to improve and design child spacing programs which in turn will improve maternal and child health. This study therefore is aimed at filling this gap by assessing birth intervals and its determinants among women of reproductive age in rural Uganda.

2. Materials and Methods

2.1. Aim of the Study. The study was aimed at identifying birth intervals and its determinants among women of reproductive age in Yumbe district in rural Uganda.

2.2. Study Design. The study employed a cross-sectional design and quantitative methods for data collection.

2.3. Study Setting. The study was conducted in Yumbe Hospital at the maternal child health (MCH) unit, outpatient department. Yumbe Hospital is located in Yumbe district which is found in the West Nile subregion of Uganda, about 600 km from the capital Kampala. The hospital is located in a rural area in the southwestern part of the district about 10 kilometres away from Yumbe town. It is a grade V hospital, and services offered at the hospital include MCH, general medicine, surgery, and community health services. The hospital also serves as the district referral hospital. Mothers who come for MCH services are predominantly the indigenous people of the district, but a few clients are from the neighboring Koboko and Arua districts as well. Maternal child health services offered at the hospital at the outpatient department include antenatal care (ANC), postnatal care (PNC), young child clinic (YCC), and family planning services.

2.4. Study Population. The study participants were women aged 15-49 years who were attending YCC at Yumbe Hospital. A total of 296 women were selected using systematic sampling method. Women who had had two successive live births were included in the study. The study excluded women who had had two successive live births whose children were very sick and needed urgent treatment.

2.5. Sampling Procedure. Systematic sampling method was used. Systematic sampling is a probability sampling technique in which the study population is arranged according to some ordering scheme and then selecting elements at regular intervals. Only the first element is selected randomly, the rest being selected according to predetermined pattern. The predetermined pattern is Kth unit which is the sampling interval $(K) = N/n$, where $N =$ population size and $n =$ sample size (Denise F pilot, 2004).

At the clinic, women and their children who were attending YCC were registered in the child health register. On data collection days, systematic sampling was achieved by sampling the Kth woman in the register after the first one had been selected at random by blind folding one of the research assistants who was asked to put her index finger on any of the names which were recorded in the register on the first day of data collection. The count started with the name of the woman at the point where her index finger touched and the third person on the list being counted downwards from the random point was considered as the first participant, and the Kth interval of 3 continued throughout the data collection period. If the Kth woman did not meet the inclusion criteria, then the next woman on the list was selected and the interval continued. Once the list was completed for a data collection day, additional participants for the following day were sampled by looping the count to the beginning of the register for that day since women were being registered for the services on every working day at the clinic. This process was continued until all the required sample size was achieved. The selected participants were informed that the interview would be done as they exited the clinic so as not to interrupt their process of receiving health care.

2.6. Determining Sampling Interval (K). N is the population sample size. n is the sample size. Time available for data collection was one month (20 working days). The average number of women received at YCC in a month was 1,020. Sampling interval $(K) = 1{,}020/296 = 3.5$. Therefore, the sampling interval was 3.

2.7. Study Variables. The outcome variable for this study was birth interval. Birth interval was measured in months using interval scale. Actual birth interval, desired birth interval, and proportion of nonfirst births that occurred before 24 months and after 24 months were measured. For actual and desired birth intervals, the last birth interval was measured.

2.7.1. Actual Birth Interval. We defined actual birth interval as the time between a live birth and successive pregnancy. Only the last birth interval was measured. This was measured by assessing the length of time between the preceding birth and the current birth and then subtracting the length of pregnancy which resulted in the current birth, since women may not know their exact date of conception. Respondents were asked how old was your second last born child when your last baby (current baby) was born? They were then asked what was the duration of your pregnancy which resulted in the birth of the last (current) baby? Therefore, the difference between the age of the second last born child at the birth of the last born (current) child and the durations of pregnancy of the last born (current) child was considered as the actual birth interval. This was measured in months, e.g., if a is the age in months of the second last born child when the last (current) baby was born and if b is the duration of pregnancy which resulted in the birth of the last (current) baby, then actual birth interval (c) would be $a - b = c$. Multiple births were treated as a single interval. Therefore, birth interval was categorized according to the WHO-recommended birth interval (24 months) and coded 1 if birth interval was ≥ 24 months and 2 if birth interval was <24 months.

2.7.2. Desired Birth Interval. This is the birth interval a woman would wish to have if all factors were favorable. This was measured in months by asking the following: at the time you became pregnant with the current baby, did you want to become pregnant then? If the woman said yes, then that was considered as her desired birth interval. If she said no, she was then asked the following: how long would you have preferred to wait from the time you gave birth to your second last born child to conception of your current baby? The length of time she mentioned was recorded as her desired birth interval.

2.7.3. Proportion of Nonfirst Births That Occurred before 24 Months. This is the number of children a woman has excluding the first birth which occurred at an interval less than 24 months. This was measured by asking the following: how many of your children were born before 2 years of the preceding birth?

2.7.4. Proportion of Nonfirst Births That Occurred after 24 Months. This is the number of children a woman has excluding the first birth which occurred at an interval more than 24 months. This was measured by asking the following: how many of your children were born after 2 years of the preceding birth?

2.8. Predictor Variables. In this study, independent variables are predisposing factors to birth intervals among women of reproductive age. This was measured by having precoded questions concerning factors that determine birth intervals ranked on an ordinal scale, and in some of the questions, the respondents were asked to choose response(s) of their choice.

2.8.1. Demographic Characteristics. Demographic characteristics which were measured include age at first birth, current age of woman, education level, occupation, religion, marital status, residence, number of living children a woman has, and sex of the second last born child.

2.8.2. Sociocultural Factors. Sociocultural factors were measured using an ordinal scale where the respondents were asked to indicate on a scale of 1 to 4 if she strongly agrees, agrees, disagrees, or strongly disagrees that the decision of her husband, mother-in-law, and significant others on when to have the next pregnancy matters a lot.

2.8.3. Behavioral Factors. Behavioral factors that were measured include plan of when to have the next child, family planning use, and couple communication about birth intervals. Plan of when to have the next child and couple communication about birth interval were measured on an ordinal scale of 1 to 3 if she never, sometimes, and always discusses with her husband and decides when to have the next child or if she makes the decision alone. Family planning use was measured by asking the respondent if she never, sometimes, or always used contraceptives between pregnancies.

2.8.4. Knowledge about Birth Intervals. Knowledge about birth intervals was measured by asking the respondents to mention the recommended birth interval. Respondents were also asked to choose precoded responses. Questions included awareness about the recommended birth intervals, dangers of short birth intervals, and the benefits of optimal birth intervals.

2.8.5. Health Facility Factors. These are health facility-related factors that influence access and utilization of services that promote healthy birth intervals. Health system factors that were measured included the following: if health workers were giving information to the women about recommended birth intervals, contraceptive information, and provision of contraceptive services.

2.9. Data Collection Tools and Procedures. We used a questionnaire as a data collection tool. The questionnaire was formulated by the authors according to the objectives of the study using literature as a source. The questionnaire contained a total number of 37 structured questions and was formulated in English and translated in the local dialect (Aringa). The questionnaire included demographic characteristics which had 12 questions, questions related to birth intervals were 6 and factors which affect birth intervals were 19 in total (knowledge about birth intervals = 8, behavioral factors = 5, social factors = 3, and health facility factors = 3). Knowledge about birth intervals was measured by asking the respondents if they were aware about the recommended birth intervals and to mention the recommended birth interval, dangers of short birth intervals, and the benefits of optimal birth intervals. On average, the interview took approximately 20 minutes per participant. To ensure reliability of the questionnaire, questions were formulated according to the research objectives. The principal investigator pretested the questionnaire on 10 women attending YCC at Midigo HCIV in Yumbe district. Adjustments were made based on the results of the pretest by rephrasing questions which were not clear to the respondents and by removing questions which did not seem to be relevant. Reliability of the questionnaire was further ensured by selecting only respondents who met the inclusion. Furthermore, the research assistants were trained for half a day before data collection to ensure reliability of the data tool. All the filled questionnaires were checked every evening after a day's data collection by the principal investigator and the research assistants to ensure completeness and correctness of data collected. The respondents were identified from the child health register among mothers who were registered on data collection days. The principal investigator or the research assistant informed the participants of the purpose and objectives of the study, and consent was sought. The principal investigator or the research assistant read the questions on the questionnaire as the respondent listened. The respondents were required to select a precoded response. Responses were ticked or filled in accordingly by the principal investigator or research assistant.

2.10. Statistical Analysis. Data analysis was completed using SPSS version 23. At univariate analysis, descriptive statistics were summarized using mean (standard deviation), median (interquartile range), and range for continuous variables and frequencies and proportion for categorical variables (Tables 1–3). At bivariate analysis, chi-square test was used to assess the association between birth interval and factor variables. All the statistic tests and their respective confidence intervals (CI) were based on a two-tailed test (Table 4). At multivariate analysis, a logistic regression model to determine the effect of factor variables on birth interval was applied for simultaneous adjustment for potential confounders. Crude and adjusted odds ratio (OR) at 95% confidence interval and predictor variables with P value ≤ 0.1 at bivariate analysis and any other plausible variables were used to measure the association between dependent and predictive variables (Table 5). Variables with P value < 0.05 were considered statistically significant for the final statistical test. Data were presented using tables.

3. Results

The study was conducted in January 2018 among 296 women aged 15-49 years who had had at least two successive live births, attending young child clinic in rural Uganda.

3.1. Sociodemographic Characteristics of Respondents. The women in the study were aged between 18 and 43 years, with a mean age of 26.82 (SD: ±5.14). Their mean age at first birth was 17.34 (SD ± 2.39). Slightly more than half of the women (156, 52.7%) were aged 25-34 years and 112 (37.8%) were aged 15-24 years. Most of the women (279, 94.3%) lived in rural areas, and only 53 (17.9%) have attended secondary education or plus. Two hundred and thirty-five (79.4%) of the women were housewives. Majority (274, 92.6%) of the women were Muslims. Two hundred and eighty-three (96%) were married, and among them, 162 (57.2%) were in monogamous marriage. Majority of the women (235, 79.4%) had had between 2 and 4 live births. One hundred and twenty-seven (42.9%) of the women wanted their pregnancy at the time of conception. Nearly half of the participants (138, 46.6%) had never used any contraceptive method before their next pregnancy. One hundred and sixteen (39.2%) of the women always decide together with their husband on when to have the next child. One hundred and forty-one (48%) of the women acknowledged that the influence of their husbands matters a lot on when to have the next child, as shown in Table 1.

3.2. Awareness about Recommended Birth Intervals. As shown in Table 2, there was universal awareness about the recommended birth intervals. All the participants had heard about the recommended birth intervals, and all of them correctly mentioned the recommended birth intervals from 24 months and above. All the participants were able to mention at least one advantage of proper birth spacing and one disadvantage of short birth intervals. The major source of information about birth intervals was from health facilities.

3.3. Birth Intervals for Women of Reproductive Age. As shown in Table 3, using the WHO-recommended birth interval of ≥24 months, 52.4% of the women had birth intervals below 24 months. The median birth interval was 22 months (IQR = 15-33) while the desired median birth interval was 36 months (IQR 36-36). Eighty-seven percent of the women desired birth intervals ≥ 24 months. Excluding the first birth for the 296 women studied, the participants had had 693 live births in total, and among them, 156 (22.5%) were born before two years of the preceding birth and 537 (77.5%) were born after two years of the preceding birth.

3.4. Bivariate Analysis. At bivariate analysis, chi-square test was used to explore the association between birth intervals and independent related variables.

As shown in Table 4, the unadjusted odds of short birth intervals were significantly higher among women aged 15-24 (COR = 5.67, 95% CI: 2.13-15.09, $P = 0.001$) and women

TABLE 1: Distribution of background characteristics of women aged 15-49 years attending YCC at Yumbe Hospital, Uganda.

Variable	Frequency ($N = 296$)	Percentage	Mean
Age			
15-24	112	37.8	
25-34	156	52.7	26.82 (SD ± 5.14)
35-44	28	9.5	
Age at first birth			17.34 (SD ± 2.39)
Residence			
Rural	279	94.3	
Urban	17	5.7	
Marital status			
Married	283	95.6	
Single & divorced	13	4.4	
Marriage status (283)*			
Polygamous	121	42.8	
Monogamous	162	57.2	
Education level			
No education	57	19.3	
Primary	186	62.8	
Secondary+	53	17.9	
Religion			
Muslim	274	92.6	
Non-Muslim	22	7.4	
Occupation			
Housewife	235	79.4	
Formal employment	20	6.8	
Informal employment	41	13.9	
Number of live births			
5+	61	20.6	
2-4	235	79.4	
Sex of the 2nd last born			
Female	147	49.7	
Male	149	50.3	
Pregnancy wanted			
No	169	57.1	
Yes	127	42.9	
Contraceptive use before the next pregnancy			
Never	138	46.6	
Sometimes	107	36.1	
Always	51	17.2	
Decide together with husband when to have next child			
Never	93	31.4	
Sometimes	87	29.4	
Always	116	39.2	
Influence of husband when to have the next baby			
No	155	52.4	
Yes	141	47.6	

*13 of the respondents were not married.

Table 2: Awareness about recommended birth intervals among women attending YCC in rural Uganda ($n = 296$).

Variable	Frequency	Percentage	Mean
Heard about recommended birth interval			
Yes	296	100	
No			
Knowledge on recommended birth intervals			
≥24 months	296	100	37.77 (SD ± 10.24)
<24 months			
Source of information			
Health facility	266	98.90	
Peers	195	65.90	
Family	136	45.90	
Radio	103	34.80	
Benefits of optimal birth intervals (≥24 months)			
Good nutrition for family	251	84.80	
Adequate time for care of children	282	95.30	
Adequate lactation	77	26.00	
Adequate time for income generation activities	213	72.00	
Good health of the mother	10	03.20	
Dangers of short birth intervals (<24 months)			
Premature birth	91	30.70	
Low birth weight	165	55.70	
Poor lactation	137	46.30	
Death of the baby	202	68.20	
Death of the mother	136	45.90	
Poor health of the child	66	22.30	

*Multiple responses.

Table 3: Birth intervals among women attending YCC at Yumbe Hospital, Uganda.

Variable	Frequency ($N = 296$)	Percentage	Median	Mean
Actual birth interval				
<24 months	155	52.4	22 (IQR: 18)	25.94 (SD ± 14.8)
≥24 months	141	47.6		
Desired birth intervals				
<24 months	40	13.3	36 (IQR: 0)	37.77 (SD ± 10.24)
≥24 months	256	86.6		
Children born before two years ($n = 693$)				
Yes	156	22.5		
No	537	77.5		

aged 25-34 (COR = 3.96, 95% CI: 1.52-10.30, $P = 0.005$) compared to women aged 35-44. Other factors which were significantly associated with short birth intervals included not planning to have the next pregnancy, not deciding together with husband about when to have the next pregnancy, and not always using contraceptives before the next pregnancy. Women who planned to have their next pregnancy were 78% less likely to have short birth intervals (COR = 0.22, 95% CI: 0.13-0.35, $P < 0.001$) compared to those who did not plan to have the next pregnancy. Women who always decide together with their husbands when to have the next child were less likely to have short birth interval (COR = 2.85, 95% CI: 0.16-0.51, $P < 0.001$). The prevalence of short birth interval was 81% lower among women who always use contraceptive before the next pregnancy compared to those who never use contraceptives (COR = 0.19, 95% CI: 0.09-0.39, $P < 0.001$).

3.5. Multivariate Analysis. After bivariate logistic regression, variables with P value ≤ 0.1 and other plausible variables were further analyzed using multivariate logistic regression to control for confounding. The OR was adjusted for the following

Table 4: Bivariate analysis of factors and short birth intervals among women attending YCC in rural Uganda.

Factors	Number (and %) of women with the birth interval <24 months N = 155 (52.4)	≥24 months N = 141 (47.6)	COR (95% CI)	P value
Age				
35-44	6 (21.4)	22 (78.6)	1.0	
25-34	81 (51.9)	75 (48.1)	3.96 (1.52-10.30)	0.005
15-24	68 (60.7)	44 (39.3)	5.67 (2.13-15.09)	0.001
Residence				
Rural	146 (52.3)	133 (47.7)	1.0	
Urban	9 (52.9)	8 (47.1)	1.02 (0.38-2.73)	0.961
Marital status				
Married	150 (53.0)	133 (47.0)	1.0	
Single & divorced	5 (38.5)	8 (61.5)	0.55 (0.18-1.74)	0.311
Education level				
No education	26 (45.6)	31 (54.4)	1.0	
Primary	104 (55.9)	82 (44.1)	1.51 (0.83-2.74)	0.174
Secondary+	25 (47.2)	28 (52.8)	1.06 (0.50-2.25)	0.870
Religion				
Muslim	145 (52.9)	129 (47.1)	1.0	
Non-Muslim	10 (45.5)	12 (54.5)	0.74 (0.31-1.77)	0.501
Occupation				
Housewife	130 (55.3)	105 (44.7)	1.0	
Formal employment	8 (40.0)	12 (60.0)	0.54 (0.21-1.37)	0.192
Informal employment	17 (41.5)	24 (58.5)	0.57 (0.29-1.12)	0.104
Number of live births				
5+	29 (47.5)	32 (52.5)	1.0	
2-4	126 (53.6)	109 (46.4)	1.28 (0.73-2.24)	0.398
Sex of the 2nd last born				
Female	68 (46.3)	79 (53.7)	1.0	
Male	87 (58.4)	62 (41.6)	1.63 (1.03-2.58)	0.037
Pregnancy wanted				
No	115 (68.0)	54 (32.0)	1.0	
Yes	40 (31.5)	87 (68.5)	0.22 (0.13-0.35)	<0.001
Contraceptive use before the next pregnancy				
Never	86 (62.3)	52 (37.7)	1.0	
Sometimes	57 (53.3)	50 (46.7)	0.69 (0.41-1.15)	
Always	12 (23.5)	39 (76.5)	0.19 (0.09-0.39)	<0.001
Decide together with husband when to have next child				
Never	54 (36.7)	28 (21.2)	1.0	
Sometimes	53 (36.1)	34 (24.8)	4.00 (0.45-1.50)	<0.001
Always	40 (27.2)	74 (54.0)	2.85 (0.16-0.51)	<0.001
Influence of husband when to have the next baby				
No	86 (58.1)	62 (41.9)	1.0	
Yes	60 (46.1)	74 (53.9)	1.70 (0.39-098)	0.033

Table 5: Predictors of short birth intervals among study respondents.

Variable	Number (and %) of women with the birth interval <24 months N = 155 (52.36)	≥24 months N = 141 (47.64)	Unadjusted OR (95% CI)	P value	AOR (95% CI)	P value
Age						
35-44	6 (21.4)	22 (78.6)	1.0		1.0	
25-34	81 (51.9)	75 (48.1)	3.96 (1.52-10.30)	0.005	3.39 (1.18-9.74)	0.024
15-24	68 (60.7)	44 (39.3)	5.67 (2.13-15.09)	0.001	4.39 (1.49-12.93)	0.007
Sex of second last born child						
Female	68 (46.3)	79 (53.7)	1		1	
Male	87 (58.4)	62 (41.6)	0.54 (0.32–0.93)	0.027	0.61 (0.35–1.05)	0.077
Pregnancy wanted						
No	115 (68.0)	54 (32.0)	1.0		1.0	
Yes	40 (31.5)	87 (68.5)	0.22 (0.13-0.35)	<0.001	0.33 (0.18-0.58)	<0.001
Decide together with husband when to have child						
Never	54 (36.7)	28 (21.2)	1.0		1.0	
Sometimes	53 (36.1)	34 (24.8)	4.43 (2.16–9.07)	<0.001	2.84 (1.32–6.11)	<0.008
Always	40 (27.2)	74 (54.0)	3.75 (1.88–7.47)	<0.001	3.10 (1.53–6.28)	0.002
Contraceptive use before next pregnancy						
Never	86 (62.3)	52 (37.7)	1.0		1.0	
Sometimes	57 (53.3)	50 (46.7)	0.69 (0.41-1.15)	0.155	0.59 (0.32-1.08)	0.085
Always	12 (23.5)	39 (76.5)	0.19 (0.09-0.39)	<0.001	0.28 (0.12-0.64)	0.003
Influence of husband on when to the next baby						
No	86 (58.1)	62 (41.9)	1.0		1.0	
Yes	60 (46.1)	74 (53.9)	2.68 (1.51–4.76)	0.001	2.59 (1.44–4.64)	0.001

variables: maternal age, sex of the second last born child, whether the last pregnancy was wanted, contraceptive use, deciding together with husband when to have the next baby, and influence of husband on when to have the next baby. Variables with $P \leq 0.05$ were considered significantly associated with birth intervals.

As shown in Table 5, factors associated with short birth intervals included young maternal age, not using contraceptives, not deciding together with husband when to have the next child, lack of husband influence on when to have the next baby, and not planning to have the next pregnancy. Women aged 15-24 years were 4 times more likely to have short birth intervals (AOR = 4.39, 95% CI: 1.49-12.93, $P =$ 0.007), and those aged 25-34 years were 3 times more likely to have short birth intervals (AOR = 3.39, 95% CI: 1.18-9.74, $P = 0.024$) compared to women aged 35-44 years. The adjusted odds of short birth intervals were lower for women who wanted the pregnancy at the time of conception (AOR = 0.33, 95% CI: 0.18-0.58, $P < 0.001$), women who always used contraceptive before the next pregnancy (AOR = 0.28, 95% CI: 0.12-0.64, $P = 0.003$), those who always decide together with their husband on the time to have the next child (AOR = 3.10, 95% CI: 1.53-6.28, $P =$ 0.002), and those who were influenced by their husband on when to have the next baby (AOR = 2.59, 95% CI: 1.44-4.64, $P = 0.001$).

4. Discussion

The aim of this study was to identify birth intervals and its determinants among women of reproductive age in rural Uganda. We measured the last birth interval for women who had had at least two live births. The study showed that slightly more than half of the study participants (52.4%) had short birth intervals. Many of the women in our study could not achieve their desired birth intervals probably because of low contraceptive prevalence where only 17.2% of the women always used contraceptives before the next pregnancy and 46.6% have never used a contraceptive method. Studies conducted in other parts of rural Uganda and Ethiopia reported similar results, where slightly more than half of the study population had short birth intervals [17, 21], unlike in Iran where only 3.8% of the women had short birth intervals [22]. Contrary to studies in Nigeria which posted higher prevalence of short birth intervals [23, 24], studies done in Uganda in general [7] and in Iran [25], Kenya [26], Bangladesh [27], and Tanzania [28] have posted lower prevalence of short birth intervals.

Median birth interval in our study was 22 months which is lower than the one recommended by WHO, yet majority of the women (86.6%) desired a birth interval of ≥24 months. These findings were consistent with studies done in Asian and Latin American countries where median birth intervals at birth order two was 25 months. Our median birth intervals were much lower than those in Ethiopia [29], in other sub-Saharan African countries [8], in South African countries [30], and in India [31]. Our study concurs with a study done in Saudi Arabia where a significantly lower proportion of the women (5.2%) desired short birth intervals [32].

Literature suggests a number of factors associated with birth intervals. In our study, the age of the woman, plan to have the next pregnancy, deciding together with husband when to have the next child, always using contraceptives before the next pregnancy, and influence of husband on when to have the next pregnancy were significantly associated with birth intervals.

Younger women were more likely to have short birth intervals compared to older women. This could probably be explained by the fact that fertility reduces with age above 35 years and older women could be having better ability to make independent decisions concerning their reproductive goals compared to the younger women. This may also be due to the fact that in this study, mean age at first birth was 17 years and older women might have been tending towards completing their family sizes. Our study findings are consistent with [22, 33], studies done in Democratic Republic of Congo and Bangladesh [27, 34], but contrast with studies done in Iraq where being younger was associated with longer birth intervals [25].

Women who planned their pregnancy were less likely to have short birth intervals compared to those who did not want the pregnancy at the time of conception. This could probably be due to the fact that women/couples who plan their pregnancy may follow the recommendations for child spacing and therefore end up with optimal birth intervals. Limited access to reproductive health services in some settings may lead to unwanted or unplanned pregnancies for those women who wish to use contraceptives at present or in the future, leading to the notion of unmet need for family planning and therefore short birth intervals [35]. Our study is consistent with a study done in the Philippines where women who had a final say about their desired birth intervals had longer birth intervals [36].

Our study found that women who always decide together with their husband on when to have the next child were less likely to have short birth intervals. This could probably be argued that proper communication between couples about reproductive goals has a positive outcome on birth spacing. The level of reproductive health decision-making among couples such as when to have the next pregnancy, family size, and family planning use among others can result in benefits which impact positively on the family in general [37]. These results are consistent with a study done in ten sub-Saharan African countries where couples who agreed about when to have the next pregnancy had significantly longer birth intervals [38].

Women whose husbands have influence on when to have the next baby were less likely to have short birth intervals. This could probably be argued that these husbands supported interventions such as contraceptive use and other interventions which promote adequate birth intervals. These findings are consistent with studies done in rural Uganda, Saudi Arabia, and Egypt [21, 32, 39] where the lack of partner support was found to be associated with short birth intervals.

Lack of contraceptive use has been documented in literature as one of the strongest predictors of short birth intervals [29]. Contraceptives delay conception after child birth and are one of the best practices that can lead to achievement of recommended birth intervals and therefore optimal maternal and child health outcomes [40]. As expected, this was demonstrated in our study. Only 17.2% of the women in our study always used contraceptives before the next pregnancy, hence the high proportion of short birth intervals. Our study is consistent with studies done in Northern Iran, Bangladesh, and Nigeria which reported significant association between contraceptive use and optimal birth intervals [18, 27, 41] but contrasts with a study done in Democratic Republic of Congo which did not show any significant association between modern contraceptive use and child spacing [34].

There was a universal awareness about recommended birth intervals in our study where all the respondents correctly mentioned the WHO-recommended birth intervals. All the respondents were able to mention at least one advantage of optimal birth intervals and one disadvantage of short birth intervals, but this knowledge was not translated into practice of optimal birth intervals by the majority of the respondents, where slightly more than half of the respondents had short birth intervals. This could probably be argued that factors other than knowledge might have resulted in this high proportion of short birth intervals. Similar results were found in Egypt where there was no significant difference in birth intervals with the control group even though the experimental group was given information about the recommended birth interval and advantages of healthy birth spacing [42].

Although literature shows that mothers' education level [21], formal employment [43], sex preference [23], and number of living children [23, 27] are associated with birth intervals, this was not demonstrated in our study. The absence of association between education level, formal employment, and birth intervals could probably be explained by less variability in the study population with only 18% of the respondents having reached secondary school level or above and only 6.8% of the study population being formally employed.

The following limitations should be considered when interpreting the results of this study. The source of data for this study was based on the self-report of mothers, and no validation of information was made with any objective sources such as health facility cards except for immunization card of the current baby. This could have introduced recall bias which was controlled by only asking the last birth interval. Respondents were also critically informed about the importance of giving accurate information by assuring the confidentiality of their responses, and it is logical to assume that biases are less likely in birth interval events than other more sensitive events. Finally, the sample size of this study may affect generalization of the results of factors to the whole population. However, a study involving a bigger sample size is necessary.

5. Conclusion

In this study, we observed relatively high prevalence of short birth intervals among rural women in Uganda despite adequate knowledge about the recommended birth intervals and the majority desiring optimal birth intervals. Factors which were likely to influence short birth intervals included younger maternal age, not using contraceptives, not planning for pregnancies, not deciding together with their husbands about when to have the next child, and lack of influence of husband on when to have the next baby. We recommend that other than imparting knowledge on recommended birth interval, Ugandan ministry of health together with other stakeholders should strengthen the existing strategies of family planning as a comprehensive package in order to promote optimal birth intervals. Specific programs should be designed to deliberately target young women and men with family planning services. A study assessing how best men can be reached with reproductive health services could be conducted in order to improve their involvement in child spacing.

Acknowledgments

This study was partly funded by Enabel (The Belgium Development Agency-Uganda) under support to the development of human resources program as part of my scholarship for master degree program. This funding was received and used at the stage of data collection. The rest of the stages of this study did not receive any funding from any organization.

References

[1] WHO, *Report of a WHO technical consultation on birth spacing*, World Health Organization, Geneva, Switzerland, 2007.

[2] J. Perin and N. Walker, "Potential confounding in the association between short birth intervals and increased neonatal, infant, and child mortality," *Global Health Action*, vol. 8, no. 1, article 29724, 2015.

[3] A. Conde-Agudelo, A. Rosas-Bermúdez, and A. C. Kafury-Goeta, "Birth spacing and risk of adverse perinatal outcomes: a meta-analysis," *JAMA*, vol. 295, no. 15, pp. 1809–1823, 2006.

[4] A. Conde-Agudelo, A. Rosas-Bermúdez, and A. C. Kafury-Goeta, "Effects of birth spacing on maternal health: a systematic review," *American Journal of Obstetrics and Gynecology*, vol. 196, no. 4, pp. 297–308, 2007.

[5] A. Conde-Agudelo, A. Rosas-Bermudez, F. Castaño, and M. H. Norton, "Effects of birth spacing on maternal, perinatal, infant, and child health: a systematic review of causal mechanisms," *Studies in Family Planning*, vol. 43, no. 2, pp. 93–114, 2012.

[6] USAID, *Healthy Timing and Spacing of Pregnancy: A Family Planning Investment Strategy for Accelerating the Pace of Improvements in Child Survival*, Washington, DC, USA, 2012.

[7] S. O. Rutstein, *Trends in Birth Spacing. DHS Comparative Reports Number 28*, ICF Macro, Calverton, MD, USA, 2011.

[8] J. Bongaarts and J. Casterline, "Fertility transition: is sub-Saharan Africa different?," *Population and Development Review*, vol. 38, no. s1, pp. 153–168, 2013.

[9] NDHS, *Nigeria Demographic and Health Survey*, ICF International, Rockville, MD, USA, 2013.

[10] ZDHS, *Zimbabwe Demographic and Health Survey*, ICF International, Rockville, MD, USA, 2015.

[11] KDHS, *Kenya Demographic and Health Survey*, ICF International, Rockville, MD, USA, 2014.

[12] TDHS, *Tanzania Demographic and Health Survey*, ICF International, Rockville, MD, USA, 2016.

[13] A. Razzaque, J. da Vanzo, M. Rahman et al., "Pregnancy spacing and maternal morbidity in Matlab, Bangladesh," *International Journal of Gynecology & Obstetrics*, vol. 89, pp. S41–S49, 2005.

[14] J. Cleland, A. Conde-Agudelo, H. Peterson, J. Ross, and A. Tsui, "Contraception and health," *The Lancet*, vol. 380, no. 9837, pp. 149–156, 2012.

[15] S. Grisaru-Granovsky, E.-S. Gordon, Z. Haklai, A. Samueloff, and M. M. Schimmel, "Effect of interpregnancy interval on adverse perinatal outcomes — a national study," *Contraception*, vol. 80, no. 6, pp. 512–518, 2009.

[16] M. Yigzaw and F. Enquselassie, "Birth spacing and risk of child mortality at Kalu district South Wollo Zone of Amhara region, Ethiopia," *Ethiopian Medical Journal*, vol. 48, no. 2, pp. 105–115, 2010.

[17] S. Yohannes, M. Wondafrash, M. Abera, and E. Girma, "Duration and determinants of birth interval among women of child bearing age in Southern Ethiopia," *BMC Pregnancy and Childbirth*, vol. 11, no. 1, p. 38, 2011.

[18] O. Fayehun, O. Omololu, and U. Isiugo-Abanihe, "Sex of preceding child and birth spacing among Nigerian ethnic groups," *African Journal of Reproductive Health*, vol. 15, no. 2, pp. 79–89, 2011.

[19] P. Rai, I. S. Paudel, A. Ghimire, P. K. Pokharel, R. Rijal, and S. R. Niraula, "Effect of gender preference on fertility: cross-sectional study among women of Tharu community from rural area of eastern region of Nepal," *Reproductive Health*, vol. 11, no. 1, p. 15, 2014.

[20] UDHS, *Uganda Demographic and Health Survey*, ICF International, Rockville, MD, USA, 2016.

[21] R. Muhindo, J. N. Okonya, S. Groves, and M. Chenault, "Predictors of contraceptive adherence among women seeking family planning services at Reproductive Health Uganda, Mityana Branch," *International Journal of Population Research.*, vol. 2015, article 574329, 8 pages, 2015.

[22] K. O. Hajian-Tilaki, N. Asnafi, and F. Aliakbarnia-Omrani, "The patterns and determinants of birth intervals in multiparous women in Babol," *Southeast Asian Journal of Tropical Medicine and Public Health*, vol. 40, no. 4, p. 852, 2009.

[23] G. Bassey, T. K. Nyengidiki, and N. D. Dambo, "Determinants of interpregnancy interval among parturient in Port Harcourt, Nigeria," *Sahel Medical Journal*, vol. 19, no. 4, pp. 180–184, 2016.

[24] C. C. Dim, E. O. Ugwu, and E. I. Iloghalu, "Duration and determinants of inter-birth interval among women in Enugu, South-Eastern Nigeria," *Journal of Obstetrics and Gynaecology*, vol. 33, no. 2, pp. 175–179, 2013.

[25] H. Fallahzadeh, Z. Farajpour, and Z. Emam, "Duration and determinants of birth interval in Yazd, Iran: a population study," *Iranian Journal of Reproductive Medicine*, vol. 11, no. 5, pp. 379–384, 2013.

[26] J. C. Fotso, J. Cleland, B. Mberu, M. Mutua, and P. Elungata, "Birth spacing and child mortality: an analysis of prospective data from the Nairobi urban health and demographic surveillance system," *Journal of Biosocial Science*, vol. 45, no. 6, pp. 779–798, 2013.

[27] U. R. Saha and A. van Soest, "Contraceptive use, birth spacing, and child survival in Matlab, Bangladesh," *Studies in Family Planning*, vol. 44, no. 1, pp. 45–66, 2013.

[28] A. Exavery, S. Mrema, A. Shamte et al., "Levels and correlates of non-adherence to WHO recommended inter-birth intervals in Rufiji, Tanzania," *BMC Pregnancy and Childbirth*, vol. 12, no. 1, p. 152, 2012.

[29] G. A. Tessema, B. M. Zeleke, and T. A. Ayele, "Birth interval and its predictors among married women in Dabat District, Northwest Ethiopia: a retrospective follow up study," *African Journal of Reproductive Health*, vol. 17, no. 2, pp. 39–45, 2013.

[30] T. A. Moultrie, T. S. Sayi, and I. M. Timæus, "Birth intervals, postponement, and fertility decline in Africa: a new type of transition?," *Population Studies*, vol. 66, no. 3, pp. 241–258, 2012.

[31] S. N. Singh, S. N. Singh, and R. K. Narendra, "Demographic and socio-economic determinants of birth interval dynamics in Manipur: a survival analysis," *Online Journal of Health and Allied Sciences*, vol. 9, p. 4, 2010.

[32] P. Rasheed and B. Al-Dabal, "Birth interval: perceptions and practices among urban-based Saudi Arabian women," *Eastern Mediterranean Health Journal*, vol. 13, no. 4, pp. 881–892, 2007.

[33] UDHS, *Uganda Demographic and Health Survey*, ICF International, Rockville, MD, USA, 2011.

[34] T. F. Chirwa, J. N. Mantempa, F. L. Kinziunga, J. D. Kandala, and N.-B. Kandala, "An exploratory spatial analysis of geographical inequalities of birth intervals among young women in the Democratic Republic of Congo (DRC): a cross-sectional study," *BMC Pregnancy and Childbirth*, vol. 14, no. 1, p. 271, 2014.

[35] T. Lutalo, R. Gray, J. Santelli et al., "Unfulfilled need for contraception among women with unmet need but with the intention to use contraception in Rakai, Uganda: a longitudinal study," *BMC Women's Health*, vol. 18, no. 1, p. 60, 2018.

[36] U. D. Upadhyay and M. J. Hindin, "Do higher status and more autonomous women have longer birth intervals?: Results from Cebu, Philippines," *Social Science & Medicine*, vol. 60, no. 11, pp. 2641–2655, 2005.

[37] H. M. Schwandt, J. Skinner, L. E. Hebert, L. Cobb, A. Saad, and M. Odeku, "Inadequate birth spacing is perceived as riskier than all family planning methods, except sterilization and abortion, in a qualitative study among urban Nigerians," *BMC Women's Health.*, vol. 17, no. 1, p. 80, 2017.

[38] T. Gebreselassie and V. Mishra, "Spousal agreement on preferred waiting time to next birth in sub-Saharan Africa," *Journal of Biosocial Science*, vol. 43, no. 4, pp. 385–400, 2011.

[39] USAID, *Optimal birth spacing: an in-depth study of knowledge, attitude and practices*, Egypt, 2004.

[40] G. Rutaremwa, A. Kabagenyi, S. O. Wandera, T. Jhamba, E. Akiror, and H. L. Nviiri, "Predictors of modern contraceptive use during the postpartum period among women in Uganda: a population-based cross sectional study," *BMC Public Health*, vol. 15, no. 1, p. 262, 2015.

[41] M. Abdel-Fattah, T. Hifnawy, T. I. El Said, M. M. Moharam, and M. A. Mahmoud, "Determinants of birth spacing among Saudi women," *Journal of Family & Community Medicine*, vol. 14, no. 3, pp. 103–111, 2007.

[42] N. Abdel-Tawab, S. F. Lūzā, and A. Zaki, *Helping Egyptian Women Achieve Optimal Birth Spacing Intervals Through Fostering Linkages Between Family Planning and Maternal/Child Health Services*, Frontiers in Reproductive Health, Population Council, 2008.

[43] A. Longwe, J. Smits, and E. de Jong, *Number and Spacing of Children and Women's Employment in Africa*, Nijmegen Cent Econ NiCE Work Pap, 2013.

27

Perspective of Traditional Birth Attendants on Their Experiences and Roles in Maternal Health Care in Rural Areas of Northern Ghana

Peter Adatara,[1] Agani Afaya,[1] Elizabeth A. Baku,[1] Solomon Mohammed Salia,[1] and Anthony Asempah[2]

[1]Department of Nursing, School of Nursing and Midwifery, University of Health and Allied Sciences, Ho, Ghana
[2]Public Affairs Unit, University of Health and Allied Sciences, Ho, Ghana

Correspondence should be addressed to Peter Adatara; padatara@uhas.edu.gh

Academic Editor: Yves Jacquemyn

Background. Traditional birth attendants play significant roles in maternal health care in the rural communities in developing countries such as Ghana. Despite their important role in maternal health care, there is paucity of information from the perspective of traditional birth attendants regarding their role on maternal health care in rural areas in Ghana. *Objective.* The aim of this study was to explore and describe the role of traditional birth attendants in maternal health care in the rural areas in Ghana. *Methods.* A qualitative explorative approach was adopted to explore the role of traditional birth attendants in maternal health care in the rural areas of Ghana. Ten (10) out of a total of twenty-seven (27) practising traditional birth attendants in the study area were purposefully selected from five (5) rural communities in the Bongo District of Ghana for the study. Data were collected through in-depth, unstructured, individual interviews using a guide. Data collected from the interviews were transcribed verbatim and analysed to identify themes. *Results.* Six main roles of traditional birth attendants on maternal health care in rural areas were identified in this study: traditional birth attendants conduct deliveries at home, they provide health education to women on nutrition during pregnancy and lactation, they arrange means of transport and accompany women in labour to health facilities, they provide psychological support and counselling to women during pregnancy and childbirth, and traditional birth attendants are not paid in cash for the services they render to women in the rural areas. *Conclusion.* Our study brought to light the critical role traditional birth attendants play in maternity in rural and remote areas in Ghana. There is a need for skilled birth attendants to collaborate with traditional birth attendants in rural and deprived communities to provide quality and culturally accepted care in the rural communities.

1. Background

One of the strategies identified as being crucial for saving the lives of pregnant women and as an indicator for progress in the reduction of maternal mortality is the utilisation of skilled birth care [1]. Although skilled birth care is identified as the ultimate strategy for saving the lives of pregnant women and infants, in rural and deprived communities in developing countries such as Ghana, women continue to deliver at home with the assistance of traditional birth attendants (TBAs) [2].

The World Health Organisation (WHO) defines a traditional birth attendant as "a person who assists the mother during childbirth and initially acquired her skills by delivering babies herself or through apprenticeship to other traditional birth attendants" [3]. Studies show that, in the rural and deprived communities in sub-Saharan Africa, TBAs constitute the greater number of childbirth care providers due to the unavailability of skilled birth attendants such as midwives, nurses, and doctors [4]. Traditional birth attendants are known to have a long history as childbirth attendants in many communities in developing countries including Ghana, although TBAs are not considered skilled birth attendants by the definition of a skilled birth attendant [5].

The picture is not different in Ghana. TBAs still continue to play significant roles in maternal health care in the rural and deprived communities where there are inadequate skilled birth attendants. Studies have shown that in Ghana women have traditionally preferred to deliver at home because it is cheaper and easier as women who deliver at home receive social support from their extended families and do not have to pay much for the delivery services [6, 7]. According to reports from the Ghana Statistical Service (GSS), 62.9% of the deliveries in the Northern Region occurred at home assisted by nonskilled attendants, while in the Central and the Upper West Regions 39.1% and 38.6% births occurred at home assisted by TBAs and relatives, respectively [7]. The above statistics explained the significant roles TBAs play in the health of women and children in rural areas in Ghana. Studies established that one of the strategies to increase utilisation of skilled birth attendants where TBAs are the predominant providers of childbirth care particularly in the rural areas involves linking TBAs with the formal health care institutions and fostering collaborative practice with TBAs [8].

Despite the importance of TBAs in maternal health care in rural and deprived communities in Ghana, there is paucity of literature regarding the exact role of TBAs in maternal health care in rural communities where many women in labour patronise their services. The aim of this study was to explore the perspective of TBAs on their roles in maternal health care in the rural and deprived communities in Ghana. The findings of the study will also be useful to the Ministry of Health and Ghana Health Service and other stakeholders involved in formulating policies on facilitating the utilisation of childbirth care services in the rural areas of Ghana to reduce maternal mortality.

2. Design and Methods

2.1. Research Design. A qualitative explorative design was used to explore and examine the role of TBAs in maternal health care from their own perspectives in the rural communities in the Bongo District of Ghana.

2.2. Research Setting. The research was carried out in the Bongo District in the Upper East Region of Ghana. This district was selected as the setting for conducting the study because it is one of the most rural and deprived districts in Ghana and has all the characteristics of a typical rural area in Ghana [7]. Also, the Bongo District was chosen because it is one of the districts with low utilisation of skilled birth care provided by skilled birth attendants [9]. The Bongo District is amongst the ten (10) districts in the Upper East Region of Ghana, with Bongo Township as its capital. According to the Bongo District Health Directorate, there is only one doctor who is the Medical Superintendent of the district hospital. He manages the hospital and sixty-five nurses in the entire district [9]. There is only one district hospital with one general practitioner (medical doctor) and few midwives providing skilled birth care. The remaining maternity units in the health facilities are manned by midwives providing primary maternity care for women during pregnancy and childbirth.

2.3. Study Population and Sampling Method. The participants for this study included men and women who practised as TBAs in the rural areas in the Bongo District of Ghana. Participants were recruited using purposeful and snowball sampling strategies. Some of the TBAs who were identified by community opinion leaders were asked to invite other TBAs to participate in this study. A total of ten (10) TBAs out of twenty-seven (27) practising TBAs in the study area were recruited from five (5) rural communities from the Bongo District of Ghana. These TBAs were chosen for the study because they met the criteria and were willing to take part in the study. The researchers strived to recruit a maximum variation sample to include diverse experiences in the study. The researchers also selected and interviewed TBAs who have requisite experience on maternal health care in the study area.

The inclusion criteria included the following:

(i) Men and women who had practised childbirth care for more than a year.

(ii) TBAs who live in the communities for more than one year.

(iii) TBAs who were still in active service and were willing to participate in the study.

2.4. Data Collection and Procedure. Data were collected through semistructured individual interviews using a guide. The interview guide contained questions that inquired about the role of TBAs in maternal health care in the rural areas. Individual interviews provided a deeper understanding of social phenomena such as the role of TBAs in maternal health care that would be obtained from questionnaires [10]. Semistructured interviews were also appropriate for this study because the researchers required detailed insights from participants [10]. The in-depth interviews allowed the researchers the opportunity to define the areas to be explored and to probe further to pursue an idea or response in detail. The interviews were done face-to-face with participants at their various homes and at their convenient time which lasted between 45 to 60 minutes. The interviews were recorded with the permission of participants.

2.5. Data Analysis. Thematic analysis approach was used to analyse the data. We examined the qualitative data, which were categorized based on prominent theme patterns expressed in the text of the individual interviews [11]. We broke down the narrative data into smaller units, coding, and naming the units according to the content they represent and grouping coded material based on shared concepts and meanings. All transcripts were read and analysed by three members of the research team in a three-stage process of data analysis and synthesis [12]. In the first stage, we used the exploratory method of holistic coding for the first coding cycle. After reading all the transcripts, the three researchers met as a group to discuss patterns and units and to develop a coding protocol. The verbatim transcripts of the individual interviews were coded into different units. In the second stage of data analysis and synthesis, the focused coding method was used for the second coding cycle. The three researchers met together and, through peer discussion and agreement, recategorized the coding units. Finally, based on the coding, the primary researcher identified themes that integrated substantial sets of the coding units. Sets of categories were created to describe the predominant themes that emerged from the text [13].

2.6. Ethical Considerations. This study is part of a research thesis carried out toward the award of a doctorate degree. The research had ethical approval from the Ethical Committee of Faculty of Health Sciences Research Technology and Innovation Committee (FRTI) at Nelson Mandela University (H14-HEA-NUR-30). The participants chosen for the interview were provided with both verbal and written information on the purpose, general content, and nature of the investigation. The participants were told that any information they provided would be kept confidential. Each participant was given time to read the letter. The consent forms were signed by each participant who could read and thumb printed by participants who could not read.

3. Results

Six (6) themes emerged from the data analysis with regard to the roles of TBAs in maternal health care:

(i) TBAs conduct deliveries at home in rural areas.

(ii) TBAs provide health education to women on nutrition during pregnancy and lactation in our community.

(iii) TBAs arrange means of transport and accompany women in labour to health facilities.

(iv) TBAs provide natural family planning to women in rural areas.

(v) TBAs provide psychological support and counselling to women during pregnancy and childbirth.

(vi) TBAs are not paid in cash for the services we render to women in the rural areas.

3.1. Profile of the Participants. The participants were made up of seven (7) women and three (3) men. All the participants had no formal education and could not read and write. Majority (8) of the participants were within the ages of 60 and 70. Only 2 of the participants were within the ages of 55 and 59. Majority of the participants have been practising childbirth care in their various communities for more than five years. All the participants apart from being childbirth care givers are also peasant farmers.

3.2. Roles of TBAs in Maternal Health Care in the Rural Communities. The TBAs during the individual interviews outlined four major roles they play in maternal healthcare in rural areas. The roles/themes are discussed below.

Theme 1: TBAs Conduct Deliveries at Home in Rural Areas. One of the major themes that emerged from this study is the role of TBAs in maternal health care in rural communities in Ghana and particularly in the Bongo District was that TBAs assist in conducting uncomplicated deliveries at home. The TBAs indicated that, due to the absence of skilled birth attendants in rural communities in the study area especially in the night and weekends, they are always called upon to assist women to deliver. These were captured in the following quotes:

> *"In the village here, we assist women to deliver at home especially in the night when they cannot go to the health facility to deliver".*

> *"I must say that I have been helping women to deliver in this village well over twenty years now. When the women are in labour and cannot go to the hospital or the clinic, they call on us and we have to assist them".*

> *"As for me I think, we have been doing the work of the nurses and doctors in this community because the trained nurses and doctors are not in this community and we are always around whether in the night or weekend we are there to attend to the women when in labour".*

The participants indicated that they always advise women to go to the health facility to deliver but sometimes they would refuse and insist that they prefer to be assisted by them.

> *"We normally advise the women to go to the health facility to deliver but they always refuse insisting that they would prefer their (TBA) services. And so, we must assist them to deliver".*

> *.... I have told many women in labour to go to the hospital where there are nurses and doctors to assist them to deliver but they would always refuse. Some would even tell us (TBA), they prefer to be assisted by us".*

Some of the participants reported that the labouring women usually prefer their services because the midwives and nurses are not in their community to conduct labour. If even at all, if women want to go to the health facility to deliver, they would have to travel more than 15 km to the nearest health facility to access skilled birth care. The participants indicated that it is more serious if the labour occurs in the night, where there is no health facility in the community or nearer. These have often compelled labouring women to rely on their services.

> *"I must say that we cannot blame the women for calling on us to assist them to deliver because there is no nurse or doctor in this community to provide the skilled birth care. And if the labouring woman wants to go to the health facility to deliver, they would have to walk more than 15 km to the nearest health facility. So, they would rely on us to help them instead of travelling that far".*

> *".... We have been assisting the women to deliver because sometimes the labour occurs in the night*

and there is no nurse or doctor in this village to assist them to deliver. We have to help them because we are their doctors and nurses in this community".

The participants indicated that even though they have been assisting them to deliver in their homes, any time they examine the woman in labour and feel that it is beyond their level, they advise the husband or relative to take her to the hospital to deliver. This was evident in the following quotes:

> *"I normally ask the husband to take the labouring woman to the hospital to deliver when I examine her and realise that it is beyond my level. We have been doing this work for many years and we are experienced even though we have not been to school to learn it".*

> *"I don't usually try to assist a woman in labour where I think based on my assessment of the woman during labour that it is beyond me. I will just be honest and tell the husband or any relative who is available to take her to the health facility for her to deliver".*

The participants reported that when they have challenges with women who are weak and pale or those delivering for the first time, they refer them to the health facilities to deliver.

> *"We have been doing this work for many years now. So, when you call on me and I see that you are delivering for the first time or the woman is looking weak or the eyes are looking whitish (pale), I know that this is not my case, I will not attempt. I will just ask the husband or whosoever is around to take her to the health facility to deliver".*

> *.........oh, I know them. I have done this work for a very long time. I am now even old, yet I still assist women to deliver. Because of my experience, when I am called and immediately I get there, I will assess the labouring woman and when I see that she has no blood or has ever delivered through operation, I will just ask her to go the hospital because I cannot give blood or operate to remove the baby".*

The participants indicated that although they have been doing this work for many years, they have never lost a woman through labour yet, they are not respected or regarded by the health personnel.

> *"I must say that since I started doing this work, I have never lost a woman or child through child birth. All the women I assisted to deliver are always happy and appreciative. Yet the nurses do not regard us.*

> *".... I assisted more than thirty (30) women to deliver since I started practising as a TBA and none of the women or the child died. But, we are not regarded or respected by the nurses. They think that we have not been to school".*

Theme 2: TBAs Provide Health Education on Nutrition during Pregnancy and Lactation. One other theme that emerged from this study regarding the role of TBAs in maternal health care in the rural areas in Ghana was that they provide health education on nutrition and natural family planning to women in their respective communities. The participants reported that although they have not been to school to learn about nutrition, their experience in childbirth care over the years has given them the opportunity to know the traditional foods that provide the right nutrition for pregnant women and nursing mothers.

> *"I must say that one of the things I do as a TBA in this community is to provide nutrition education to pregnant women and nursing mothers for healthy growth of the foetus or the baby. Many of the pregnant women especially the younger ones do not know what to eat and what not to eat during pregnancy. So, I mostly engage them with their mothers-in-law to educate them on what to eat and what they need to avoid when you are pregnant or nursing your baby".*

> *"Teaching mothers on the kind of food to eat during pregnancy and when nursing a baby has been part of my duties in this community. I have been doing this work for some time now and the women in this community know about it and would always seek my advice on nutrition when pregnant or after delivery".*

The participants also explained that even though they have not been to school they are much aware of the traditional food stuff that are available in their community that mothers do not have to spend lots of money to buy unlike nurses who usually advise and prescribe certain diets for women who cannot afford to buy them. These were captured in the following quotes:

> *"As I said earlier, we live in this community and we know the food stuff in this community that are good for pregnant women or the nursing mother. We usually do not advise or prescribe certain food stuff that are not available in this community unlike what the nurses have been doing. Most of the women in the community do not have money to go to market to buy all those things the nurses have been asking to do".*

> *".... hmmm, as for me, I usually advice the pregnant or nursing mothers based on what they have in the family, so that they won't go out looking for money to buy. There are nutritious food stuffs in this community far better than what is sold in the market"*

One of the participants of this study mentioned the food stuff in the community that are usually recommended or prescribed for pregnant and nursing mothers for the purposes of healthy growth of the foetus and the pregnant mother herself, thereby enhancing breast milk production in the case of nursing mothers and boosting the immunity of the mother.

"The food stuff that I usually recommend for pregnant mothers which are available in this community and everyone can afford them include 'Kolgo' in Frafra, also known as dawadawa (locust bean boiled and fermented), smoked guinea fowl, beans, dry okro soup and bitor soup (local vegetable soup) and bitter-leaf soup. All the above-mentioned foods are equally good for nursing mothers, but we usually add 'zoomkom and pusakoom'. Zoomkom is local drink prepared from millet flour and fruit, tooro (baobab tree fruits) to provide energy and facilitate breast milk production for the nursing mothers".

Some of the participants indicated that there are certain foods that are to be avoided because they are not good for the mother and the child.

"We usually recommend that pregnant women should not be eating too much pepper, certain types of fish such as swordfish and king mackerel. I realised throughout the years of my practice that any time pregnant women eat these types of foods they encounter problems. So, we advise them to avoid them".

Majority of the participants reported that although there are taboos in the community prohibiting pregnant women from eating certain foods, there are always alternatives available.

"I must acknowledge that in this community, women especially pregnant women are prohibited from eating chicken, snails, dog meat, cat meat and monkey meat. But, we can always find alternatives to these foods".

Theme 3: TBAs Arrange Means of Transport and Accompany Women in Labour to Health Facilities. This study revealed that TBAs arrange means of transport and accompany women in labour to health facilities to give birth. The participants indicated during the interviews that there were occasions where they (TBAs) had to arrange transport for labouring women and accompanied them to health facilities to give birth.

"I must indicate that there were times, I personally had to arrange for a taxi cab or motor cycle to transport women in labour to a health facility to give birth. In many of such occasions, I had to personally accompany the labouring woman to the health facility to give birth because none of the relatives was around to do that"

Another participant also indicated how she accompanied a labouring woman to a health facility and had to pay for a drug that was prescribed but was not in the health facility.

"We do a lot of things for women especially during labour in this community. There was a day I had to accompany a labouring woman to give birth in the hospital. When we got to the hospital, the doctor prescribed a drug for her to buy but she didn't have money. I had to use my own money to buy the drug for her"

The participants reported that, because of the long distance that women had to travel to health facilities in the study area to give birth, relatives of labouring women usually prefer TBAs to accompany labouring women in case they deliver on the way to the health facility.

"The reason why we (TBAs) accompany labouring women to health facilities to give birth is because of the long distance that labouring woman would have to travel to the health facility to give birth. So, we go with them to the health facility especially if the means of transport is a taxi cab and in case the baby is coming out on the way to the health facility, we can assist her to give birth".

Moreover, participants reported that, apart from the relatives asking them (TBAs) to accompany labouring women to health facilities to give birth, midwives working in the health facilities usually plead with them to always accompany labouring women to health facilities to give birth especially if it was in the night.

"We were advised by the midwives in the health facilities to accompany labouring women to the health facilities to deliver especially if it is in the night".

"I was personally told by the midwives in the health facilities that I should always support and accompany labouring women to health facilities to give birth. So, because of the advice from the midwives, I had to always arrange transport and accompany labouring women to the health facility to give birth".

It was also revealed in this study during interviews with the study participants that TBAs were motivated by midwives in the health facilities in the study area to always accompany labouring women to give birth in the health facilities. TBAs are usually given a bar of soap and sometimes some money by midwives to motivate them to accompany women to health facilities to deliver.

"The midwives in the health facilities motivate us to accompany labouring women to the health facilities to give birth. Anytime I accompany a labouring woman to a health facility to give birth, the midwives give me a bar of key soap to wash my clothes and sometimes, they give me some money to buy whatever I want to buy".

Theme 4: TBAs Offer Education to Couples on Natural Family Planning Methods. Apart from education on nutrition during pregnancy and lactation, TBAs offer education to couples on natural family planning methods.

"One thing I also do as part of my work in this community is to educate young couples how to space their childbirths. I have done this over the years in this village and couples especially women patronize my services a lot and it is helping them".

"We also educate married women on how to study their menstrual cycle to avoid pregnancy if the child is not yet three years or more. This has helped many of them to avoid giving birth every year to create problems for themselves and their children".

Some of the participants indicated that the couples patronise their education on family planning because it has no side effects and they do not pay any money for it as compared to what the nurses offer to them in the health facilities.

".... what I have heard from the women who patronize our services on family planning is that they don't experience any problem using the natural family planning unlike the drugs and injections the nurses give them. Apart from that they don't pay any money for our services".

The women like our services because they have nothing to lose. They won't pay money for it and they will not experience any problem after they have used the natural family planning method".

Although participants indicated that the natural family planning methods have no side effects, it is sometimes difficult for some couples to strictly follow the instructions. Some women miscalculate their menstrual cycle and end up becoming pregnant.

"I can't say that we have been achieving 100% results in our education on natural family planning methods as a way of spacing childbirth. There are times we give instructions to women and they end up not following it. And when that happens, they end up becoming pregnant when the child is less than one or two years".

"I must say that some women fail to follow instructions and they become pregnant unaware. But when they become pregnant as married couples and the baby is still less than two years, we counsel them to keep the pregnancy and take good care of the child. Our tradition does not permit a woman especially a married woman to abort pregnancy".

Theme 5: TBAs Provide Psychological Support and Counselling to Women during Pregnancy and Childbirth. The interviews with the participants revealed that one of the roles that the TBAs play in maternal healthcare in rural and deprived communities is the provision of psychological support and counselling to women during pregnancy and childbirth. The participants said the provision of psychological support to women during pregnancy and childbirth is what makes their childbirth services patronised by women in their communities.

"We usually provide psychological support and counselling to women during pregnancy and childbirth. Labour is a painful thing and therefore, women going through the pain need support and advice to go through the delivery process with confidence".

"We sometimes provide psychological support to labouring women to have confidence to tolerate the pain especially the young mothers who are delivering for the first time that they can make it.

Participants indicated that the psychological supports they provide to labouring women and pregnant women range from massaging their back to praising them for their efforts during labour. They explained that the psychological support is supposed to encourage women to put up their best in the labour process and to have a positive attitude toward the delivery process.

"We massage them and keep patting their back and encourage them that they can make it with little effort. We encourage them to have a positive attitude toward the labour".

"One of the things I usually do to women when they are in labour is to keep on praising them in whatever they do and inform them they need to do more for the baby to come out early so that they can rest. Sometimes, I have to join other women to sing for the labouring woman to help her minimize the labour pain and to encourage them to push harder for the baby to come out".

The participants explained that providing psychological support to women during labour is one of the major roles that makes them enjoy their services. The participants indicated providing psychological support is what is lacking in the health facilities that make some of the women in the rural areas not patronising the birth care services of skilled birth attendants in rural areas.

"I must say that things like singing for women during labour, praising them, massaging their back, encouraging them during labour and not shouting at them is what makes our services different from what is done in the health facilities. These things are not done in the health facilities. And it is the more reason why some women do not like going to deliver in the health facility".

"............Psychological support is very important in labour management. We usually do that to motivate the labouring women to deliver without so much stress. One reason why most of the women do not like going to health facilities to deliver but keep on calling us anytime they are in labour is because of the support we provide them".

Some of the participants indicated that labour is a natural life event that birth care providers need to understand and encourage labouring women to go through it successfully without any problem. They recommended that skilled birth attendants should cultivate the habit of supporting labouring women psychologically and allowing relatives to assist them when they are busy.

> *"I know nurses and doctors are always busy and are not able to provide the needed psychological support to labouring women. But, what they need to understand is the fact that labour is a natural life event and therefore, labouring women should be encouraged to go through it successfully without any problem or complaint".*

> *"It is bad to hear that in the health facilities, nurses shout at women who are in labour. Labour is a natural life event and sometimes the labouring women do not know what they are doing and so, they need encouragement and not insults and shouting at them. If the nurses are always busy they can allow relatives to assist them provide the support the labouring woman needs".*

Some of the participants indicated that there were times they accompanied labouring women to a health facility to be attended by the healthcare professionals and instead of appreciating and encouraging them to do more, they rather blame them for detaining the woman for a long time before bringing her to the health facility.

> *"I felt very bad when I had to accompany a woman who was in labour and came to me to take her to a health facility. Upon getting to the health facility, the midwife after receiving the woman, did not even examine her to know the stage of the labour process or the progress of the labour but just started blaming me for keeping the woman for a long time before bringing her. She would not listen to me for any explanation. And I really felt bad that day and since then I did not accompany any labouring woman to a health facility again".*

> *"I must say that the nurses do not want to appreciate what we the TBAs do to help labouring women in the community. Instead of they (the midwives) allowing us to work together to see how we can help these women they are rather blaming us for causing problems for them. The midwives think that because we haven't been to school, so we don't know anything about assisting women to deliver. But, you are not available in this community to help them when they are in labour and need you. Is half a loaf of bread not better than nothing"?*

Theme 6: TBAs Are Not Paid in Cash for the Services We Render to Women in the Rural Areas of Ghana. The TBAs indicated that although they have been assisting women in maternal health related care in the rural areas of Ghana, they are not paid in cash for the services they render to the women in the rural communities in the study area. Although TBAs are usually paid in kind by the husband or relatives in the forms gifts such as soap, guinea fowls, fowls, and goats, they are not paid any allowance by government or anybody for the care they render to women in rural areas. Their services are on sacrificial basis and not for a fee. This practice has often left them struggling to take care of their own needs although what they do put so much stress on them.

> *"....... As for our work, it is not a paid work, I do it for free and I have never charged any woman before assisting her to deliver. So, we don't benefit anything from what we do in terms of money but just the joy you get when you are able to see a woman deliver successfully."*

> *"......I must say that we don't benefit anything from this work we are doing. We are not paid any money for rendering any service to women in this village. It's our challenge because we do this work and sometimes, the women are so poor that majority of them are not able to afford to buy soap for us to wash our clothes".*

Participants mentioned that although they render the services in maternal health care in the rural areas that should have been done by trained skilled birth attendants such as midwives and doctors who are paid by the government, they are not given anything by the health sector neither are they recognised.

> *"We have been doing the work of the nurses who are paid monthly to do that and yet the government does not give us anything. They don't even recognise that we are doing their work for them".*

> *"I must say that some of the nurses who come to this community to work do not have anything to do because we do their work for them and yet we are not paid a penny".*

Participants suggested that there is the need for the government to support them with logistics and some allowances to motivate them to put up their best in helping and supporting the poor women in the rural communities who cannot afford to travel long distances to access skilled birth care. These suggestions were captured in the following quotes:

> *".... I think government should support us by giving small money and supporting with things such as gloves, detergents and aprons to enable us do our best to assist these poor women who usually rely on us for assistance".*

> *"I do not understand why, the government and the health care managers in Bongo would not support us. We are doing all this work for them at least they should give us something small if not every month may be every three months to motivate us to put up our best".*

4. Discussion

Our study sought to explore and describe the role of traditional birth attendants in maternal health care in the rural areas in Ghana. TBAs have long been practising as traditional midwives in rural areas of Ghana and yet, there is a lack of recent empirical evidence on the roles TBAs play in maternal health care in rural areas of Ghana. The present study found that one of the roles TBAs play in maternal health care in the rural communities in Ghana is that they conduct deliveries at home. The participants indicated that although they have not been formally trained to conduct deliveries, they have been assisting women deliver at home in their communities over the years. The results depict that TBAs in the rural communities of Ghana are highly utilised in childbirth care because there are no skilled birth attendants in the rural areas especially during the nights and weekends to attend to women who are in labour. It should be noted that, in the absence of a skilled birth attendant in the community, labouring women would have no options than to patronise the services of TBAs. After all, half a loaf of bread is better than nothing. The present finding is consistent with findings from recent studies, which have shown that TBAs continue to assist women in labour to deliver in some rural communities in developing countries [14, 15], for instance, in a qualitative study to assess stakeholder views/on the incorporation of TBAs into the formal health systems of low- and middle-income countries. It was concluded that TBAs are involved in the provision of pregnancy care [16]. These findings imply that healthcare managers in developing countries need to develop strategies of training TBAs and facilitating a collaborative practice amongst TBAs and midwives in rural communities as a short-term solution till such a time where there are adequate midwives in the rural communities to reduce maternal mortality. This study findings point to the fact that, in rural communities in developing countries such as Ghana, although the strategy of encouraging the utilisation of skilled birth attendants during childbirth is a laudable idea, it is difficult to achieve in a situation where the skilled birth attendants are not available in the community and TBAs are the only care providers available. There is the need for skilled birth attendants to partner with TBAs in rural areas to provide woman-centred childbirth care.

Moreover, the present findings suggest that, apart from the traditional role of assisting women to deliver in rural communities, TBAs equally perform critical and important functions such as providing education on nutrition during pregnancy and lactation. These roles are often performed by TBAs taking into consideration the cultural values and tradition of the women and the community at large, thereby wining the confidence of the labouring women and their family. Recent studies have highlighted that because TBA-client relationships are often positive and incorporate shared values and belief, the flexible attitudes of TBAs regarding payment are the factors that usually influence many home births in rural communities in developing countries [8, 16, 17]. What is interesting about the present findings is the fact that TBAs provide education on nutrition during pregnancy and lactation based on the available local nutritious foods that would meet the nutrition needs of the pregnant women or the lactating mothers and could be afforded by most families. This is an important finding that could be adopted and be practised by midwives when educating pregnant women and lactating mothers during antenatal and child welfare clinics to ensure women practise it. Healthcare managers of the institutions in developing countries need to know how these practices could be integrated into the skilled birth care organisation in ways that would ensure women's needs are better met.

It was also revealed in this study that one of the maternal health care roles of TBAs was to arrange means of transport and accompany labouring women to health facilities to give birth. It was reported in previous studies that TBAs play important role in improving maternal health care in rural areas by referring women in labour and at times, accompanying them to health facilities for childbirth [18, 19]. Companionship during child birth by TBAs offers physical and social support to labouring women as they are always anxious about the unknown outcome of the childbirth. The finding of this study implies that TBAs could be used as referral agents in rural communities to promote skilled birth care and provide social and psychological support. Also, it was discovered in this study that TBAs provide counselling and education on natural family planning to women in rural communities in the study area. It was revealed that although some of the women in this study knew about modern family planning contraceptives, some of them still seek education on natural family methods such as the calendar method and abstinence from sexual intercourse as a form family planning from TBAs. This finding is consistent with previous studies that indicated that TBAs offer services such as traditional methods of family planning to couples who do not want to use modern contraceptives in rural areas [14]. This implies that TBAs could also be used to educate women on the use of modern family planning methods to prevent unwanted pregnancies and sexual transmitted infections in the rural areas.

Providing psychological support and counselling to women during pregnancy and childbirth was found in this study to be other important role TBAs play in maternal health care in the study area. Previous studies reported psychological support and counselling to women during pregnancy and childbirth as one of the reasons accounting for home births in developing countries such as Ghana [20, 21]. For instance, in a qualitative study conducted to identify the reasons that accounted for home births and use of traditional birth attendants in rural Zambia, it was found that most women utilised the birth services provided by TBAs because they perceived them to be respectful, skilled, friendly, and trustworthy and they provide psychological support to women during childbirth [21].

Although TBAs play important roles regarding maternal health care in the rural communities of Ghana, it came to light in our study that they are not paid in cash for the services they render to women in the rural areas of Ghana. Although, TBAs are usually paid in kind by the husbands or relatives in the form of gifts such as soap, guinea fowls, fowls, and goats, TBAs are not supported with logistics and allowances to motivate them to hold the fort in rural and hard to reach communities till such time that midwives are posted to those communities. It is important for healthcare managers and policy planners to identify all available childbirth care providers in rural communities and support them in terms of logistics and some allowances as a form of motivation to enable them to perform their roles. Skilled birth attendants should foster collaboration with TBAs in the rural communities to ensure that some refresher training is given to TBAs with regular monitoring and supportive supervision to ensure that they work within their limits and those that are beyond their level are quickly referred to health facilities for expert management. The training of TBAs is found in literature to be an effective way of enhancing their roles in rural areas [22].

4.1. Limitation of the Study. Although this study had some unique findings, it also had some limitations. This qualitative research about TBA focused particularly on their viewpoints and the roles they play in maternal health care in rural areas in Ghana. Including the viewpoints of other stakeholders such as skilled birth attendants on the roles of TBAs in rural communities would have enriched the findings. Also, the interviews were conducted with 10 participants which are not adequate to generalise the findings of this study.

5. Conclusion

It was concluded from this study that TBAs play critical role in maternal health in rural and remote areas in Ghana. This study identified the roles of TBAs in maternal health care in rural areas to include assisting women during delivery, providing health education on nutrition during pregnancy and lactation, providing natural family planning to women and providing psychological support, and counselling to women during pregnancy and childbirth. There is need for skilled birth attendants to collaborate with traditional birth attendants in rural and deprived communities to provide culturally accepted care in health facilities to facilitate the utilisation of birth care service.

6. Implication for Nursing Practice

The findings of this study have implications for nursing practice. The findings of this study call for collaborative practice between skilled birth attendants and traditional birth attendants to ensure that TBAs are supported in terms of training needs, logistics and motivation in the form of allowances to put up their best in maternal health care in rural and hard to reach communities where there are no or few skilled birth attendants. There is also the need for health care providers and policy makers to develop strategies of training TBAs especially on complications of labour and referral to health facility for expert's management.

References

[1] World Health Organisation, ICM, and FIGO, *Making Pregnancy Safer: The Critical Role of Skilled Attendants: Statement*, World Health Organization, Geneva, Switzerland, 2004.

[2] World Health Organization, *Traditional Birth Attendants: A Joint WHO/UNICEF/UNFPA Statement*, World Health Organization, Geneva, Switzerland, 1992.

[3] M. Carlough and M. McCall, "Skilled birth attendance: What does it mean and how can it be measured? A clinical skills assessment of maternal and child health workers in Nepal," *International Journal of Gynecology and Obstetrics*, vol. 89, no. 2, pp. 200–208, 2005.

[4] World Health Organization, *Trends in Maternal Mortality: 1990 to 2010. Estimates by WHO, UNICEF, UNFPA, The World Bank and the United Nations Population Division*, World Health Organization, Geneva, Switzerland, 2011.

[5] F. A. Akum, "A qualitative study on factors contributing to low institutional child delivery rates in Northern Ghana: the case of bawku municipality," *Journal of Community Medicine & Health Education*, vol. 3, article 236, 2013.

[6] C. A. Moyer, P. B. Adongo, R. A. Aborigo, A. Hodgson, and C. M. Engmann, "'They treat you like you are not a human being': Maltreatment during labour and delivery in rural northern Ghana," *Midwifery*, vol. 30, no. 2, pp. 262–268, 2014.

[7] Ghana Statistical Service, "Ghana multiple indicator cluster survey with an enhanced malaria module and biomarker," Final Report, Ghana Statistical Service, Accra, Ghana, 2012.

[8] L. M. Sibley, T. A. Sipe, and M. Koblinsky, "Does traditional birth attendant training increase use of antenatal care? A review of the evidence," *Journal of Midwifery & Women's Health*, vol. 49, no. 4, pp. 298–305, 2004.

[9] Bongo District Health Directorate, "Annual health report," Tech. Rep., Bongo District Health Directorate, 2015.

[10] D. Silverman, *Doing Qualitative Research: A Practical Handbook*, Sage, London, UK, 4th edition, 2013.

[11] M. B. A. Miles, M. Huberman, and J. Saldana, *Qualitative Data Analysis: A Methods Sourcebook*, Sage, Thousand Oaks, Calif, USA, 2014.

[12] J. W. Creswell, *Educational Research: Planning, Conducting, and Evaluating Quantitative and Qualitative Research*, Pearson, Upper Saddle River, NJ, USA, 4th edition, 2012.

[13] J. Saldaña, *Fundamentals of Qualitative Research: Understanding Qualitative Research*, Oxford University Press, New York, NY, USA, 2010.

[14] B. T. Shaikh, S. Khan, A. Maab, and S. Amjad, "Emerging role of traditional birth attendants in mountainous terrain: A qualitative exploratory study from Chitral district, Pakistan," *BMJ Open*, vol. 4, no. 11, Article ID e006238, 2014.

[15] O. O. Owolabi, C. Glenton, S. Lewin, and N. Pakenham-Walsh, "Stakeholder views on the incorporation of traditional birth attendants into the formal health systems of low-and middle-income countries: A qualitative analysis of the HIFA2015 and CHILD2015 email discussion forums," *BMC Pregnancy and Childbirth*, vol. 14, article 118, 2014.

[16] M. K. Dodzo and M. Mhloyi, "Home is best: Why women in rural Zimbabwe deliver in the community," *PLoS ONE*, vol. 12, no. 8, Article ID e0181771, 2017.

[17] C. Pfeiffer and R. Mwaipopo, "Delivering at home or in a health facility? health-seeking behaviour of women and the role of traditional birth attendants in Tanzania," *BMC Pregnancy and Childbirth*, vol. 13, article 55, 2013.

[18] C. Wilunda, G. Dall'Oglio, C. Scanagatta et al., "Changing the role of traditional birth attendants in Yirol West County, South Sudan," *PLoS ONE*, vol. 12, no. 11, Article ID e0185726, 2017.

[19] P. C. Chi and H. Urdal, "The evolving role of traditional birth attendants in maternal health in post-conflict Africa: A qualitative study of Burundi and northern Uganda," *SAGE Open Medicine*, vol. 6, Article ID 20503, 2018.

[20] T. Miller and H. Smith, "Establishing partnership with traditional birth attendants for improved maternal and newborn health: A review of factors influencing implementation," *BMC Pregnancy and Childbirth*, vol. 17, article 367, 2017.

[21] C. Sialubanje, K. Massar, D. H. Hamer, and R. A. C. Ruiter, "Reasons for home delivery and use of traditional birth attendants in rural Zambia: a qualitative study," *BMC Pregnancy and Childbirth*, vol. 15, article 216, 2015.

[22] S. Hernandez, J. B. Oliveira, and T. Shirazian, "How a training program is transforming the role of traditional birth attendants from cultural practitioners to unique health-care providers: a community case study in rural Guatemala," *Frontiers in Public Health*, vol. 5, article 111, 2017.

28

Maternal Mortality in Dodoma Regional Referral Hospital, Tanzania

Mzee M. Nassoro,[1] Paul Chetto,[1] Enid Chiwanga,[1] Athanase Lilungulu,[2] Deogratius Bintabara,[3] and Jacquiline Wambura[1]

[1]*Department of Obstetrics and Gynaecology, Dodoma Regional Referral Hospital, Dodoma, Tanzania*
[2]*Department of Obstetrics and Gynaecology, University of Dodoma, College of Health Sciences, Dodoma, Tanzania*
[3]*Department of Public Health, College of Health Sciences, University of Dodoma, Dodoma, Tanzania*

Correspondence should be addressed to Mzee M. Nassoro; mzeemasumbuko@gmail.com

Academic Editor: Daniel Vaiman

Background. Maternal mortality has remained a challenge in Tanzania. The Tanzania Demographic and Health Survey 2015-16 has shown that the problem has been increasing despite various strategies instituted to curb it. It has been shown that most of the maternal deaths occurring in health facilities, whether direct or indirect, have other contributing factors. The objective of this study was to analyse causes and associated factors for maternal deaths in Dodoma Regional Referral Hospital (DRRH). *Methods.* A retrospective review of all files of the women who died in 2018 and were classified as maternal deaths. *Results.* A total of 8722 women gave birth in DRRH, out of which 35 died and were confirmed as maternal deaths. The number of live births was 8404 making the maternal mortality ratio of 417 per 100,000 live births. The leading causes of maternal death were eclampsia (9), sepsis (6), ruptured uterus (5), and haemorrhage (5). The third-phase delay was the leading contributing factor to 19 maternal deaths. This includes delays in referral from another facility as well as delays in getting treatment at DRRH and inadequate skills of providers at both the referring facilities and DRRH. The first-phase and second-phase delays contributed to 7 and 6 deaths, respectively. Furthermore, poor antenatal care contributed to 2 deaths. *Conclusion.* Maternal mortality is still high in Dodoma Regional Referral Hospital. Eclampsia was the leading cause of maternal deaths in 2018 followed by sepsis and obstetric haemorrhage. Delays associated with health system factors (third-phase delay) contributed much more to maternal mortality than the first-phase delay. Mentorship programmes on management of obstetric complications need to be instituted in order to reduce maternal deaths in Dodoma Regional Referral Hospital.

1. Introduction

The World Health Organisation defines maternal death as death of a woman while pregnant or within 42 days of termination of pregnancy, irrespective of the duration and site of the pregnancy, from any cause related to or aggravated by the pregnancy or its management but not from accidental or incidental causes [1]. In this context, one has to be conversant with identifying such deaths; otherwise, there might be undernotification of maternal deaths in health facilities where a woman of reproductive age may die in a medical or surgical ward with an undiagnosed obstetric complication.

Maternal death is an indicator of a poor quality of care. It is for this reason that reduction of these deaths has been a global and national agenda for all countries. During the era of MDGs, goal number 5 was to improve maternal health whereby target number one was to reduce maternal deaths by three-quarters between 1995 and 2015. This target was generally not achieved because there was only 44% decline in the global maternal mortality ratio from 384 to 216 for every 100,000 live births. Ninety-nine percent of these deaths occur in low-income countries and half of these in sub-Saharan Africa [2, 3]. In these countries, the risk of women dying of pregnancy-related complications is 1 in 180, compared to 1 in 4900 for high-income countries [3].

In Tanzania, trends of maternal mortality have remained high. According to TDHS which uses the sisterhood method to estimate maternal mortality, the ratio was 578 per 100,000 live births in 2004-2005 which went down slightly to 454 per 100,000 live births in 2010. However, in TDHS-MIS 2015-16, the ratio had again gone up to 556 per 100,000 live births, a trend which shows that strategies for reduction of maternal mortality have not worked [4, 5].

Dodoma region has been implementing several strategies to reduce maternal deaths as directed in Tanzania Maternal and Perinatal Death Surveillance and Response guidelines, including notifying these deaths within 48 hours and discussing them within 7 days. During such discussions, action plans are devised for identified gaps. In the year 2018, there were 68 maternal deaths recorded in the region, which was 8 more deaths from those of 2017 [6]. Thirty-five of these women died at DRRH.

When complications arise, immediate and appropriate interventions are needed to save the women. By virtue of its status of being a referral centre for the whole region, DRRH sometimes receives women in late stages of obstetric complications due to delays either from home or referring health facilities where care was inadequate. These delays can be categorised in three areas as depicted by Sereen Thaddeus and Deborah Maine. The first-phase delay is at the family level where there is late decision to seek care. This can be due to lack of knowledge of the danger signs, lack of funds to transport the woman to a health facility, or inability of the woman to decide as to where she wants to give birth. The second-phase delay is on the way to reach the health facility. This can be due to lack of transport to a health facility or bad roads. The third-phase delay is when the woman cannot get immediate and adequate care at a health facility either due to shortage or inadequate skills of the staff and shortage of equipment, medicine, or medical supplies [7]. A delayed referral from one health facility to another is also classified as a third-phase delay. These delays are the main contributing factors to maternal deaths. Research has shown that most of the maternal deaths in Tanzania are due to the third-phase delays [8].

As per national guidelines, maternal deaths occurring in DRRH are discussed in order to identify the causes and delays. Unfortunately, these sessions are not attended by all members as outlined in the guidelines on Maternal and Perinatal Death Surveillance and Response. This makes follow-up on the action plans to be difficult. Moreover, no annual analysis of causes of these deaths has ever been done. Despite the small numbers that had occurred in the year 2018, we have decided to make this analysis on the causes and the associated factors and suggest interventions which can help the hospital in reducing these deaths because every one of them counts.

2. Methods

2.1. Study Design. This is a retrospective case review of all maternal deaths that occurred in Dodoma Regional Referral Hospital in 2018.

2.2. Study Setting. The study setting was at Dodoma Regional Referral Hospital in Dodoma city. This is the oldest public hospital in Dodoma region serving as a referral centre for all councils in Dodoma with a population of 2.2 million people. It also serves patients from neighbouring districts of neighbouring regions (Gairo, Morogoro; Kiteto, Manyara; and Manyoni, Singida).

The obstetrics and gynaecology department has five units, namely, antenatal ward, labour and delivery ward, postnatal ward, postcaesarean section ward, and gynaecological ward. There is also a theatre specifically for obstetrics and gynaecology and an intensive care unit which is shared by all departments.

The antenatal and postnatal wards are under the same roof with 32 beds. This ward admits pregnant women at gestation age of 28 weeks onwards with pregnancy-related or any other illness as well as postnatal women with their newborns. The labour and delivery ward admits women in labour either from home, from the antenatal ward, or from other health facilities. There are 5 delivery rooms at the labour ward with 5 delivery beds.

The postcaesarean section ward has 32 beds. It admits patients who had delivered by caesarean section or patients with postpartum complications either from home or from other facilities.

When a patient with obstetric or gynaecological problem is very sick, she is kept in the intensive care unit where doctors from the obstetrics and gynaecology department visit her during the rounds.

The department of obstetrics and gynaecology has five specialists and three registrars. There are also intern doctors who rotate in the department after every three months. The nursing staff consists of registered nurses and nurse midwives. Total deliveries range from 30 to 40 in 24 hours with a caesarean section rate of 22%.

In early November 2018, the department shifted to a new building where all units are now under one roof.

2.3. Data Collection. In DRRH, all maternal death files are kept under lock and key after being discussed in Maternal and Perinatal Death Surveillance and Response meetings. The nurse in charge of the department is the custodian of the keys to that locker. All maternal death files from 1st January 2018 to 31st December 2018 were retrieved and analysed. A checklist was used to collect information from the case files. The information collected included age, education status, parity, number of live births, marital status, booking status, referral status, referral diagnosis, length of hospital stay, mode of delivery, interventions in the hospital before death, cause of death, and associated factors.

2.4. Data Analysis. Data collected was entered into a computer using Excel programme, and analysis of the entered data was made.

2.5. Ethical Considerations. This review was approved by the Dodoma Regional Referral Hospital research committee. Anonymity of the deceased was maintained as required by guidelines when discussing maternal deaths.

3. Results

During the year 2018, a total of 8722 women delivered at DRRH and out of them 35 died and were confirmed as maternal deaths. Many of the deceased were 35 years old and above, married, and peasants with no formal education. There were15 grand multipara followed by primigravida (9). Majority of them were admitted as referrals from other health facilities (32) (Table 1).

The main reasons for admission were eclampsia (9), sepsis (6), and ruptured uterus (5). Others were postpartum haemorrhage, anaemia, and peripartum cardiomyopathy, each contributing to 3 admissions. Heart disease in pregnancy, antepartum haemorrhage, abruptio placentae, and intrauterine fetal death contributed to one admission each. Two admissions were due to abortion complications. The leading causes of maternal death were eclampsia (9), sepsis (6), ruptured uterus (5), and haemorrhage (5) (Table 2).

The third-phase delay (delayed referral from other facilities, delay in getting treatment in DRRH, and inadequate skills of providers at a referring facility as well as at DRRH) was the leading contributing factor to 19 maternal deaths. This was followed by delayed decision at the family level contributing to 7 deaths and delays to reach a health facility contributing to 6. Another contributing factor was poor antenatal care (2 deaths) (Table 3).

Table 1: General information.

Characteristic	Number
Number of all women who delivered	8722
Number of maternal deaths	35
Number of women who delivered at DRRH	13
Number of women who were referred after childbirth	15
Number of women who died undelivered	4
Mode of delivery at DRRH:	
SVD	2
CS	8
Laparotomy for ruptured uterus	3
Age (years)	
≤15-19	4
20-24	7
25-29	4
30-34	7
35 and above	13
Level of education	
No formal education	18
Primary	14
Secondary	1
College	2
Marital status	
Single	2
Married/cohabiting	33
Occupation	
Housewife	13
Peasant	17
Petty trade	3
Employed (formal)	2
Parity	
1	9
2	6
3	3
4	2
5+	15
Source of admission	
Home	3
Referred from another health facility	32

Of 8722 women who delivered at DRRH, there were 8404 live births and 35 maternal deaths. This makes MMR for 2018 to be 417 per 100,000 live births. Most of the deceased were of age 35 and above and with no formal education. Housewives and petty traders made majority of these women. A great majority of the women who had died were referred from other health facilities.

4. Discussion

Maternal mortality is one of the indicators of quality of care in a country and a nation as a whole. It is for this reason that it was in both the Millennium Development Goals (MDGs) and the Sustainable Development Goals (SDGs).

Various methods are used to assess maternal mortality and quality of maternity care in Tanzania. Of these, the Demographic and Health Survey has been used frequently to measure the country's progress in improving maternal and child health. However, these are community-based surveys and information is collected from relatives of the deceased [5]. Moreover, they do not seek to identify the causes of maternal deaths. On the other hand, facility-based analyses go further beyond the numbers and try to establish the cause of maternal death as well as other associated factors including gaps in provision of care and delays.

In the period of this analysis, a total of 8722 women delivered at DRRH and 35 died from causes directly or indirectly related to the pregnancy, delivery, or their management. Moreover, most of these deaths were associated with other factors. Among the deliveries, there were 8404 live births [6]. If extrapolated to the standard reporting of maternal mortality ratio, this is equal to 417 deaths for every 100,000 live births. This ratio is almost similar to that of other referral hospitals such as Shinyanga with the rate 449 per 100,000 live births in 2014 and Kilimanjaro Christian Medical Centre which was 492.1/100,000 as a ten-year trend. Comparably, the national hospital, Muhimbili, has even a higher ratio of 1541/100,000 for the year 2011 [9–11]. These ratios are high and reflect poor quality of obstetric care.

This analysis shows that majority of the deaths occurred in women aged 35 years and above (13 deaths) followed by age groups of 30 to 34 and 20 to 24, both of which contributed to 14 deaths. However, if aggregated, it is obvious that most deaths occurred in women who were 30 years and above (20 deaths). The adolescents and those aged 25 to 29 years had the least contribution to the deaths, each making

Table 2: Reason for admission and causes of death.

Reason for admission	Number
IUFD	1
Antepartum haemorrhage	1
Abruptio placentae	1
Ruptured uterus	5
PPH	3
Eclampsia	9
Sepsis	6
Anaemia in pregnancy	3
Heart disease in pregnancy	1
Abortion	2
Peripartum cardiomyopathy	3
Cause of death	
Direct causes obstetric	31
Haemorrhage	5
Ruptured uterus	5
Eclampsia	9
Sepsis	6
Abortion complications	4
Peripartum cardiomyopathy	2
Indirect causes	4
Anaemia	2
HIV and AIDS	1
Valvular heart disease	1

There were a variety of causes of admissions, but eclampsia, sepsis, and uterine rupture were the top most. However, if uterine rupture is included in the cause of death due to haemorrhage, then obstetric haemorrhages is the leading reason of admission for those who had died. All haemorrhages (obstetric haemorrhage and ruptured uterus) caused 10 maternal deaths.

Table 3: Associated factors contributing to deaths.

Factor	Number
Delayed decision at the family level	7
Delays in reaching the health facility	6
Delayed referral	6
Delay in getting treatment at DRRH	6
Inadequate skills of providers at DRRH	5
Inadequate skills of providers at a referring facility	2
Poor antenatal care	2

Delay in receiving care at the facility level was the leading associated factor. This includes delayed referral from peripheral facilities to DRRH, delayed treatment at DRRH, and inadequate skills of providers at peripheral health facilities as well as at DRRH.

up 4 deaths. This contradicts the general theory that adolescent pregnancy carries more risks of death because of more unfavourable obstetric risk factors inherent with this age group. These findings are similar to those from a study by Nove et al. and that by Blanc et al. [12, 13].

Grand multiparity has long been established as a risk factor for maternal death. In this analysis, 15 of the deceased were women who were para 5 and above. However, this finding does not correlate with those of Shinyanga Regional Referral Hospital and Muhimbili National Hospital (MNH) where the grand multipara made up 28.3 and 12.1, respectively [9, 10]. This difference could be due to numbers of grand multipara becoming pregnant, especially for big cities like Dar es Salaam.

The major cause of maternal deaths was eclampsia which was responsible for 9 of all maternal deaths. This corresponds to the findings in a study conducted at Bugando hospital in Mwanza where severe preeclampsia and eclampsia caused the majority of deaths [14]. Deaths from eclampsia can be prevented at different levels in the continuum of obstetric care. At the antenatal clinic, blood pressure recordings and urinalysis for proteinuria can identify women with hypertensive disorders and appropriate management can be initiated before worsening of the condition and leading to eclampsia and possible death. However, this is not the case in most of the antenatal clinics in Dodoma. Inadequate antenatal care in detection of hypertensive disorders of pregnancy has also been reported in a research conducted in Dar es Salaam [15].

The prevailing situation in Dodoma is that of unavailability of sphygmomanometers in most of the antenatal clinics where most pregnant women with hypertensive disorders in pregnancy are missed. There is also shortage of these machines in the antenatal and labour wards of some of the lower health facilities leading to delays in identifying women with hypertensive disorders in pregnancy. Furthermore, all facilities caring for pregnant women are supposed to have staff trained in seven signal functions of basic emergency obstetrics and newborn care, one of which is to administer magnesium sulphate for prevention or treatment of eclampsia. However, shortage of skilled staff has had a negative effect on this intervention which is further compounded by delayed referrals of eclamptic patients.

Sepsis caused 6 of maternal deaths at Dodoma Regional Referral Hospital in 2018. This complication occurs if principles of infection prevention and control are not adhered to during provision of obstetric care. In their study on causes and risk factors for maternal mortality in rural Tanzania, Illah et al. found that sepsis was among the top 3 causes of maternal mortality in Rufiji district. In another study conducted at MNH, sepsis ranked fourth in direct causes of maternal deaths [10, 16].

These findings underscore the importance of ensuring that all health care workers attending pregnant and delivering women should strictly adhere to the infection prevention and control practices.

Obstetric haemorrhage and ruptured uterus contributed to 5 deaths each. Despite several interventions in place to prevent and treat obstetric haemorrhage, deaths caused by this condition have become persistent. In the Global Burden of Disease study conducted in 2015, Kassebaum et al. found that obstetric haemorrhage was the leading cause of direct maternal deaths worldwide [17]. In another study conducted in Ifakara, Tanzania, obstetric haemorrhage ranked second as a cause of maternal death [18]. As haemorrhage due to uterine atony is the leading cause of all obstetric haemorrhages, the hospital needs to ensure that active management of the third stage of labour is instituted to every woman during delivery.

Likewise, the health care workers should always be ready and work as a team to intervene in an event of obstetric haemorrhage. This can be achieved if every health care worker at the maternity ward is taught simple life-saving manoeuvres such as abdominal aortic compression, bimanual compression of the uterus, and intrauterine balloon tamponade. There should also be a standard operating procedure for following up women who underwent emergency obstetric surgeries. Availability of safe blood at any time cannot be overemphasised.

Uterine rupture causes death due to haemorrhage. Grand multiparity, fetal malposition, malpresentation, and fetopelvic disproportion are risk factors for uterine rupture especially in grand multipara. A previous uterine scar is another significant predisposing cause for uterine rupture. In this analysis, all maternal deaths caused by uterine rupture either had been referred from other facilities or were from home where they had been labouring for more than 24 hours. There is a need to educate multiparous women as well as those with previous uterine scars not to try to deliver at home. The antenatal clinics and facilities without operating theatres should refer patients with risks of uterine rupture much earlier to higher facilities for continuum of care. The use of partograph should also be emphasised in order to detect any deviation in the progress of labour and take appropriate action.

Complications of abortion still have a significant contribution to maternal deaths. In this analysis, 4 women died from such complications. There were no clues as to whether these abortions were induced or not. These findings are similar to those of Shinyanga Regional Referral Hospital and MNH though with different frequencies [9, 10]. They also correspond to the findings of a study on patterns of hospital-based maternal mortality in Tanzania conducted by Bwana et al. [19].

The third-phase delay, which occurs at the health facility level, contributed to most of the deaths which occurred at DRRH. Delayed referral from the other health facilities, delay in getting treatment at DRRH, inadequate skills of providers at a referring facility, and inadequate skills of providers at DRRH are all third-phase delays. Although delayed referral from another facility could be due to unavailability of transport, the health care providers may also lack the ability to realise the criteria needing referral for continuation of care that is not available at that particular lower facility. This could be contributed to shortage of experienced staff because currently there are so many newly employed health care providers working in lower level facilities. Apart from delayed referral, inadequate skills of a health care provider also contributed to deaths. In one of the cases, a poorly repaired lower segment of the uterus continued bleeding and the patient arrived late at DRRH. Deaths due to inadequate skills also occurred in DRRH where in some of the deaths a junior doctor performing caesarean section failed to control bleeding in uterine atony which led to subtotal hysterectomy; unfortunately, the woman died. In their analysis of maternal deaths in Hunan province in China, Lili et al. also found that improper knowledge and skills of county institutions contributed to most of the avoidable maternal deaths [20]. In another study on contributing factors to maternal deaths in health facilities conducted in Nigeria, Burkina Faso, Gambia, Guinea, Senegal, and Sierra Leone, the third delay was found to have a significant contribution [21]. These findings emphasise the importance of adequate skilled staff and availability of equipment in order to prevent avoidable maternal deaths. Availability of means of transport for timely referral is also of paramount importance.

In this analysis, delayed decision at the family level (first-phase delay) contributed to only 7 maternal deaths. This contribution is lower compared to other studies. In a study conducted in Varanasi, India, the first delay was found to have caused 90% of maternal deaths which occurred in that area [22]. Though we could not find the reasons for the first-phase delay in our setting, a study conducted in Bangladesh identified several causes such as delivery conducted by the untrained birth attendant or family members, delays in understanding about maternal complications, delays in decision-making to transfer the mother, and lack of proper knowledge and education, and traditional myth influenced the maternal deaths [23]. These reasons are closely related to lack of women empowerment and also contributed to the delay in reaching a health facility which, in our study, caused 6 deaths. Further contributors to the delay in reaching health facility were lack of funds and transport. Continued advocacy, incentives to traditional birth attendants to bring pregnant women to health facilities, and individual birth plans may reduce maternal deaths caused by the first- and second-phase delays.

5. Conclusion

Maternal mortality is still high in Dodoma Regional Referral Hospital. Eclampsia, sepsis, and obstetric haemorrhage were the leading causes. Delays associated with health system factors (third-phase delay) contributed much more to the maternal deaths than the delay in decision-making at a family level (first delay). Delayed referral from other health facilities, delay in getting treatment at DRRH, and inadequate skills of providers at both DRRH and referring facilities have been featured out as the leading associated factors. In order to reduce these delays, timely feedback to all referring facilities needs to be strengthened as well as mentorship programmes to health care workers of these facilities. The hospital should conduct job trainings and regular drills on management of all obstetric emergencies. The senior doctors should also supervise the junior doctors, especially in women with obstetric emergencies requiring surgical intervention. The antenatal, postnatal, and labour wards should have trays with all medicine and medical supplies essential for management of obstetric emergencies such as haemorrhage and eclampsia. All lower health facilities should have clearly structured referral protocols for transportation of women with obstetric emergencies to Dodoma Regional Referral Hospital. A further study on trends of maternal deaths at this hospital is needed to follow up on progress of the interventions instituted.

Authors' Contributions

Mzee M. Nassoro conceptualised the study while Paul Chetto, Enid Chiwanga, Athanase Lilungulu, and Deogratius Bintabara reviewed the manuscript. Jacquiline Wambura assisted in availing the files and in data collection.

Acknowledgments

We acknowledge the assistance provided by the nurse in charge of the maternity block at Dodoma Regional Referral Hospital and the staff.

References

[1] WHO, *International statistical classification of diseases and related health problems. Tenth revision*, WHO, Geneva, 1992.

[2] World Health Organisation, UNICEF, and United Nations Population Fund and the World Bank, *Trends in Maternal Mortality: 1990 to 2015*, WHO, Geneva, 2015.

[3] UN Maternal Mortality Estimation Inter Agency Group, "Global, regional and national levels trends in maternal mortality between 1990 and 2015, with scenario based projections to 2030; a systematic analysis".

[4] National Bureau of Statics, *Dar es Salaam Tanzania; Tanzania Demographic and Health Survey 2010*, ICF Macro Calverton, Maryland, USA, 2011.

[5] Ministry of Health, Community Development, Gender, Elderly and Children(MoHCDGEC), Ministry of Health Zanzibar, National Bureau of Statistics (NBS), Office of the Chief Government Statistician (OCGS) and ICF, *2015 - 16 TDHS-MIS Key Findings*, MoHCDGEC, MoH, NBS, OCGS and ICF, Rockville, Maryland, USA, 2016.

[6] Dodoma Regional Health Management Team, "Reproductive and Child Health Coordinator's report, 2018".

[7] S. Thaddeus and D. Maine, "Too far to walk: maternal mortality in context," *Social Science & Medicine*, vol. 38, no. 8, pp. 1091–1110, 1994.

[8] E. Urassa, S. Massawe, H. Mgaya, G. Lindmark, and L. Nyström, "Female mortality in reproductive ages in Dar es Salaam, Tanzania," *East African Medical Journal*, vol. 71, no. 4, pp. 226–231, 1994.

[9] O. E. Mapunda, S. E. Msuya, N. A. Kapologwe, B. John, D. J. Damian, and M. J. Mahande, "Assessment of maternal mortality and its associated causes at Shinyanga Regional Hospital in Tanzania," *Women's Health Bulletin*, vol. 4, no. 2, 2016.

[10] A. B. Pembe, C. Paulo, B. S. D'mello, and J. van Roosmalen, "Maternal mortality at Muhimbili National Hospital in Dar-es-Salaam, Tanzania in the year 2011," *BMC Pregnancy and Childbirth*, vol. 14, no. 1, 2014.

[11] E. W. Maro, N. R. Mosha, M. J. Mahande, J. Obure, and G. Masenga, "Ten years trend in maternal mortality at Kilimanjaro Christian Medical Center Tanzania, 2003–2012: a descriptive retrospective tertiary hospital based study," *Asian Pacific Journal of Reproduction*, vol. 5, no. 3, pp. 214–220, 2016.

[12] A. Nove, Z. Matthews, S. Neal, and A. V. Camacho, "Maternal mortality in adolescents compared with women of other ages: evidence from 144 countries," *The Lancet Global Health*, vol. 2, no. 3, pp. e155–e164, 2014.

[13] A. K. Blanc, W. Winfrey, and J. Ross, "New Findings for Maternal Mortality Age Patterns: Aggregated Results for 38 Countries," *PLoS One*, vol. 8, no. 4, article e59864, 2013.

[14] M. Magoma, A. Massinde, C. Majinge, R. Rumanyika, A. Kihunrwa, and B. Gomodoka, "Maternal death reviews at Bugando Hospital north-western Tanzania: a 2008–2012 retrospective analysis," *BMC Pregnancy and Childbirth*, vol. 15, no. 1, 2015.

[15] D. P. Urassa, A. Carlstedt, L. Nyström, S. N. Massawe, and G. Lindmark, "Eclampsia in Dar es Salaam, Tanzania — incidence, outcome, and the role of antenatal care," *Acta Obstetricia et Gynecologica Scandinavica*, vol. 85, no. 5, pp. 571–578, 2006.

[16] E. Illah, G. Mbaruku, H. Masanja, and K. Kahn, "Causes and risk factors for maternal mortality in rural Tanzania-case of Rufiji Health and Demographic Surveillance Site (HDSS)," *African Journal of Reproductive Health*, vol. 17, no. 3, pp. 119–130, 2013.

[17] Global Burden of Disease 2015 Maternal mortality collaborators, "Global, regional, and national levels of maternal mortality, 1990–2015: a systematic analysis for the Global Burden of Disease Study 2015," *The Lancet*, vol. 388, no. 10053, pp. 1775–1812, 2016.

[18] A. K. Manyeh, R. Nathan, and G. Nelson, "Maternal mortality in Ifakara health and demographic surveillance system: spatial patterns, trends and risk factors, 2006 - 2010," *PLoS One*, vol. 13, no. 10, article e0205370, 2018.

[19] V. M. Bwana, S. F. Rumisha, I. R. Mremi, E. P. Lyimo, and L. E. G. Mboera, "Patterns and causes of hospital maternal mortality in Tanzania: a 10-year retrospective analysis," *PLoS ONE*, vol. 14, no. 4, article e0214807.

[20] X. Lili, H. Jian, Z. Mengjun et al., "Epidemiological analysis of maternal deaths in Hunan province in China between 2009 and 2014," *PLoS One*, vol. 13, no. 11, article e0207920, 2018.

[21] N. Gunawardena, G. Bishwajit, and S. Yaya, "Facility-based maternal death in Western Africa: a systematic review," *Frontiers in Public Health*, vol. 6, p. 48, 2018.

[22] K. Kumari, R. K. Srivastava, M. Srivastava, and N. Purwar, "Maternal mortality in rural Varanasi: delays, causes, and contributing factors," *Indian Journal of Community Medicine*, vol. 44, no. 1, pp. 26–30, 2019.

[23] A. Biswas, M. A. Halim, K. Dalal, and F. Rahman, "Exploration of social factors associated to maternal deaths due to haemorrhage and convulsions: analysis of 28 social autopsies in rural Bangladesh," *BMC Health Services Research*, vol. 16, no. 1, p. 659, 2016.

29

Dysmenorrhea among University Health Science Students, Northern Ethiopia: Impact and Associated Factors

Teshager Aklilu Yesuf, Nigist Assefa Eshete, and Eskinder Ayalew Sisay

Department of Pharmacy, College of Health Sciences, Mekelle University, P.O. Box 1871, Mekelle, Ethiopia

Correspondence should be addressed to Teshager Aklilu Yesuf; teshe27@gmail.com

Academic Editor: Robert Gaspar

Background. It is estimated that more than half of all women in adolescence age suffer from dysmenorrhea and it often interferes with their daily physical and emotional aspects. It is the leading cause of short-term school absenteeism and is associated with a negative impact on academic and daily activities. *Objectives.* To investigate impacts of dysmenorrhea, factors associated with it, and its self-management strategies used by health science students. *Methods.* A cross-sectional institution based study was conducted among 246 Mekelle University health science students selected by stratified random sampling technique. Data were collected using self-administered semistructured questionnaire. Data were analyzed using SPSS 16. *Results.* The prevalence of dysmenorrhea was 71.8%. Participants who had long menstrual cycle interval, long menses flows, and positive family history and who were alcohol users were more likely to had dysmenorrhea. Participants reported that 28.6% feel depressed, 16.2% are absent from class, and 22.9% had poor personal relationship due to dysmenorrhea and 78.2% of them practiced self-medication. *Conclusion.* Dysmenorrhea is common among Mekelle University health science students and it is major problem representing the cause of feeling depressed, poor personal relationship, and class absenteeism. Majority of the study participants used self-medication to treat dysmenorrhea.

1. Introduction

The term dysmenorrhea refers to severe painful cramping sensation in the lower abdomen often accompanied by sweating, tachycardia, headache, nausea, vomiting, diarrhea, and tremulousness occurring just before or during the menses. It is a common gynecological problem among adolescent females which is severe enough to affect their functioning [1–3].

Since the pain results from uterine vasoconstriction and contractions mediated by prostaglandins, the most reliable and effective treatment of dysmenorrhea is to inhibit prostaglandin synthesis using nonsteroidal anti-inflammatory drugs (NSAIDs) [4]. If symptoms do not respond to NSAIDs for three menstrual periods, combined oral contraceptive pills for three menstrual cycles can be tried [5, 6].

Several studies have shown that prevalence of dysmenorrhea varies greatly depending on methods of data collection. According to a study done in Jordan, the prevalence of dysmenorrhea was 90.1% [7]. In China, dysmenorrhea occurred on 37% of the menstrual dates on average and was unrelated to irregularity of menstrual cycles [8]. The symptoms of primary dysmenorrhea begin a few hours before menstruation begins and may peak during the heaviest flow during menstruation [9]; the most common symptoms are stomach cramp (78.0%), backache (58.9%), and mood change (56.9%) [10].

Younger age, low body mass index, smoking, early menarche, prolonged or aberrant menstrual flow, premenstrual somatic complaints, pelvic infections, psychological disturbance, genetic influence, and a history of sexual assault influence the prevalence and severity of dysmenorrhea [3, 11]. A study conducted in Jordan indicated that underweight, having a low family income, living in a rural area, and family history of dysmenorrhea were associated with dysmenorrhea [9]. A study conducted in Vietnam showed mean age and age at menarche, educational status, and religion were associated with dysmenorrhea [12]. A study conducted in Turkey showed that dysmenorrhea was significantly higher in coffee consumers, females with menstrual bleeding duration greater than or equal to seven days, and those who had a family history of dysmenorrhea [13]. Prevalence of dysmenorrhea decreased with increase in age [14, 15]. An experimental study conducted in Iran showed that regular physical activity significantly reduced dysmenorrhea [16].

Dysmenorrhea affects the physical, psychological, and social status of female adolescents. According to study conducted in India among female medical students who reported dysmenorrhea, 31.67% and 8.68% were frequently missing college and classes, respectively [17]. A study done in South India showed that ibuprofen was taken by 80.95% of students [2] while a study done in Taiwan and Ghana showed that paracetamol was the most effective strategies in relieving dysmenorrhea [15, 18]. According to Egyptian study, fresh ginger was effective in relieving menstrual pain [19].

The objective of this study was to determine the prevalence of dysmenorrhea and assess its impact and management strategies used among Mekelle University health science students.

2. Methods and Participants

2.1. Study Design. A cross-sectional study was conducted from April to May 2014 in Mekelle University, College of Health Sciences, Northern Ethiopia. There were a total of 535 health science female students (medicine, pharmacy, public health, nursing, and dentistry). Considering 95% confidence interval, 5% margin of error, 10% contingency for nonresponse rate, and 50% expected prevalence of dysmenorrhea, a sample of 246 students was calculated using single proportion formula. A two-step stratified random sampling technique was used to select study participants: sampling from each department and then sampling from each academic year based on appropriate proportion of the respective field of study.

Pretested self-administered semistructured questionnaire which was prepared in English was used to collect data. Ethical clearance was obtained from the institutional review board of Mekelle University and consent was sought from each participant. Data were coded and entered using SPSS 16 (SPSS Inc., Chicago, USA) for analysis. Frequencies, means, and standard deviations were calculated where appropriate for each of the variables. Binary logistic regression was done to determine factors associated with dysmenorrhea and p value less than 0.05 was considered statistically significant.

3. Results

3.1. Participants' Background Information. Out of a total of 246 participants recruited to the study, 4 were excluded because of failure to complete the questionnaire, resulting in a response rate of 98%. The mean age of the study participants was 20.5 ± 1.16 years. Most participants were freshman accounting 74 (30.6%) (Table 1).

Majority of participants 173 (71.8%) experienced dysmenorrhea. More than half of the students (54.4%) reported having a family history of dysmenorrhea (Table 2).

Multivariate logistic regression analysis showed that field of study, alcohol use, family history of dysmenorrhea, and duration of menses flow as well as menstrual cycle interval were significantly associated with dysmenorrhea (Table 3).

Most participants have lower abdominal pain (67%). The majority of participants who had dysmenorrhea experienced

TABLE 1: Demographic characteristics of participants.

Variables	Frequency	Percent
Department		
Medicine	95	39.3
Pharmacy	24	9.9
Public health	25	10.3
Nursing	81	33.5
Dentistry	17	7.0
Academic year		
First year	74	30.6
Second year	56	23.1
Third year	70	28.9
Fourth Year	36	14.9
Fifth year	6	2.5
Religion		
Orthodox	179	74.0
Muslim	28	11.6
Protestant	31	12.8
Other	4	1.7
Marital status		
Unmarried	222	92.9
Married	17	7.1
Mothers' educational level		
Unable to read and write	26	11.0
Able to read and write	65	27.4
High school	40	16.9
Diploma and above	106	44.7

TABLE 2: Menstrual characteristics of participants, 2014.

Variable	Frequency	Percent
Menstruation cycle		
21 days or less	37	15.4
23 to 34 days	188	78.3
35 or greater days	15	6.2
Menstruation cycle regularity		
Regular	163	67.4
Irregular	79	32.6
Menstruation bleeding duration		
2-3 days	54	22.4
4-5 days	155	64.3
6-7 days	32	13.3
Experience of dysmenorrhea		
Yes	173	71.8
No	68	28.2
Family history of dysmenorrhea		
Yes	129	54.4
No	108	45.6

TABLE 3: Factors associated with dysmenorrhea, 2014.

Variables	AOR (95.0% CI)	p value
Field of study		**0.047***
Medicine	Reference	
Pharmacy	1.95 (0.479, 7.90)	0.352
Public health	1.86 (0.55, 6.30)	0.321
Nursing	0.52 (0.19, 1.38)	0.188
Dentistry	0.05 (0.01, 0.85)	0.039
Alcohol use		**0.016***
Yes	0.06 (0.01, 0.59)	
No	Reference	
Menstrual cycle		**0.030***
Less than or equal to 21 days	5.62 (1.01, 31.37)	0.049
22–34 days	1.36 (0.31, 5.99)	0.685
Greater than or equal to 35 days	Reference	
Duration of menses		**0.033***
2-3 days	4.20 (1.01, 17.61)	0.050
4-5 days	1.34 (0.36, 5.01)	0.663
6-7 days	Reference	
Family history of dysmenorrhea		**0.001***
Yes	0.27 (0.13, 0.59)	
No	Reference	
Constant	0.06	0.529

*Statistically significant at p value < 0.05; AOR: adjusted odds ratio.

TABLE 4: Dysmenorrhea associated symptoms and sites of pain, 2014.

Symptoms	Frequency	Percent
Lower abdominal pain	163	67.4
Back pain	126	52.0
Thigh pain	20	8.3
Headache	94	19.8
Dizziness	131	27.5
Nausea, vomiting, and diarrhea	50	10.5
Decreased concentration	87	18.3
Loss of appetite	114	23.9

their symptoms at the onset of menstruation flow (36.4%). Dizziness was the commonest associated symptom, reported by 27.5% respondents, and loss of appetite was the second commonest associated symptom reported by 23.9% respondents (Table 4).

Most participants, 225 (94.1%), did not smoke cigarettes. There were 27 (11.2%) participants who use alcohol. Majority of participants, 137 (56.8%), in this study have habit of drinking coffee. Participants reported that 28.6% of them feel depressed, 16.2% were absent from class, and 22.9% had poor personal relationship because of dysmenorrhea (Table 5).

Ibuprofen was used by 48% of participants. The majorities of the study participants use bed rest (33.6%) and drink more water or tea (31.6%) as a homemade remedy for dysmenorrhea (Table 6).

TABLE 5: Impacts of menstrual pain, 2014.

Impact of menstrual pain	Frequency	Percent
Poor concentration at class	62	11.0
Absent from class	91	16.2
Poor personal relationship	129	22.9
Feel depressed	161	28.6
Limitation of sleeping	36	6.5
Limit your exercise	83	14.8

TABLE 6: Medications and home remedies used for managing dysmenorrhea, 2014.

Management strategies	Frequency	Percent
Ibuprofen	137	48.0
Paracetamol	34	12
Diclofenac	72	25.3
Oral contraceptive pills	2	0.7
Apply pad	71	16
Bed rest	150	33.6
Drink more water or tea	141	31.6
Massage the site of pain	69	15.5
Drink different fluids such as soft drinks especially coca cola	15	3.4
None	40	14

4. Discussion

In this study, the prevalence of dysmenorrhea was 71.8%. This is similar to what is previously reported by Ghanaian adolescent girls, 74.4% [18]. But dysmenorrhea was diagnosed based solely on a girls' perception of pain, which is difficult to quantify and could be related to nonmenstrual events.

Previous studies showed that the prevalence of dysmenorrhea decreases with increasing age and it is significantly associated with early age of menarche [3, 10, 11]. But age at first menarche had no association in our study. Length of menstrual cycle ($p = 0.03$) and duration of menses ($p = 0.033$) were found to be associated with dysmenorrhea. In China, increased menstrual flows (median 4 days and $p < 0.05$) have been reported to be associated with an increase in the severity of dysmenorrhea [8].

Positive family history of dysmenorrhea ($p < 0.01$) was significantly associated with dysmenorrhea. A similar result was obtained from India [2]. The fact that family history was shown to be a risk factor for dysmenorrhea may be related to the risk for related conditions such as endometriosis and genetic factors [13]. Alcohol drinking was also associated with dysmenorrhea ($p = 0.016$). In this study, regular exercise was not associated with experience of dysmenorrhea. But an experimental study done in Turkey found that participating in physical activity decreased the length of menstruation pain and volume of bleeding [16]. Menstrual pain may result from increased contraction of uterine muscle which is innervated by the sympathetic nervous system. Stress is supposed to increase the sympathetic activity which may lead to the increase of menstrual pain by enhancing the intensity of uterine contraction. So, due to the fact that exercise reduces stress, the sympathetic activity may be decreased. Physical activity also leads to the release of endorphins which are produced by brain and may enhance the pain threshold [16].

Dysmenorrhea is a cause of recurrent short-term school absenteeism in adolescent girls and a cause of work absenteeism in women of reproductive age. An estimated 10–15% of women experience monthly menstrual pain severe enough to prevent normal daily function at school, work, or home [18]. In this study, 28.6% of participants reported they feel depressed which could affect their concentration in class and 16.2% of them reported missing classes. Although dysmenorrhea is not a life-threatening condition on its own, monthly recurrence of severe symptoms represents a significant morbidity.

Primary dysmenorrhea is attributable to increased endometrial synthesis of prostaglandins during menstruation. About 2–4 days before the onset of menstruation, prostaglandins proceed into the uterine muscle and cause uterine contractions that help in the expulsion of the endometrium. NSAIDs are the best established initial therapy for dysmenorrhea as they have direct analgesic effect through inhibition of prostaglandin synthesis and they also decrease the volume of menstrual flow [2]. The practice of self-medication appears to be widespread in the adolescent population with dysmenorrhea. In this study, 78.2% of participants reported self-medication. This result is higher than findings from Ghana (51.5%) [18]. Only 5.8% of the study participants had consulted a physician in our study.

NSAIDs are highly effective in treating dysmenorrhea when they are taken before the onset of menses and continued through day two [18]. But our finding indicated that 73.7% of participants reported taking these medications when pain starts indicating the need for professional consultation.

5. Conclusion

Dysmenorrhea is a major problem representing the leading cause of class absenteeism. Females with long menstrual bleeding duration and long menstrual cycle interval, positive family history of dysmenorrhea, and alcohol drinking habit are more likely to experience dysmenorrhea. It is very important to create awareness about the causes and treatment of dysmenorrhea via the education system and media. Health professional consultation must be promoted to help students who have dysmenorrhea.

References

[1] M. Poureslami and F. Osati-Ashtiani, "Assessing knowledge, attitudes, and behavior of adolescent girls in suburban districts of Tehran about dysmenorrhea and menstrual hygiene," *Journal of International Women's Studies*, vol. 3, no. 2, pp. 51–61, 2002.

[2] B. Kiran, T. Sandozi, L. Akila, A. Chakraborty, Meherban, and RJ. Rani, "Study of the prevalence, severity and treatment of dysmenorrhea in medical and nursing students," *International Journal of Pharma and Bio Sciences*, vol. 3, no. 1, pp. 161–170, 2012.

[3] E. M. Mohamed, "Epidemiology of dysmenorrhea among adolescent students," *Life Science Journal*, vol. 9, no. 1, pp. 348–353, 2012.

[4] R. N. Okoro, H. Malgwi, C. K. Ngong, and G. O. Okoro, "Dysmenorrhoea: ways of management among nigerian university students," *Actual Gynecology and Obstetrics*, vol. 4, pp. 106–113, 2012.

[5] C. Liong, "The association of primary dysmenorrhea with the perception of pain, work stress and lifestyles of nurses," *Hong Kong Medical Journal*, vol. 23, no. 5, pp. 267–272, 2010.

[6] A. K. Gupta, A. K. Jaiswal, and S. Kumar, "Assessment of university campus student's awareness and attitude towards analgesics (NSAIDS)," *Journal of Pharmaceutical Sciences and Research*, vol. 5, no. 2, pp. 612–618, 2014.

[7] T. L. Mukattash, L. Tahaineh, N. AlRawi, A. Jarab, H. Hammad, and K. Nuseir, "Behaviors and attitudes towards dysmenorrhea; a crosssectional survey of 2,000 jordanian university students," *Jordan Medical Journal*, vol. 47, no. 1, pp. 26–34, 2013.

[8] H. Zhou, Z. Yang, and S. Group, "Prevalence of dysmenorrhea in female students in a Chinese university: a prospective study," *Health*, vol. 2, no. 4, pp. 311–314, 2010.

[9] J. E. Memmott, *The Effect of Music-Assisted Progressive Muscle Relaxation on the Self-Reported Symptoms of Women with*

Primary Dysmenorrhoea, The University of Kansas, 2009, http://dissertations.umi.com/ku:10242.

[10] K. Tangchai, V. Titapant, and D. Boriboonhirunsarn, "Dysmenorrhea in thai adolescents: prevalence, impact and knowledge of treatment," *Journal of the Medical Association of Thailand*, vol. 87, supplement 3, pp. S69–S73, 2004.

[11] F.-F. Chung, C.-C. C. Yao, and G.-H. Wan, "The associations between menstrual function and life style/working conditions among nurses in Taiwan," *Journal of Occupational Health*, vol. 47, no. 2, pp. 149–156, 2005.

[12] I. A. Jang, M. Y. Kim, S. R. Lee, K. A. Jeong, and H. W. Chung, "Factors related to dysmenorrhea among Vietnamese and Vietnamese marriage immigrant women in South Korea," *Obstetrics & Gynecology Science*, vol. 56, no. 4, pp. 242–248, 2013.

[13] A. Unsal, U. Ayranci, M. Tozun, G. Arslan, and E. Calik, "Prevalence of dysmenorrhea and its effect on quality of life among a group of female university students," *Upsala Journal of Medical Sciences*, vol. 115, no. 2, pp. 138–145, 2010.

[14] A. Polat, H. Celik, and B. Gurates, "Prevalence of primary dysmenorrhea in young adult female university students," *Archives of Gynecology and Obstetrics*, vol. 279, pp. 527–532, 2009.

[15] H.-F. Cheng and Y.-H. Lin, "Selection and efficacy of self-management strategies for dysmenorrhea in young Taiwanese women," *Journal of Clinical Nursing*, vol. 20, no. 7-8, pp. 1018–1025, 2011.

[16] N. Mahvash, A. Eidy, K. Mehdi, M. T. Zahra, M. Mani, and H. Shahla, "The effect of physical activity on primary dysmenorrhea of female university students," *World Applied Sciences Journal*, vol. 17, no. 10, pp. 1246–1252, 2012.

[17] S. Amita, "Prevalence and severity of dysmenorrhea among first and second year female medical students," *Indian Journal of Physiology and Pharmacology*, vol. 52, no. 4, pp. 389–397, 2008.

[18] S. Gumanga and A. Kwame, "Prevalence and severity of dysmenorrhea among some adolescent girls in a secondary school in Accra, Ghana," *Postgraduate medical journal of Ghana*, vol. 1, no. 1, 2012.

[19] H. Awed, T. El-Saidy, and T. Amro, "The use of fresh Ginger herbs as a home remedy to relieve primary dysmenorrhea," *Journal of Research in Nursing and Midwifery*, vol. 2, no. 8, pp. 104–113, 2013.

Permissions

All chapters in this book were first published by Hindawi Publishing Corporation; hereby published with permission under the Creative Commons Attribution License or equivalent. Every chapter published in this book has been scrutinized by our experts. Their significance has been extensively debated. The topics covered herein carry significant findings which will fuel the growth of the discipline. They may even be implemented as practical applications or may be referred to as a beginning point for another development.

The contributors of this book come from diverse backgrounds, making this book a truly international effort. This book will bring forth new frontiers with its revolutionizing research information and detailed analysis of the nascent developments around the world.

We would like to thank all the contributing authors for lending their expertise to make the book truly unique. They have played a crucial role in the development of this book. Without their invaluable contributions this book wouldn't have been possible. They have made vital efforts to compile up to date information on the varied aspects of this subject to make this book a valuable addition to the collection of many professionals and students.

This book was conceptualized with the vision of imparting up-to-date information and advanced data in this field. To ensure the same, a matchless editorial board was set up. Every individual on the board went through rigorous rounds of assessment to prove their worth. After which they invested a large part of their time researching and compiling the most relevant data for our readers.

The editorial board has been involved in producing this book since its inception. They have spent rigorous hours researching and exploring the diverse topics which have resulted in the successful publishing of this book. They have passed on their knowledge of decades through this book. To expedite this challenging task, the publisher supported the team at every step. A small team of assistant editors was also appointed to further simplify the editing procedure and attain best results for the readers.

Apart from the editorial board, the designing team has also invested a significant amount of their time in understanding the subject and creating the most relevant covers. They scrutinized every image to scout for the most suitable representation of the subject and create an appropriate cover for the book.

The publishing team has been an ardent support to the editorial, designing and production team. Their endless efforts to recruit the best for this project, has resulted in the accomplishment of this book. They are a veteran in the field of academics and their pool of knowledge is as vast as their experience in printing. Their expertise and guidance has proved useful at every step. Their uncompromising quality standards have made this book an exceptional effort. Their encouragement from time to time has been an inspiration for everyone.

The publisher and the editorial board hope that this book will prove to be a valuable piece of knowledge for researchers, students, practitioners and scholars across the globe.

List of Contributors

Simon Byonanuwe, Emmanuel Nzabandora, Maxwell Okello, Yarine Fajardo and Baltazar Nyongozi
Department of Obstetrics and Gynaecology, Kampala International University Teaching Hospital, Uganda

Theophilus Pius
Department of Medical Laboratory Science, Kampala International University Teaching Hospital, Uganda

David Santson Ayebare
Interdisciplinary Research & Development Center Limited, Mbarara, Uganda

Collins Atuheire
Department of Public Health, Kampala International University-Western Campus, Uganda

Wilson Mugizi
Postgraduate Studies & Research Directorate, Kampala International University-Western Campus, Uganda

Martin Nduwimana
Department of Paediatrics, Kampala International University Teaching Hospital, Uganda

Robinson Ssebuufu
Department of Surgery, Kampala International University Teaching Hospital, Uganda

Chisolum Ogechukwu Okafor and Michael Echeta Aronu
Department of Radiology, Nnamdi Azikiwe University, The Light Specialist Hospital, Nnewi Campus, Nnewi, Nigeria

Charles Ikechukwu Okafor and Ikechukwu Innocent Mbachu
Department of Obstetrics and Gynaecology, Nnamdi Azikiwe University, The Light Specialist Hospital, Nnewi Campus, Nnewi, Nigeria

Izuchukwu Christian Obionwu
Radiology Unit, The Light Specialist Hospital, Anambra State, Nnewi, Nigeria

Tariku Tesfaye Bekuma, Melese Girmaye Negero, Gemechu Kejela and Haile Bikila
Department of Public Health, Institute of Health Sciences, Wollega University, Ethiopia

Belaynesh Firrisa
Department of Nursing, Nekemte Specialized Hospital, Ethiopia

Richard Michael Blay, Nii Koney-Kwaku Koney and Benjamin Arko-Boham
Department of Anatomy, University of Ghana Medical School, College of Health Sciences, University of Ghana, Korle Bu, Accra, Ghana

Abigail Duah Pinamang and Ewurama Dedea Ampadu Owusu
Department of Medical Laboratory Sciences, School of Biomedical and Allied Health Sciences, College of Health Sciences, University of Ghana, Korle Bu, Accra, Ghana

Augustine E. Sagoe
Central Medical Laboratory, Immunology Unit, Korle-Bu Teaching Hospital, Korle Bu, Accra, Ghana

Alison Maclean, Rafah Alnafakh, Nicola Tempest and Dharani K. Hapangama
Department of Women's and Children's Health, Institute of Translational Medicine, University of Liverpool, Member of the Liverpool Health Partnership, Liverpool Women's NHS Foundation Trust, Liverpool L8 7SS, UK

Areege Kamal
Department of Women's and Children's Health, Institute of Translational Medicine, University of Liverpool, Member of the Liverpool Health Partnership, Liverpool Women's NHS Foundation Trust, Liverpool L8 7SS, UK
Pathology Department, Oncology Teaching Hospital, Baghdad Medical City, Baghdad, Iraq

Meera Adishesh
Department of Women's and Children's Health, Institute of Translational Medicine, University of Liverpool, Member of the Liverpool Health Partnership, Liverpool Women's NHS Foundation Trust, Liverpool L8 7SS, UK
Lancashire Teaching Hospitals NHS Foundation Trust, Chorley, UK

Saheed Olanrewaju Afolabi, Joy Folahan, Olalekan Agede and Olufunke Olorundare
Department of Pharmacology and Therapeutics, University of Ilorin, Ilorin, Nigeria

Adugna Dufera
Department of General Public Health, College of Medicine and Health Science, Ambo University, Ambo, West Shoa, Ethiopia

Elias Teferi Bala, Habtamu Oljira Desta and Kefyalew Taye
Department of Public Health College of Medicine and Health Science, Ambo University, Ambo, Ethiopia

Mulatu Agajie, Wagari Kelbessa, Dula Ayana and Solen Abera
Assosa University, College of Health Science, Department of Public Health, Ethiopia

Eshetu Yimer and Gizachew Yaregal
Benishangul Gumuz Regional Health Bureau, Ethiopia

Amir Muhidin
Assosa General Hospital, Ethiopia

Debebe Shaweno
School of Health and Related Research, University of Sheffield, Sheffield, England, UK

Gebrehiwot Gebremariam Weldeargeawi
Department of Public Health, College of Medicine and Health Science, Adigrat University, Ethiopia

Zenawi Negash
JSI/Research and Training Institute, Inc., Tigray, Ethiopia

Alemayehu Bayray Kahsay
School of Public Health, Mekelle University, Ethiopia

Yemane Gebremariam
School of Public Health, Mekelle University, Tigray, Ethiopia

Kidanemaryam Berhe Tekola
Department of Nutrition, School of Public Health, Mekelle University, Ethiopia

Meseret Jeldu and Temesgen Arusi
Wolkite University, Ethiopia

Tadios Asres
Saint Paul's Millennium Medical College, Ethiopia

Muluken Gunta Gutulo
Wolaita sodo univesrsity, Ethiopia

Elli Anagnostou, Despina Mavrogianni, Ilectra-Niki Prifti, Evangelia Dimitroulia, Athanasios Protopapas, Peter Drakakis and Dimitrios Loutradis
1st Department of Obstetrics and Gynecology, Division of Human Reproduction, IVF Unit, Alexandra Hospital, Medical School of National Kapodistrian University of Athens, Athens, Greece

Charles Festo, Jackline Mrema and Ester Elisaria
Department of Impact Evaluation, Health System and Policy Analysis, Ifakara Health Institute, Dar es Salaam, Tanzania

Winfrida B. Lyoba
Department of Impact Evaluation, Health System and Policy Analysis, Ifakara Health Institute, Dar es Salaam, Tanzania
Department of Global Health and Bio-Medical Sciences, College of Life Science and Bioengineering, The Nelson Mandela Institution of Science and Technology, Arusha, Tanzania

Joyce D. Mwakatoga
Department of Agricultural Extension and Community Development, College of Agriculture, Sokoine University of Agriculture, Morogoro, Tanzania

Shewangizaw Hailemariam and Amare Genetu
Department of Midwifery, College of Health Science, Mizan-Tepi University, Mizan-Teferi, Ethiopia

Ermiyas Sahile
Department of Midwifery, College of Health Science, Kotebe Metropolitan University, Addis Ababa, Ethiopia

Haileyesus Gedamu
Nursing Department, Bahir Dar University, Bahir Dar, Ethiopia

Yilkal Tafere
Public Health Department, Debretabor University, Debretabor, Ethiopia

Liyew Agenagnew
Department of Psychiatry, Faculty of Medical Sciences, Institute of Health, Jimma University, Jimma, Ethiopia

Bosena Tebeje
School of Nursing, Faculty of Health Sciences, Institute of Health, Jimma University, Jimma, Ethiopia

Ruth Tilahun
Department of Midwifery, College of Health Sciences and Medicine, Dilla University, Dilla, Ethiopia

Ifeyinwa Mary Asuzu
Department of Pathology and Forensic Medicine, University of Abuja, Abuja 902101, Nigeria

Olaejirinde Olaniyi Olaofe
Department of Morbid Anatomy & Forensic Medicine, Obafemi Awolowo University, Ile-Ife 220282, Nigeria

Oche Mansur Oche, Habibullah Adamu, Aisha Abubakar, Munira Sahabi Aliyu and Abubakar Shehu Dogondaji
Department of Community Health, Usmanu Danfodiyo University, Sokoto, Nigeria

Medhin Girmay Reda
College of Medicine and Health Sciences, Adigrat University, Adigrat, Ethiopia

Girma Tenkolu Bune and Mohammed Feyisso Shaka
School of Public Health, College of Health Sciences and Medicine, Dilla University, Dilla, Ethiopia

Kefyalew Amogne Azanaw
Department of Nursing, Debre Tabor Health Science College, Ethiopia

Abebaw Addis Gelagay
Department of Reproductive and Child Health, College of Medicine and Health Sciences, University of Gondar, Gondar, Ethiopia

Ayenew Molla Lakew and Destaw Fetene Teshome
Department of Epidemiology and Biostatistics, College of Medicine and Health Sciences, University of Gondar, Gondar, Ethiopia

Kenneth Setorwu Adde, Eugene Kofuor Maafo Darteh and Akwasi Kumi-Kyereme
Department of Population and Health, College of Humanities and Legal Studies, University of Cape Coast, Cape Coast, Ghana

Hubert Amu
Department of Population and Behavioural Sciences, School of Public Health, University of Health and Allied Sciences, Hohoe, Ghana

Felister Apili
Department of Nursing, College of Health Sciences, Makerere University, Kampala, Uganda
Faculty of Health Sciences, Lira University, Lira, Uganda

Charles Peter Osingada and Scovia Nalugo Mbalinda
Department of Nursing, College of Health Sciences, Makerere University, Kampala, Uganda

Stephen Ochaya
Department of Clinical Pathology, Academic Hospital, Uppsala, Sweden
Department of Immunology and Microbiology, Gulu University, Gulu, Uganda

David Mukunya
Center for Intervention Science in Maternal and Child Health, University of Bergen, Bergen, Norway

Grace Ndeezi and James K. Tumwine
Department of Paediatrics and Child Health, College of Health Sciences, Makerere University, Kampala, Uganda

Huda Mossa Omran
Department of Molecular Medicine, College of Medicine and Medical Sciences, Princess Al-Jawhara Center for Genetics and Inherited Diseases, Arabian Gulf University, Manama, Bahrain
Pulse Health Training Center, Manama, Bahrain

Moiz Bakhiet
Department of Molecular Medicine, College of Medicine and Medical Sciences, Princess Al-Jawhara Center for Genetics and Inherited Diseases, Arabian Gulf University, Manama, Bahrain

Volker Ehemann
Institute of Pathology, University Hospital Heidelberg, Heidelberg, Germany

Mengstu Melkamu Asaye
Women and Family Health Department, School of Midwifery, College of Medicine and Health Sciences, University of Gondar, Ethiopia

Kirubel Minsamo Mishore
School of Pharmacy, Haramaya University, Harar, Ethiopia

Abebaw Demissie Woldemariam
Department of Anesthesia, Harar Health Sciences College, Harar, Ethiopia

Solomon Assefa Huluka
Department of Pharmacology and Clinical Pharmacy, School of Pharmacy, Addis Ababa University, Addis Ababa, Ethiopia

Habtamu Gebrehana Belay, Tewachew Muche Liyeh, Habtamu Abie Tassew, Abeba Belay Ayalew, Yitayal Ayalew Goshu and Gedefaye Nibret Mihretie
Department of Midwifery, College of Health Science, Debre Tabor University, Debre Tabor, Ethiopia

M. Aleni
Department of Nursing and Midwifery, Muni University, 725 Arua, Uganda

R. Muhindo
Department of Nursing and Midwifery, Muni University, 725 Arua, Uganda
Department of Nursing, Makerere University, 7062 Kampala, Uganda

S. N. Mbalinda
Department of Nursing, Makerere University, 7062 Kampala, Uganda

Peter Adatara, Agani Afaya, Elizabeth A. Baku and Solomon Mohammed Salia
Department of Nursing, School of Nursing and Midwifery, University of Health and Allied Sciences, Ho, Ghana

Anthony Asempah
Public Affairs Unit, University of Health and Allied Sciences, Ho, Ghana

Mzee M. Nassoro, Paul Chetto, Enid Chiwanga and Jacquiline Wambura
Department of Obstetrics and Gynaecology, Dodoma Regional Referral Hospital, Dodoma, Tanzania

Athanase Lilungulu,
Department of Obstetrics and Gynaecology, University of Dodoma, College of Health Sciences, Dodoma, Tanzania

Deogratius Bintabara,
Department of Public Health, College of Health Sciences, University of Dodoma, Dodoma, Tanzania

Teshager Aklilu Yesuf, Nigist Assefa Eshete and Eskinder Ayalew Sisay
Department of Pharmacy, College of Health Sciences, Mekelle University, Mekelle, Ethiopia

Index